GENETIC POLYMORPHISMS

Edited by **Narasimha Reddy Parine**

Genetic Polymorphisms
http://dx.doi.org/10.5772/66548
Edited by Narasimha Reddy Parine

Contributors

Israel Gomy, Huma Mehboob, Beata Kaleta, Arjumand Warsy, Maha Daghestani, Fatima Al-Makinzy, Sooad Al-Daihan, Sophia Alam, Yamin Liu, Zhao Li, Xiaofan Guo, Jing Xiong, Xueli Zhang, Hua Shao, Yufan Guan, Roselle Abraham, Xi-Dai Long, Xue-Min Wu, Xiao-Ying Huang, Jin-Guang Yao, Chao Wang, Chun-Ying Luo, Bing-Chen Huang, Wen-Pei Yang, Qiang Xia, Zhi-Feng Xi, Jun Lu, Xing-Zhizi Wang, Tian-Qi Zhang, Qun-Qing Xu, Yasemin Baskin, Gizem Calibasi Kocal, Abdullah Tuncay Demiryürek, Seniz Demiryürek, Igor A. Sobenin, Urszula Kaczor, Francesco Fedele, Paolo Severino, Mariateresa Pucci, Cadiele Oliana Reichert, Joel Da Cunha, Débora Levy, , Luciana Morganti Ferreira Maselli, Sérgio Bydlowski, Celso Spada

Published by InTech

Janeza Trdine 9, 51000 Rijeka, Croatia

Publishing Process Manager Nina Kalinic
Technical Editor SPi Global
Cover InTech Design team

First published September, 2017
Printed in Croatia
Legal deposit, Croatia: National and University Library in Zagreb

Additional hard copies can be obtained from orders@intechopen.com

Genetic Polymorphisms , Edited by Narasimha Reddy Parine
p. cm.
Print ISBN 978-953-51-3515-9
Online ISBN 978-953-51-3516-6

For EU product safety concerns:
IN TECH d.o.o., Prolaz Marije Krucifikse Kozulić 3, 51000 Rijeka, Croatia,
info@intechopen.com or visit our website at intechopen.com.

Meet the editor

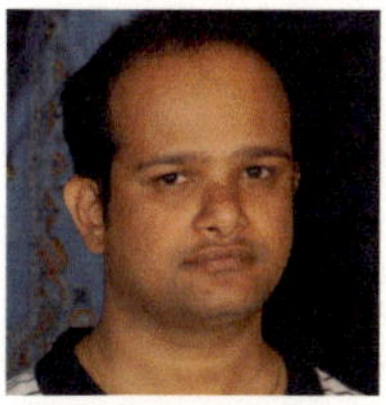

Dr. Narasimha Reddy Parine is an assistant professor at the Department of Biochemistry, College of Science, King Saud University in Saudi Arabia. He received his PhD degree from Andhra University, India. After 16 years of biomedical research, he is a well-known figure who routinely applies molecular biology techniques in his lab. His research interest has focused on studying the molecular targets, particularly DNA damage and DNA repair, Wnt signaling pathway, inflammation, epigenetic modifications, long noncoding RNA, and microRNAs. He has more than 50 publications, serves on editorial boards of 5 journals, and regularly reviews for 15 journals and 2 granting bodies. His achievements have been recognized by several awards and honors.

Contents

Preface

With the advancement of recent technologies, the search for cancer genes has tremendously improved. We plan to use such high-throughput methods, e.g., next-generation DNA sequencing (NGS) and mutation detection techniques, to study genes involved in human and disease development.The in-depth coverage of the sequencing allowed by next-generation sequencing technologies makes it possible to index all classes of mutations in human diseases. Nonetheless, identifying driver mutations is a major task of disease genome analysis. Most of the recent genome analysis studies of sporadic and hereditary diseases have targeted the whole genome and specific genes to enhance the chances of identifying new and novel driver mutations. Genetic variation plays a critical role in most of the diseases. Cells contain somatic mutations, such as single-nucleotide variants, deletions, insertions, and copy-number variations in their genomes. Most of the recent reports revealed that the overwhelming majority of diseases are caused by novel variants that affect the function of individual proteins. About 85% of the disease-inducing variants are normally found in the exome regions. Genome-wide association studies (GWAS) of SNPs in human diseases have identified approximately 300 frequent variants related with risk alleles, which are contributing to cause a wide range of diseases. So far, most of the reported rare mutations conveyed small effects on disease risk; furthermore, even in enormously large studies, most of the genetic factors to disease risk remain unexplained. GWAS studies proved that independently rare mutations with comparatively large effect may account for a vast proportion of this missing variance. In fact, studies describing about the unexplained disease risk have reported about the occurrence of individually rare variants with relatively large effect.

This *Genetic Polymorphisms* book, composed of research studies and review chapters from a group of international researchers, covers the basics of genetic polymorphisms, their role in human disease, and utilization as biomarkers. The book provides useful information to all life science researchers, educators, students, and others who are interested in applications of molecular markers.

I thank the InTech book department and its publication manager **Ms. Nina Kalinić** for the book editing opportunity and help during the entire editorial process of this book. I am thankful to all the authors of the book chapters for their chapter contributions and cooperation.

Dr. Narasimha Reddy Parine
College of Science, King Saud University,
Saudi Arabia

Section 1

Genetic Polymorphisms in Human Health

Chapter 1

Polymorphisms in Pharmacogenetics of Personalized Cancer Therapy

Gizem Calibasi Kocal and Yasemin Baskin

Additional information is available at the end of the chapter

http://dx.doi.org/10.5772/intechopen.69207

Abstract

Therapy process of personalized cancer management covers surgery, chemotherapy, radiation therapy and targeted therapies. The choice of cancer chemotherapeutic agents and doses depends upon the location and stage of tumor, as well as the general state of the patient. On the chemotherapy, radiotherapy, and targeted therapy processes, pharmacogenetics offers customized solutions according to the personal genetic information. Especially for clinicians, genetic information obtained from polymorphism-based pharmacogenetic tests is highly crucial for the better prediction ability of drug response and life-threatening toxic reactions due to the narrow therapeutic index of cancer chemotherapeutic agents. Pharmacogenotyping utilizes different examination strategies, such as single nucleotide polymorphism analysis, somatic/germline mutation analysis and partial/full genome sequencing. The promising effect of pharmacogenetics on the solving of the individual variability in drug response and toxic reactions is being observed with the accumulation of the information that unravel the human genomic variations from large-scale population and multi-parameter-based pharmacogenetic studies of the post-genomic era. Polymorphisms contribute wide variations in human genome and may define how individuals respond to medications, either by changing the pharmacokinetics and pharmacodynamics of drugs or by altering the cellular response to therapeutic agents. To define the effect of polymorphisms on the targets of chemotherapeutics is necessary for the prediction of altered pharmacokinetics of therapeutic agents.

Keywords: personalized medicine, pharmacogenetics, polymorphisms

1. Introduction

1.1. Genetic polymorphisms

1.1.1. Mutation or polymorphism

Genetic and environmental factors are the two main reasons that cause human phenotype variations. If the genomic DNA sequences of two individuals are compared, substantial sequence variations can be detected at different points of the whole genome. There are many forms of these genetic variations [1]. Polymorphism term, arose from the combination of the Greek words 'poly' (meaning as multiple) and 'morph' (meaning as form), is used in genetics to describe multiple forms of a single gene that exist in a population. Polymorphisms are genetic variants and refer to the occurrence of various phenotypes in a certain population. A polymorphism is a DNA sequence variation and does not classify as mutation. In genetic polymorphisms, there are two or more equally acceptable sequence of a gene and the common allele must have a frequency of 1% or more in the population. If the frequency is lower than 1%, the allele is accepted as a mutation. On the other hand, a mutation is a change in DNA sequence away from normal allele and forms abnormal variant [2].

1.1.2. Nomenclature

The unique and universal nomenclature to refer specific single nucleotide polymorphisms (SNPs) is that using the rs number (reference sequence). It stands for Reference SNP cluster ID. The rs number allows the precise identification of a polymorphic variation in the numerous databases (NCBI, HapMap, SNP500 Cancer, etc.). For instance, a SNP causes a replacement of an amino acid by another amino acid; this can be defined by the name and the position of the replaced amino acid, followed by the name of the novel amino acid. As an example, a common SNP in the *DPYD* gene is identified as rs 1801160 [V732I or Val732Ile]. SNPs are also identified by the name and position of nucleotide in the reference DNA sequence. The same SNP in the *DPYD* gene, presented with rs 1801160, is identified as 2194G>A. The letters A, T, C, and G can be used for both nucleotides and amino acids, and this can cause confusion [3].

1.1.3. Types of polymorphisms

Developments in next generation sequencing technologies under the "Human Genome Project," simplify to investigate the allelic variants of a gene taken from different people of a population [4]. These various genetic polymorphisms include minor changes on DNA sequence, as substitutions, deletions, insertions, and repeats. These changes influence the three-dimensional structure, expression and activity of the proteins encoded by these genes. Alterations called as single nucleotide polymorphisms (SNPs, pronounced snip) are the most common form of polymorphisms on a gene sequence. They occur when alleles reveal only a single base pair (bp) change—A, T, C or G—in the genome sequence between individuals. For example, one variant may have an A nucleotide at a certain position and other has a G nucleotide (**Figure 1**). This type of change generates single nucleotide variants (SNVs). SNPs can affect gene function due to the change of protein but can also occur in noncoding parts of the gene so they would not be seen in the protein product [5, 6].

1.1.4. Polymorphisms and ethnicity

Intrinsic factors and extrinsic factors cause variability in drug response. Extrinsic factors such as food and concomitant medications may be controllable, but intrinsic factors such as gender, ethnicity, age, renal or hepatic function, and genetic differences in the expression of enzymes need advance knowledge to control [7]. Ethnicity is one of the key factors that can explain the observed variability in both pharmacokinetics (PK) and pharmacodynamics (PD) of therapeutics, resulting in differences in response to drug therapy as well as chemotherapeutics. United States Food and Drug Administration (FDA) guidelines pay attention to "ethnically sensitive situations" for some drugs and suggests the types of solutions that may control such ethnic sensitivity. One of the most important factors that may contribute to this ethnic sensitivity of a drug, include genetic polymorphisms in metabolic pathways of drugs [7, 8]. To define the variability on the response or metabolism of specific therapeutics or drug targets, drug companies and prestigious research groups are biobanking DNA samples [9]. Although the clinical relevance of some variants is well characterized, the relevance of some variant alleles is as yet unknown.

1.1.5. Allele frequency and Hardy-Weinberg principle

There are some challenges on the use of disease-associated polymorphism knowledge. One of these challenges is the lack of the unique information regarding the frequency of specific polymorphism in the targeted population. Without a unique presenting style of the

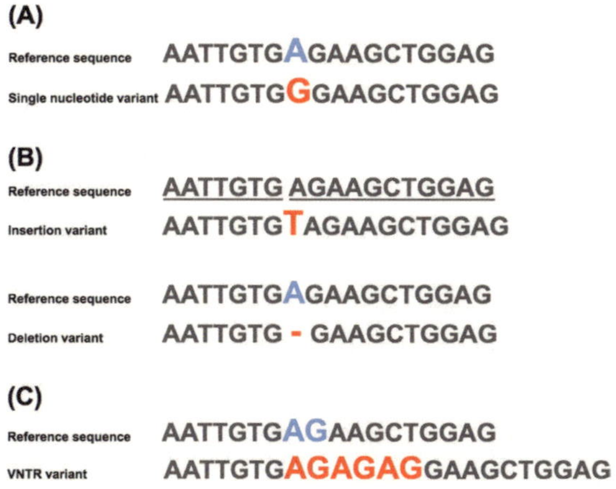

Figure 1. Classes of DNA variation affecting a single nucleotide position. (A) Single nucleotide variant (SNV) in which two variants differ by having a G nucleotide or a C nucleotide (B) Insertion variation in which variant 1 has exactly same reference sequence, variant 2 has one more T nucleotide; Deletion variation in which variant 1 has a A nucleotide, variant 2 does not have; (C) Variable number of tandem repeats (VNTR) in which two variants differ by having repeats of nucleotides.

polymorphism-related data, prevention of the risk for disease and drugs remain unknown. In addition, determining the factors that may affect the association of the allele with disease or drugs, such as ethnicity, may not be possible without population-based allele frequencies [10–12]. SNPs can be assigned with an allele frequency—the ratio of chromosomes in the population carrying the less common variant to those with the more common variant. It is important to note that there are variations among different populations, so a common SNP allele may be much rare in one geographical or ethnic group than another [13, 14]. The Hardy-Weinberg principle can be used to calculate allele frequencies [15]. The Hardy-Weinberg principle (also known as the Hardy-Weinberg equilibrium, equation, theorem, or law) states that allele frequencies in a population will remain stable from generation to generation in the absence of other evolutionary factors, such as mutation, polymorphisms, genetic drift, gene flow, meiotic drive, and mate choice. Hardy-Weinberg principle describes that the ideal condition against the effects of these factors can be analyzed. The principle is named after Godfrey Harold Hardy and Wilhem Weinberg, who first demonstrated it mathematically. If Hardy-Weinberg principle is violated, the key interferences of a genetic polymorphisms-based study may be compromised. Thus, accumulating evidence suggests that Hardy-Weinberg principle-based reporting may be optimal in genetic and nongenetic journals, because variability in the analyzed data can cause errors or peculiarities [15].

2. Polymorphisms-based pharmacogenetics applications and personalized cancer therapy

Most of the chemotherapeutic agents for cancer treatment affect a minority of cancer patients and have a narrow therapeutic index that frequently causes life-threatening toxicities and even death. Even specific molecule-targeted therapies, which are safer than cytotoxic drugs, are associated with severe adverse events. Thus, novel treatment strategies that can increase the effectiveness of therapy and decrease the rate of adverse events will be developed. Under this approach, the aim of personalized medicine is to tailor the therapy options according to patient's molecular profile [16, 17]. Establishing the relation between molecular characteristics of patient and drug outcomes is crucial for the identification of predictive biomarkers and understands the base of personalized therapy. Personalized medicine can also be called as P4 medicine due to the various contents as predictive, personalized, preventive, and participatory medicine (P4); it separates patients into different groups with an individual's molecular profile. Thus, personalized medicine covers the determination of the safest and most effective chemotherapeutic agents [18]. The goal of discipline of pharmacogenetics, first used in the late 1950s, is to make 'personalized medicine' as applicable to various patient groups. It can be defined as the study of patients' genotype affecting drug response. In some patient groups, certain drugs work well but not as well in others. Pharmacogenetics-based studies (between genotype of patients and the response of therapeutics) allow designing more effective and population-specific therapeutic treatments (**Figure 2**). Polymorphism analysis, mutation analysis and genome sequencing are the backbones of discipline of pharmacogenetics.

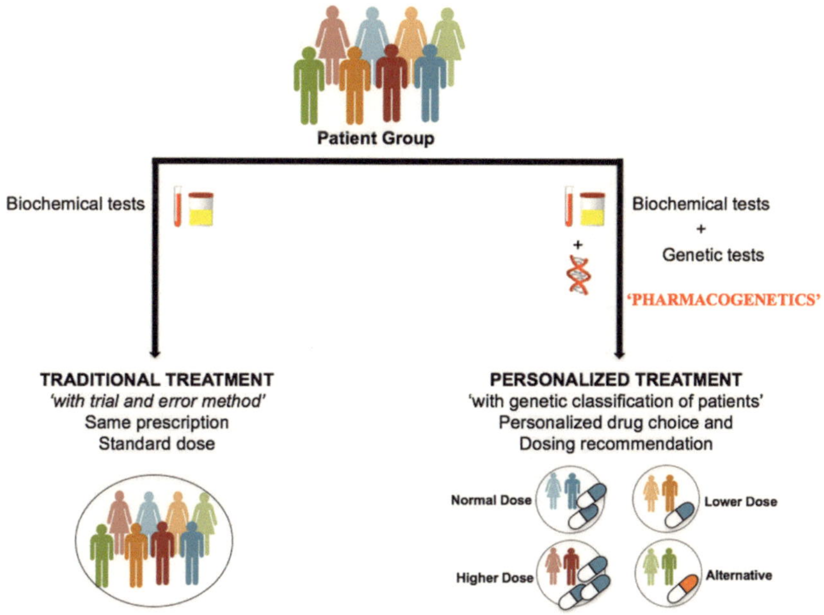

Figure 2. The traditional prescribing approaches in clinical therapies, such as 'trial and error', 'one drug fits all' and 'one dose fits all', have limits due to the drug safety. Pharmacogenetics combines standard biochemical tests with molecular genetics based tests to detect DNA variations in the human genome for the application of genomic-based prescribing.

Polymorphisms and their association with diseases should be handled based on gene as biomarkers, due to the relatively large frequency in the human genome. To learn, how to use and interpret the polymorphisms analysis and which test(s) should be chosen is essential.

2.1. Methods for polymorphism detection

After the deep sequencing of human genome with Human Genome Project, the detection of population-based DNA polymorphisms, especially that effect the development and the progress of diseases, is the second phase of human genomics. High-throughput polymorphism genotyping process includes fast and cost-effective identification of polymorphisms in different individuals and lead to the determination of associations between genotype and phenotype. Generally, genotyping steps start with the isolation of starting material as DNA from patient; it follows with amplification to increase the sample amount and then finalize with polymerase chain reaction (PCR), sequencing or array-based technologies. A number of good polymorphism genotyping technologies are currently in use to meet the needs of clinics and researches, but only one genotyping method is not ideal for all applications (**Table 1**). Slow speed of assays due to the time-consuming protocols, high instrument and consumable costs, and requirements on the performing multiple assays in parallel are the main challenges of polymorphism genotyping technologies. Studies on ideal polymorphism genotyping technologies are on development process [19–21].

Method	Advantages	Disadvantages
Allele-specific single-base primer extension	High success rate; High accuracy; Quantitative; Adaptation to multiplexing.	High instrument cost; Relatively long protocol; Tricky multiplex PCR.
Allele-specific enzymatic cleavage – restriction fragment length polymorphism (RFLP)	High accuracy; SNP at a restriction endonuclease recognition sequence.	High instrument cost; Long protocol; Difficult adaptation for high-throughput genotyping
Pyrosequencing	Provides sequence information surrounding the polymorphism; Real-time scoring; Quantitative.	High instrument and consumable cost; Long protocol; Limited throughput
Mass spectrometry	High accuracy (as long as the sample is very pure); Fast genotyping reactions in seconds; Allows thousands of reactions in a day.	High instrument and consumable cost; Long protocol; Limited throughput; Requires very pure sample for accuracy.
Invader assay	No PCR for amplification; Simple protocol; Isothermal reaction	Requires large amount of genomic DNA; Requires optimizations for each SNP; Key enzyme is not suitable for general research use.

Table 1. A summary of popular polymorphism detection methods with their advantages and disadvantages [19–21].

2.2. Polymorphisms as biomarkers for drug response and toxicity

Variations in the metabolism of a chemotherapeutic agent due to genetic alterations may cause significant differences in terms of efficacy and toxicity. Such pharmacological effects occur since oncologists schedule the dosing of chemotherapeutic agents according to patient's body surface area and other nongenetic factors. Genetic differences due to the polymorphisms are thought as one of the strongest reasons in adverse drug reactions (ADRs). Genetic polymorphisms are considered as molecular biomarkers in pharmacogenetic-based studies both in clinic and research to predict the ADRs and apply the medications as personal. The main objective of pharmacogenetics is to understand the nature of various responses including adverse drug reactions (ADRs) to drugs [22]. Pharmacogenetic associations are important in cancer chemotherapy due to the extremely narrow chemotherapeutic index of anticancer drugs given for cancer management. Polymorphisms in both patient's genome and tumor genome affect the regulation of drug transport, retention and efflux of anticancer drugs, determining the penetration into tumor tissue. Genetic information of tumors is not stabile as somatic tissues; new alterations on genetic material (as mutation or chromosomal loss) can occur continuously. Therefore, drug-related toxicities depend on the genotype of nontumor tissue. Thus, the tumor genome possesses most of the polymorphisms that influence the sensitivity or resistance of drugs (KRAS and EGFR, KIT, TS polymorphisms, etc.); hence, treatment efficacy and tumor genome will have a key role as a dose limiting factors in cancer management. Polymorphisms on the host genome, which tumor genome does not present, are the main determinants of toxicity risk (e.g. polymorphisms on the genes of drug metabolism such as *dihydropyrimidine dehydrogenase gene (DPYD), thiopurine-S-methyltransferase (TPMT), UDP-glucuronosyltransferase (UGT),* etc.) [23]. Genotyping studies have revealed that the gene encoding a specific protein can have a number of differences in sequence at the nucleotide level. These differences especially called as polymorphisms, sometimes do not cause significant alterations on the final product, but may have an effect on the substrate specificity and activity of the product (especially for enzymes) or other characteristics and functions. For example, polymorphisms in *cytochrome P450 2D6 (CYP2D6)* are one of the cytochrome P450 enzymes of the liver that can influence how humans metabolize cancer drugs, although the enzymes are basically the same sequence and structure. Polymorphisms in CYP2D6 have been seen in the general population about 10% and it has been associated with poor-metabolizer phenotype of enzyme. This is important for codeine-based pain medications due to the activation of codeine to morphine and includes CYP2D6-dependent step [24].

Pharmacogenetic tests based on the determination of genetic variants for drug efficacy or toxicity has begun to use in the 2000s, although genetic-based studies began in the 1950s. FDA has been working to improve pharmacogenetic technologies in the development, regulation and use of medications and revised drug labels in terms of pharmacogenetic biomarkers in oncology area (**Table 2**) [25, 26].

It is important to describe important gene polymorphisms and their clinical meaning in oncology field that may determine the optimum pharmacological treatment in terms of treatment outcomes, tolerability and the occurrence of serious, even life-threatening adverse reactions.

Pharmacogenetic biomarker	Drugs	Labeling	Outcome
UGT1A1	Irinotecan Belinostat Nilotinib Pazopanib	Dose determination and administration; Warnings and precautions, clinical pharmacology	Toxicity
DPYD	Capecitabine Fluorouracil	Warnings and precautions, patient counseling information	Toxicity
TPMT	Cisplatin	Adverse reactions	Toxicity
	Mercaptopurine Thioguanine	Dose determination and administration; Warnings and precautions; Adverse reactions; Clinical pharmacology	Toxicity
G6PD	Rasburicase Dabrafenib	Warnings and precautions; Contraindications; Adverse reactions; Patient counseling information	Toxicity
CYP2D6	Tamoxifen Rucaparib	Dose determination and administration; Clinical pharmacology	Toxicity

Table 2. FDA-approved pharmacogenetic biomarkers for anti-cancer drug labeling [26].

2.2.1. *Uridinediphosphate glucuronosyl transferase 1A1 (UGT1A1)*

The UGT super family includes four main UGT families, namely UGT1, UGT2, UGT3, and UGT8. The *UGT1* and *UGT2 genes*, encode 16 functional proteins, have been extensively studied and well characterized. A phase II metabolic enzyme, UGT1A1 is the most studied UGT enzyme due to its main role in glucuronidation of exogenous and endogenous substrates, including bilirubin. UGT1A1 also appears in the metabolism processes of most of the anti-cancer drugs, such as topoisomerase I inhibitor irinotecan, the topoisomerase II inhibitor etoposide [27]. Alterations on the glucuronidation activity of UGT1A1 caused by genetic or environmental factors may have significant physiological and pharmacological results on the metabolism of anticancer agents. Allelic variations have been identified in the promoter region and exon 5 of UGT1A1 region. The wild-type allele of *UGT1A1* gene (known as *UGT1A1*1*) has six thymine- adenine (TA) repeats in the promoter region of gene (TATA box). Allelic differences vary from five (*UGT1A1*36*, proficient allele) to eight (*UGT1A1*37*, deficient allele) TA repeats, and these differences affect the UGT1A1-mediated glucuronidation of SN-38 (7-ethyl-10-hydroxycamptothecin), active metabolite of anticancer drug irinotecan both *in vitro* and *in vivo*. Increasing number of TA repeats has been associated with decreased transcription of gene and overall UGT1A1 activity (**Table 3**) [28]. Patients (allele frequency in Caucasians 8–20% are homozygous, 40–50% are heterozygous) with seven TA repeat sequence (named UGT1A1*28) have severe toxicity risk after irinotecan treatment because of decreased gene expression and overall UGT1A1 activity (30% enzyme activity in *28 relative to *1 allele). These patients [with $(TA)_7$ repeats] have fourfold relative toxicity risk compared with patients with six repeat sequences [29]. *UGT1A1*60* (in linkage disequilibrium with TATA box variants) and *UGT1A1*93* are the other variants located in the promoter region. Both of them are found homozygous in around 10% of Caucasians [30]. *UGT1A1*6* and *UGT1A1*27* are located in coding region exon 1. *UGT1A1*6* is the most frequent variant in Asian populations (not found in Caucasians) and associated with ~30% decreased enzyme activity in homozygous patients. *UGT1A1*27* is almost completely eradicated enzyme activity. Nearly 3% of Asian people, are homozygous for both *6 and *27 variant [28, 31].

2.2.2. *Dihydropyrimidine dehydrogenase gene (DPYD)*

The pyrimidine antimetabolites 5-fluorouracil and its oral prodrug capecitabine are widely used chemotherapeutic agents in the management of variety of tumor types, including colorectal, breast, and head and neck cancers. They activate metabolically and inhibit thymidylate synthase enzyme, which takes role in cellular replication. However, 5-FU leads significant toxicities, such as myelosuppression, mucositis, hand-foot syndrome, and diarrhea. On the other hand, accumulation of knowledge on 5-FU mechanism has developed new strategies that increase the treatment efficacy and response [32, 33]. 5-FU is metabolized by dihydropyrimidine dehydrogenase (DPD) enzyme, and it converts the fluoropyrimidine to its inactive metabolite dihydrofluorouracil (**Figure 3**). DPD enzyme, which is encoded by *DPYD* gene, is a rate-limiting enzyme of 5-FU catabolism and is also used for evaluating the variability of 5-FU metabolism among patients [34]. SNPs in the *DPYD* gene are responsible for insufficient production of DPD enzyme; therefore, low levels of enzyme increase the half-life of the drug,

http://dx.doi.org/10.5772/intechopen.69207

Genotype	Ref SNP	HGVS Region	Drug	Enzymatic activity Clinical phenotype
*UGT1A1*1*	Common allele-Wild type	(TA) 6TA	Irinotecan	Normal enzyme activity
*UGT1A1*28*	rs 8175347	(TA) 7 TA TATA box	Irinotecan	Reduced enzyme activity *1/*28 Irinotecan dosing based on clinical findings *28/*28 Dose reduction recommended.
*UGT1A1*36*	rs 8175347	(TA) 5 TA TATA box	Irinotecan	Normal enzyme activity *Irinotecan dosing recommendations are less clear.*
*UGT1A1*37*	rs 8175347	(TA) 8 TA TATA box	Irinotecan	Normal enzyme activity *Irinotecan dosing recommendations are less clear.*
*UGT1A1*60*	rs 4124874	c.-3279T>G Promoter region	Irinotecan	Normal enzyme activity *Standard irinotecan dosing*
*UGT1A1*93*	rs10929302	c.-3156G>A Promoter region	Irinotecan	Normal enzyme activity *Standard irinotecan dosing*
*DPYD*9A*	rs1801265	c.85T>C, p.Cys29Arg Exon 2	5-fluorouracil Capecitabine	Normal enzyme activity *Standard irinotecan dosing*
*DPYD*2A*	rs3918290	IVS14 + 1G>A Intron 14 and exon 14	5-fluorouracil Capecitabine	Reduced enzyme activity *Increased toxicity risk*
*DPYD*13*	rs55886062	c.1679T>G, p.Ile560Ser Exon 13	5-fluorouracil Capecitabine	Reduced enzyme activity *Increased toxicity risk*
TYMS 2R/2R, TYMS 2R/3RG, TYMS 3RG/3RG,	rs34743033	28bp VNTR (2R; 3R) Promoter enhancer region	5-fluorouracil Capecitabine	Enzyme activity based on the repeats *2R/2R: Decreased TYMS expression, increased 5-FU responsiveness, increased risk of toxicity* *2R/3RG, 3RG/3RG: Increased TYMS expression, decreased 5-fluorouracil, capecitabine responsiveness, poor prognosis.*

Genotype	Ref SNP	HGVS Region	Drug	Enzymatic activity Clinical phenotype
TYMS 3RG/3RC, *TYMS 2R/3RC,* *TYMS 3RC/3RC*	rs2853542	G>C SNP in 2nd repeat of 3R allele (3RC) Promoter enhancer region	5-fluorouracil Capecitabine	Enzyme activity based on the repeats *3RG/3RC: Increased TYMS expression, decreased 5-FU responsiveness, poor prognosis* *2R/3RC or 3RC/3RC: Decreased TYMS expression, increased 5-FU responsiveness, increased risk of toxicity*
MTHFR, 677C>T	rs1801133	c.677C>T, p.Ala222Val Exon 4	Methotrexate	Reduced enzyme activity *Homozygosity: Risk for toxicity from drugs and requirement for dosing adjustments/ discontinuation* *Heterozygosity: Associated with intermediate enzyme activity* *Lower dose requirements for methotrexate*
MTHFR, 1298A>C	rs1801131	c.1298A>C; p.Glu429Ala Exon 7	Methotrexate	Reduced enzyme activity *Homozygosity/Heterozygosity: Associated with intermediate enzyme activity. Lower dose requirements for methotrexate.*
*TPMT*1*	Common allele-Wild type	Common allele-Wild type	6-mercaptopurine; Azathioprine; Thioguanine	Normal enzyme activity
*TPMT*2*	rs1800462	c.238G>C, p.Ala80Pro Exon 5	6-mercaptopurine; Azathioprine; Thioguanine	Poor activity Homozygosity: very low/absent enzyme activity Heterozygosity: intermediate activity *Low/Absent Activity: Increased risk for developing life-threatening side effects at a standard dose of a thiopurine drug.* *Intermediate (Reduced) Activity: Increased risk for toxicity at a standard dose of a thiopurine drug.*

Genotype	Ref SNP	HGVS Region	Drug	Enzymatic activity Clinical phenotype
*TPMT*3A*	rs1800460 rs1142345	c.[460G>A;719A>G], p.[Ala154Thr;Tyr240Cys] Exon 7, 10	6-mercaptopurine; Azathioprine; Thioguanine	Poor activity *Homozygosity—Low/Absent Activity: Increased risk for developing life-threatening side effects from a standard dose of a thiopurine drug.* *Heterozygosity- Intermediate (Reduced) Activity: Increased risk for toxicity from a standard dose of a thiopurine drug.*
*TPMT*3B*	rs1800460	c.460G>A, p.Ala154Thr Exon 7	6-mercaptopurine, Azathioprine, Thioguanine	Poor activity Homozygosity—*Low/Absent Activity: Increased risk for developing life-threatening side effects at a standard dose of a thiopurine drug.* Heterozygosity—*Intermediate (Reduced) Activity: Increased risk for toxicity at a standard dose of a thiopurine drug.*
*TPMT*3C*	rs1142345	c.719A>G, p.Tyr240Cys Exon 10	6-mercaptopurine, Azathioprine, Thioguanine	Poor activity *Homozygosity—Low/Absent Activity: Increased risk for developing life-threatening side effects from a standard dose of a thiopurine drug.* *Heterozygosity—Intermediate (Reduced) Activity:* *Increased risk for toxicity from a standard dose of a thiopurine drug.*
*CYP2D6*1*	Common allele-Wild type	Common allele-Wild type	Tamoxifen	Normal activity *Extensive metabolizer*
*CYP2D6*2*	rs16947	c.584G>c, p.Arg296Cys Exon 2	Tamoxifen	Normal enzyme activity
*CYP2D6*4*	rs3892097	1846G>A Exon 3—Junction of intron 3 and exon 4 (Not applicable variant occurs in a noncoding region)	Tamoxifen	Inactive enzyme

Genotype	Ref SNP	HGVS Region	Drug	Enzymatic activity Clinical phenotype
*CYP2D6*5*		Whole gene deletion On allele	Tamoxifen	Inactive enzyme
*CYP2D6*6*	rs5030655	c.1707delT, p.Trp152Gly Exon 3	Tamoxifen	Inactive enzyme
*CYP2D6*9*		AGA deletion at 2613-2615, p.Lys281 del	Tamoxifen	Reduced enzyme activity (Partially functioning)
*CYP2D6*10*	rs1065852	c.188C>T, p.Pro34Ser Exon 1	Tamoxifen	Reduced enzyme activity
*CYP2D6*17*	rs28371706 rs16947	c.320C>T, p.Thr107Ile; c.886T>C, p.Cys296Arg Intron 1	Tamoxifen	Reduced enzyme activity
*CYP2D6*41*	rs28371725	c.2988G>A Intron 6 (Not applicable variant occurs in a noncoding region)	Tamoxifen	Reduced enzyme activity

Note: Guidelines for the description and nomenclature of gene variations are available from the Human Genome Variation Society (HGVS): http://www.hgvs.org/content/guidelines.

Table 3. Biological impact of the important pharmacogenetic biomarker variants [28, 42–46].

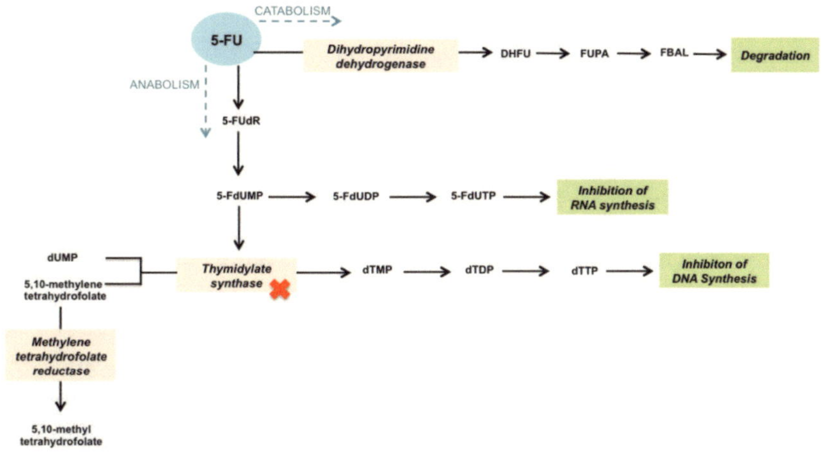

Figure 3. Metabolism of 5-fluorouracil (5-FU). The initial and rate-limiting enzyme of 5-FU is dihydropyrimidine dehydrogenase (DPD), catalysing the conversion of 5-FU into 5,6-dihydrofluorouracil (DHFU). DHFU is degraded into fluoro-beta-ureidopropionic acid (FUPA) and fluoro-beta-alanine (FBAL) through degradation cascade. 5-Fluoro-2′-deoxyuridine-5′-monophosphate (5-FdUMP), is the cytotoxic product resulting from a multi-step activation of 5-FU, inhibits the enzyme thymidylate synthase (TS) enzyme. This inhibition leads to accumulation of deoxy-uridine-monophospate (dUMP) and depletion of deoxy-thymidine-monophosphate (dTMP), which leads to inhibition of DNA synthesis. 5-FU can also inhibit RNA synthesis in a pathway that involves 5-fluorouridine monophosphate (5-FUMP) and subsequent conversion to 5-fluorouridine triphosphate (5-FUTP) via 5-fluorouridine diphosphate (5-FUDP).

thus, resulting in excess drug accumulation and toxicity due to the inefficient catabolism of drug. Genetic testing of polymorphisms is being used for the classification of patients who would be at high risk for severe or fatal toxicity when receiving fluoropyrimidine-based chemotherapy (**Table 3**) [35]. Complete deficiency of DPD has been seen in approximately 5% of the overall population and also 3–5% of the population has a partial DPD deficiency due to sequence variations in DPYD gene [36].

The IVS14+ 1G>A change with the combination of a mutation in intron 14 and a deletion at 5′-splice consensus sequence of exon 14, the most known and frequent variant (known as DPYD*2A), is resulting the formation of a truncated enzyme product lacking activity. The estimated incidence of homozygous genotype of this allelic variant is 0.1% and heterozygous genotype is 0.5–2.0% in Caucasians [37, 38]. Other variants, which are associated with increased toxicity risk, include 496A>G in exon 6, T1679G (DPYD*13) in exon 13 and 2846A>T in exon 22 [39–41]. Genetic mutations in *DPYD* can be analyzed by highly sensitive methods even for heterozygous variants such as pyrosequencing. But determination of the 5-FU and dihydrofluorouracil concentration ratio in plasma by high-pressure liquid chromatography (HPLC) may be more reliable predictor test for toxicity [35]. Besides *DPYD*, there are some other pharmacogenetic biomarkers that are being used for the determination of the efficacy and toxicity of fluoropyrimidine-related therapies, such as *thymidylate synthase gene (TYMS)*.

2.2.3. Thymidylate synthase gene (TYMS)

The main intracellular target of fluoropyrimidine-related therapies is to inhibit thymidylate synthase (TS) enzyme (encoded by the *TYMS* gene) that catalyzes the transformation of dUMP, which is essential for DNA replication (**Figure 3**) [47]. Fluorodeoxyuridylate (5-FdUMP), an activated metabolite from 5-FU, forms stable complexes with TS enzyme and folate to stop DNA synthesis over blocking the conversion of dUMP to dTMP. Therefore, low expression levels of TS enzyme in colorectal patients receiving 5-FU-based treatment were associated with desired drug response as well as to longer survival [47]. Polymorphisms, which lead *TYMS* variations (2R/2R, 2R/3R, or 3R/3R) by forming double-tandem repeat (2R) or a triple-tandem repeat (3R) on the *TYMS* promoter enhancer region (generally abbreviated as *TSER*), influence the translation of TYMS mRNA and toxicity (**Table 3**). It has been showed that homozygous 3R/3R cells overexpressed *TYMS* mRNA compared with homozygous 2R/2R cells [48]. Apart from these repeats, a G>C SNP has been showed on the 12th nucleotide of the second repeat at 3R allele, and it is causing a tri-allelic locus as 2R, 3RG, and 3RC. The 3RC allele has similar transcriptional activity of the 2R allele [49]. Another genetic polymorphism of the *TYMS* gene has been identified as a 6 basepair deletion at position 1494 in the 3′-untranslated region (3′-UTR). It was demonstrated that there is a strong association between the 6-bp deletion and low *TYMS* mRNA expression in colorectal tumor tissue [50, 51].

2.2.4. *Methylene tetrahydrofolate reductase (MTHFR)*

Methylene tetrahydrofolate reductase (MTHFR) a regulatory enzyme is involved in folate metabolism that redirects folate metabolites from pyrimidine synthesis towards methionine synthesis (**Figure 3**). Most of the *MTHFR* gene variants of enzyme contain polymorphisms that lead loss-of-function in the enzyme (**Table 3**). The level of loss-of-function depends on the type and number of polymorphisms in coding gene. Therefore, *MTHFR* polymorphisms affect drug metabolism, such as methotrexate, may be more likely to experience toxicity. c.677C>T (p.A222V) and c.1298A>C (p.G429A) are the most common polymorphisms of *MTHFR* gene that forms abnormal forms of enzyme. Both polymorphisms are associated with reduced MTHFR enzyme activity. Adjustment drug dosages and prediction of the toxicity risk, *MTHFR* polymorphism test may be performed for a patient who is treated with methotrexate [23].

2.2.5. *Thiopurine-S-methyltransferase (TPMT)*

Thiopurine-S-methyltransferase (TPMT) enzyme, encoding by *TPMT* gene, catalyzes the S-methylation of thiopurine drugs (such as 6-mercaptopurine, azathioprine, and thioguanine) for drug inactivation. The purine antimetabolites are converted to active thioguanine nucleotides that can be incorporated into DNA or RNA to block the DNA replication. During this activation process, purine antimetabolites cause cellular toxicity for both malign and benign cells. TPMT catalyzes inactivation of the formed thioguanine nucleotides [52]. It is known that some patients have low enzyme activity due to germline genetic variations. There are several *TPMT* polymorphisms that caused more than 20 variant alleles of *TPMT* gene (from *TPMT*2* to *TPMT*20*) and have different effects on TPMT function (**Table 3**). Among these variant alleles *TPMT*2*, *TPMT*3A*, *TPMT*3B*, and *TPMT*3C* have been determined as responsible for enzyme deficiency. Among these alleles TPMT*2, TPMT*3A and TPMT*3C are deficient alleles that present poor enzyme activity [45]. Accumulation of cytotoxic thiopurine nucleotides leading to severe toxicity has been shown in people with deficient *TPMT* alleles, after receiving a standard dose thiopurine-based treatment. Patients with low TPMT activity expose more activated thioguanine nucleotides and more treatment toxicity as well as efficacy. Patient's genotype predicts thiopurine nucleotide levels and treatment outcomes in thiopurine drug metabolism that shows tri-modal distribution with 89–94% of patients having high enzyme activity, 6–11% of them having intermediate activity (as heterozygous), and 0.3% of them having low or no activity (as homozygous) [53].

2.2.6. Glucose-6-phosphate dehydrogenase (G6PD)

Glucose-6-phosphate dehydrogenase (G6PD) is a metabolic enzyme involved in pentose phosphate pathway that is important in red blood cell metabolism. The *G6PD* gene is highly polymorphic with more than 300 variants. *G6PD* gene deficiency is a common disease-causing enzymopathy and is associated with low levels of G6PD enzyme. The most remarkable symptom of *G6PD* gene deficiency is hemolytic anemia caused by the ingestion of drugs and food substances that result in oxidative stress. The excess peroxide due to deficiency has a risk for both hemolytic and methemoglobinemia. Rasburicase is a recombinant urate oxidase that has been used for the initial management of plasma uric acid in pediatric and adult patients with leukemia, lymphoma and solid tumors who are receiving chemotherapeutic agents and are expected for tumor lysis syndrome. Rasburicase is contraindicated in patients with *G6PD* gene deficiency; therefore, FDA recommends screening for G6PD deficiency before beginning rasburicase treatment. Dabrafenib is a kinase inhibitor that blocks the growth and spread of cancer cells in the body. Dabrafenib consists of a sulfonamide moiety and contains hemolytic anemia risk in patients with G6PD deficiency. Thus, FDA recommends monitoring for patients with G6PD deficiency started with dabrafenib [54–56].

2.2.7. Cytochrome P450 2D6 (CYP2D6)

Cytochrome P450 2D6 (CYP2D6) deficiency is the first discovered pharmacogenetic deficiency with the characterization of decreased enzyme expression-related polymorphisms. Decreased mRNA levels of *CY2D6* were determined as the reason of reduced metabolism and adverse reactions to an anti-hypertensive drug, debrisoquine. These findings based on molecular technologies display the importance of genotyping on the pharmacological phenotyping involved in drug metabolism [35]. CYP2D6 is a highly polymorphic enzyme (**Table 3**). According to increased or decreased enzyme activity due to SNPs, duplications or deletions, genetic variants of CYP2D6 were classified into four metabolic phenotypes: ultra-rapid metabolizer, extensive metabolizer, intermediate metabolizer and poor metabolizer (**Table 4**). This classification system has been used to control treatment recommendations for several drugs, including tamoxifen [57].

Tamoxifen is a selective estrogen receptor modulator, which is used in the treatment of estrogen receptor-positive breast cancer. Tamoxifen is a weak estrogen antagonist by itself, but it is converted into its main active metabolite, antiestrogenic endoxifen, by CYP2D6. CYP2D6 genotype is predictive of endoxifen exposure that is critical in determining treatment outcome [59]. Increased endoxifen exposure is associated with increased treatment efficacy and toxicity [60, 61].

Phenotype	Genotype
Poor metabolizer	Two inactive alleles
Intermediate metabolizer	Two active alleles
Extensive metabolizer	One active and one inactive alleles; Two decreased activity alleles; One decreased activity and one inactive allele
Ultra-rapid metabolizer	More than two copies of active allele

Notes: Active alleles: **1, *2, *33, *35;* decreased activity alleles: **9, *10, *17, *29, *36, *41;* inactive alleles: **3, *4, *5, *6, *7, *8, *11-*16, *19-*21, *38, *40, *42.*

Table 4. CYP2D6 phenotypes according to activity status of *CYP2D6* alleles (adapted from Swen JJ., et al. 2011) [58].

2.3. Biomarker discovery studies for pharmacogenetic applications

Pharmacogenetics and its backbone studies in terms of polymorphisms present new developments and trends in the field of tailored medications and advancements in the modification of therapeutic choices utilizing genotypic information from polymorphism analysis. Pharmacogenetic biomarker studies have multiple processes from discovery to clinical implementation (**Figure 4**). The ultimate aim of the biomarker studies is to find a clinically accessible decision-maker biomarker to improve patient outcomes. However, many of the valid associations cannot be achieved for clinical implementation due to the lack of sufficient robustness or clinical importance for the question. Biomarker discovery studies should be performed as the screening of genotype-phenotype relations in large cohorts with statistical and bioinformatics tools. The most significant markers obtained from discovery studies are replicated for analytical validation in different cohorts with the evaluation of assay reproducibility and robustness. After successful analytical validity, the biomarker and assay must be evaluated to confirm its performance in diagnosing the clinical phenotype or predicting outcome of

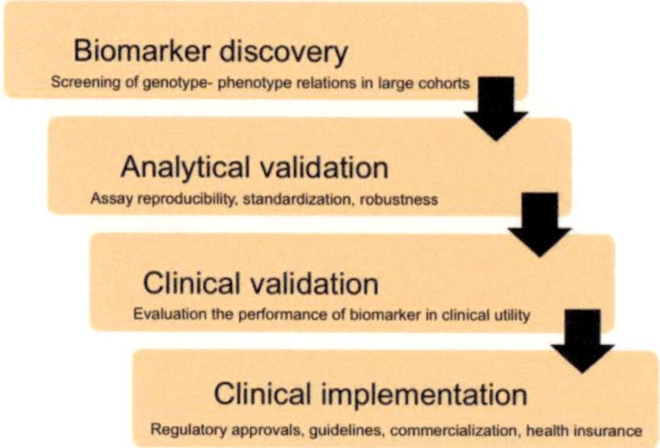

Figure 4. Schematic presentation of pharmacogenetic biomarker studies from development to clinical implementation.

interest. A clinically valid biomarker assay can undergo translation through prospective confirmation of clinical utility to improve patient outcomes. And finally, analytically and clinically validated biomarker assay is ready for implementation phase that includes regulatory approval and incorporation in clinical practice guidelines, commercialization and coverage by health insurance [52, 62].

2.4. Future directions and conclusion

After "Human Genome Project," science world began to use individual genotypic information to predict the risk of diseases, to prognose the disease, to guide therapeutic decision-making, and to develop targeted medications. Especially, the better prediction ability for drug response and life-threatening toxic reactions is highly crucial for clinicians due to the narrow therapeutic index of many cancer chemotherapeutic agents. The aim of personalized medicine is to prescribe a convenient chemotherapeutics to the right patients with right dose to achieve maximal therapeutic benefit with minimal toxicity. Deep observation of the human genome is still ongoing, and it will help to discover new targets and select the most efficacious drug for each patient's tumor, which is named as genomic prescribing system, the next evolution of systemic cancer management. Genetic polymorphisms, as significant biomarkers, have provided significant and crucial information in the management of toxicity and dosing of cancer treatments. So far the achievements have been limited due to the multifactorial challenges on the polymorphism-based personalized cancer management. Especially reliable clinical data for the effects of genetic alterations on the disease pathogenesis, drug metabolism and response are not always available; and performing the large-scale prospective clinical studies, to understand the associations of polymorphisms and the application of chemotherapeutics, is often laborious. However, these prospective studies are required for establishing possible relations for evaluating the utility and cost-effectiveness of polymorphism-based pharmacogenetic tests and personalized medicine. Ethical, social, and regulatory issues relevant with pharmacogenetic-based personalized medicine are the other complex and challenging factors to establish the relations between genetic polymorphisms and personalized drug responses.

The main application of genetic polymorphism knowledge is improving the futuristic health care through gene therapy, discovery of new drugs and drug targets and upgrade the discovery processes with advanced technologies. The use of single candidate genes can be useful as a part of initial treatment, but in near future, it will never be enough to provide fully tailored treatment decisions on the cancer management. Other omics technologies will complement the genotype-phenotype association-based pharmacological-pathway approach, such as transcriptomics, epigenomics, and miRNAomics.

2.4.1. Polymorphism and pharmacogenetics facts

- Humans share about 99.9% sequence identity. The other 0.1% are mostly SNPs.
- SNPs are the most common polymorphism type and occur about every 1000 bases.

- SNPs can be silent—99% of them are not in coding regions and not in genes and thus cause harmless, harmful, latent changes.
- Genetic polymorphisms are one of the most important factors that may contribute to ethnic sensitivity of a drug.
- FDA recommends for following guidelines relating to "ethnically sensitive situations" for some drugs and suggests solutions that may control such ethnic sensitivity in the context of therapeutic applications and study designs.
- The Hardy-Weinberg principle can be used to calculate allele frequencies.
- Hardy-Weinberg principle-based reporting may be optimal in genetic polymorphism-based studies.
- Personalized medicine separates patients into different groups with an individual's molecular profile and covers the determination of the safest and most effective chemotherapeutic agents.
- The aim of pharmacogenetics is to make 'personalized medicine' as applicable to various patient groups.
- Although a number of good polymorphism genotyping technologies are currently in use to meet the needs of clinics and researches, not only one genotyping method is ideal for all applications. Studies on ideal polymorphism genotyping technologies are still ongoing.
- FDA has been working to improve pharmacogenetics technologies in the development, regulation and use of medications and revise drug labels in terms of pharmacogenetic biomarkers in oncology area.
- Polymorphism in the *DPYD* gene is responsible for insufficient production of DPD enzyme; therefore, low levels of enzyme increase drug accumulation and toxicity due to the inefficient catabolism of drug.
- Allelic differences of *UGT1A1* affect the glucuronidation of SN-38, active metabolite of irinotecan both *in vitro* and *in vivo*.
- *TPMT* polymorphisms have different effects on function of TPMT that inactivates thioguanine nucleotides. Patients with low TPMT activity expose more activated thioguanine nucleotides and more treatment toxicity as well as efficacy.
- FDA recommends screening for G6PD deficiency before the beginning of rasburicase treatment.
- *CYP2D6* deficiency is the first discovered pharmacogenetic deficiency. Genetic variants of CYP2D6 are classified into ultra-rapid metabolizer, extensive metabolizer, intermediate metabolizer, and poor metabolizer.
- Biomarker development studies involve multiple steps, as biomarker assay development, analytical validation, clinical validation, and clinical implementation.

Author details

Gizem Calibasi Kocal[1] and Yasemin Baskin[1,2,3]*

*Address all correspondence to: yasemin.baskin@deu.edu.tr

1 Department of Basic Oncology, Institute of Oncology, Dokuz Eylul University, Izmir, Turkey

2 Personalized Medicine and Pharmacogenomics/Genomics Research Centre-BIFAGEM, Dokuz Eylul University, Izmir, Turkey

3 Faculty of Medicine, Department of Medical Informatics and Biostatistics, Dokuz Eylul University, Izmir, Turkey

References

[1] Bosch TM, Meijerman I, Beijnen JH, Schellens JH. Genetic polymorphisms of drug-metabolising enzymes and drug transporters in the chemotherapeutic treatment of cancer. Clinical Pharmacokinetics. 2006;**45**(3):253-285. DOI: 10.2165/00003088-200645030-00003

[2] Lander ES. Initial impact of the sequencing of the human genome. Nature. 2011;**470**(7333):187-197. DOI: 10.1038/nature09792

[3] Robert J, Le Morvan V, Giovannetti E, Peters GJ; PAMM Group of EORTC. On the use of pharmacogenetics in cancer treatment and clinical trials. European Journal of Cancer. 2014;**50**(15):2532-2543. DOI: 10.1016/j.ejca.2014.07.013

[4] Karki R, Pandya D, Elston RC, Ferlini C. Defining "mutation" and "polymorphism" in the era of personal genomics. BMC Medical Genomics. 2015;**8**:37. DOI: 10.1186/s12920-015-0115-z

[5] Strachan T, Goodship J, Chinner P. Principles of genetic variation. In: Strachan T, Goodship J, Chinner P, editors. Genetics and Genomics in Medicine. 1st ed. New York: Garland Science Taylor and Francis Group; 2015. pp. 79-116. DOI: 978-0-8153-4480-3

[6] Chakravarti A. Single nucleotide polymorphisms: To a future of genetic medicine. Nature. 2001;**409**:822-823. DOI: 10.1038/35057281

[7] Huang SM, Temple R, Throckmorton DC, Lesko LJ. Drug interaction studies: Study design, data analysis, and implications for dosing and labeling. Clinical Pharmacology & Therapeutics. 2007;**81**(2):298-304. DOI: 10.1038/sj.clpt.6100054

[8] Andersson T, Flockhart DA, Goldstein DB, Huang SM, Kroetz DL, Milos PM, Ratain MJ, Thummel K. Drug-metabolizing enzymes: Evidence for clinical utility of pharmacogenomic tests. Clinical Pharmacology & Therapeutics. 2005;**78**(6):559-581. DOI: 10.1016/j.clpt.2005.08.013

[9] Bjornsson TD, Callaghan JT, Einolf HJ, Fischer V, Gan L, Grimm S, Kao J, King SP, Miwa G, Ni L, Kumar G, McLeod J, Obach RS, Roberts S, Roe A, Shah A, Snikeris F,

Sullivan JT, Tweedie D, Vega JM, Walsh J, Wrighton SA; Pharmaceutical Research and Manufacturers of America (PhRMA) Drug Metabolism/Clinical Pharmacology Technical Working Group.; FDA Center for Drug Evaluation and Research (CDER). The conduct of in vitro and in vivo drug-drug interaction studies: A Pharmaceutical Research and Manufacturers of America (PhRMA) perspective. Drug Metabolism and Disposition. 2000;**31**(7):815-832. DOI: 10.1124/dmd.31.7.815

[10] Galvan A, Ioannidis JP, Dragani TA. Beyond genome-wide association studies: Genetic heterogeneity and individual predisposition to cancer. Trends in Genetics. 2010;**26**(3):132-141. DOI: 10.1016/j.tig.2009.12.008

[11] Dadd T, Dadd T, Weale ME, Lewis CM. A critical evaluation of genomic control methods for genetic association studies. Genetic Epidemiology. 2009;**33**(4):290-298. DOI: 10.1002/gepi.20379

[12] Wang K. Testing for genetic association in the presence of population stratification in genome-wide association studies. Genetic Epidemiology. 2009;**33**(7):637-645. DOI: 10.1002/gepi.20415

[13] Guan W, Liang L, Boehnke M, Abecasis GR. Genotype-based matching to correct for population stratification in large-scale case-control genetic association studies. Genetic Epidemiology. 2009;**33**(6):508-517. DOI: 10.1002/gepi.20403

[14] Yesupriya A, Evangelou E, Kavvoura FK, Patsopoulos NA, Clyne M, Walsh MC, Lin BK, Yu W, Gwinn M, Ioannidis JP, Khoury MJ. Reporting of human genome epidemiology (HuGE) association studies: An empirical assessment. BMC Medical Research Methodology. 2008;**8**:31. DOI: 10.1186/1471-2288-8-31

[15] Salanti G, Amountza G, Ntzani EE, Ioannidis JP. Hardy-Weinberg equilibrium in genetic association studies: An empirical evaluation of reporting, deviations, and power. European Journal of Human Genetics. 2005;**13**(7):840-848. DOI: 10.1038/sj.ejhg.5201410

[16] Keefe DM, Bateman EH. Tumor control versus adverse events with targeted anticancer therapies. Nature Reviews Clinical Oncology. 2011;**9**(2):98-109. DOI: 10.1038/nrclinonc.2011.192

[17] Sim SC, Kacevska M, Ingelman-Sundberg M. Pharmacogenomics of drug-metabolizing enzymes: A recent update on clinical implications and endogenous effects. Pharmacogenomics Journal. 2013;**13**(1):1-11. DOI: 10.1038/tpj.2012.45

[18] Tian Q, Price ND, Hood L. Systems cancer medicine: Towards realization of predictive, preventive, personalized and participatory (P4) medicine. Journal of Internal Medicine. 2012;**271**(2):111-121. DOI: 10.1111/j.1365-2796.2011.02498.x

[19] Twyman RM. Single nucleotide polymorphism (SNP) genotyping techniques—an overview. In: Fuchs J, Podda M, editors. Encyclopedia of Diagnostic Genomics and Proteomics. New York: Marcel Dekker Inc; 2005. pp. 1202-1207. DOI: 10.1081/E-EDGP 120020761

[20] Kwok PY. Methods for genotyping single nucleotide polymorphisms. Annual Review of Genomics and Human Genetics. 2001;**2**:235-258. DOI: 10.1146/annurev.genom.2.1.235

[21] Kim S, Misra A. SNP genotyping: Technologies and biomedical applications. Annual Review of Biomedical Engineering. 2007;**9**:289-320. DOI: 10.1146/annurev.bioeng.9.060906.152037

[22] Pirmohamed M, Park BK. Genetic susceptibility to adverse drug reactions. Trends in Pharmacological Sciences. 2001;**22**:298-305. DOI: 10.1016/S0165-6147(00)01717-X

[23] Ulrich CM, Robien K, McLeod HL. Cancer pharmacogenetics: Polymorphisms, pathways and beyond. Nature Reviews Cancer. 2003;**3**(12):912-920. DOI: 10.1038/nrc1233

[24] Rogers JF, Nafziger AN, Bertino Jr JS. Pharmacogenetics affects dosing, efficacy, and toxicity of cytochrome P450-metabolized drugs. American Journal of Medicine. 2002;**113**(9):746-750. DOI: 10.1016/S0002-9343(02)01363-3

[25] Crews KR, Hicks JK, Pui CH, Relling MV, Evans WE. Pharmacogenomics and individualized medicine: Translating science into practice. Clinical Pharmacology & Therapeutics. 2012;**92**(4):467-475. DOI: 10.1038/clpt.2012.120

[26] United States Food and Drug Administration. Table of Pharmacogenomic Biomarkers in Drug Labeling [Internet]. 2017. Available from: https://www.fda.gov/Drugs/ScienceResearch/ResearchAreas/Pharmacogenetics/ucm083378.htm [Accessed: March 14, 2017]

[27] Bosma PJ, Seppen J, Goldhoorn B, Bakker C, Oude Elferink RP, Chowdhury JR, Chowdhury NR, Jansen PL. Bilirubin UDP-glucuronosyltransferase 1 is the only relevant bilirubin glucuronidating isoform in man. Journal of Biological Chemistry. 1994;**269**(27):17960-17964

[28] Etienne-Grimaldi MC, Boyer JC, Thomas F, Quaranta S, Picard N, Loriot MA, Narjoz C, Poncet D, Gagnieu MC, Ged C, Broly F, Le Morvan V, Bouquié R, Gaub MP, Philibert L, Ghiringhelli F, Le Guellec C; Collective work by Groupe de Pharmacologie Clinique Oncologique (GPCO-Unicancer).; French Réseau National de Pharmacogénétique Hospitalière (RNPGx). UGT1A1 genotype and irinotecan therapy: General review and implementation in routine practice. Fundamental & Clinical Pharmacology. 2015;**29**(3):219-237. DOI: 10.1111/fcp.12117

[29] Iyer L, Das S, Janisch L, Wen M, Ramírez J, Karrison T, Fleming GF, Vokes EE, Schilsky RL, Ratain MJ. UGT1A1*28 polymorphism as a determinant of irinotecan disposition and toxicity. Pharmacogenomics Journal. 2002;**2**(1):43-47. DOI: 10.1038/sj/tpj/6500072

[30] Innocenti F, Grimsley C, Das S, Ramírez J, Cheng C, Kuttab-Boulos H, Ratain MJ, Di Rienzo A. Haplotype structure of the UDP-glucuronosyltransferase 1A1 promoter in different ethnic groups. Pharmacogenetics. 2002;**12**(9):725-733. DOI: 10.1097/00008571-200212000-00006

[31] Gagne JF, Montminy V, Belanger P, Journault K, Gaucher G, Guillemette C. Common human UGT1A polymorphisms and the altered metabolism of irinotecan active metabolite 7-ethyl-10-hydroxycamptothecin (SN-38). Molecular Pharmacology. 2002;**3**:608-617. DOI: 10.1124/mol.62.3.608

[32] Longley DB, Harkin DP, Johnston PG. 5-fluorouracil: Mechanisms of action and clinical strategies. Nature Reviews Cancer. 2003;**3**(5):330-338. DOI: 10.1038/nrc.1074

[33] Baskin Y, Amirfallah A, Unal OU, Calibasi G, Oztop I. Dihydropyrimidine dehydrogenase 85T>C mutation is associated with ocular toxicity of 5-fluorouracil: A case report. American Journal of Therapeutics. 2015;**22**(2):e36–e39. DOI: 10.1097/MJT.0b013e31829e8516

[34] van Staveren MC, Guchelaar HJ, van Kuilenburg AB, et al. Evaluation of predictive tests for screening for dihydropyrimidine dehydrogenase deficiency. Pharmacogenomics Journal. 2013;**13**:389-395. DOI: 10.1038/tpj.2013.25

[35] Aiello M, Vella N, Cannavò C, Scalisi A, Spandidos DA, Toffoli G, Buonadonna A, Libra M, Stivala F. Role of genetic polymorphisms and mutations in colorectal cancer therapy (Review). Journal of Molecular Medicine. 2011;**4**(2):203-208. DOI: 10.3892/mmr.2010.408

[36] Amstutz U, Froehlich TK, Largiadèr CR. Dihydropyrimidine dehydrogenase gene as a major predictor of severe 5-fluorouracil toxicity. Pharmacogenomics. 2011;**12**(9):1321-1336. DOI: 10.2217/PGS.11.72

[37] Loganayagam A, Arenas Hernandez M, Corrigan A, Fairbanks L, Lewis CM, Harper P, Maisey N, Ross P, Sanderson JD, Marinaki AM. Pharmacogenetic variants in the DPYD, TYMS, CDA and MTHFR genes are clinically significant predictors of fluoropyrimidine toxicity. British Journal of Cancer. 2013;**108**(12):2505-2515. DOI: 10.1038/bjc.2013.262

[38] Offer SM, Fossum CC, Wegner NJ, Stuflesser AJ, Butterfield GL, Diasio RB. Comparative functional analysis of DPYD variants of potential clinical relevance to dihydropyrimidine dehydrogenase activity. Cancer Research. 2014;**74**(9):2545-2554. DOI: 10.1158/0008-5472.CAN-13-2482

[39] Mattison LK, Ezzeldin H, Carpenter M, Modak A, Johnson MR, Diasio RB. Rapid identification of dihydropyrimidine dehydrogenase deficiency by using a novel 2-13C-uracil breath test. Clinical Cancer Research. 2004;**10**(8):2652-2658. DOI: 10.1158/1078-0432.CCR-03-0374

[40] Gross E, Ullrich T, Seck K, Mueller V, de Wit M, von Schilling C, Meindl A, Schmitt M, Kiechle M. Detailed analysis of five mutations in dihydropyrimidine dehydrogenase detected in cancer patients with 5-fluorouracil-related side effects. Human Mutation. 2003;**22**(6):498. DOI: 10.1002/humu.9201

[41] van Kuilenburg AB, De Abreu RA, van Gennip AH. Pharmacogenetic and clinical aspects of dihydropyrimidine dehydrogenase deficiency. Annals of Clinical Biochemistry. 2003;**40**(Pt 1):41-45. DOI: 10.1258/000456303321016150

[42] Marcuello E, Altés A, Menoyo A, Del Rio E, Gómez-Pardo M, Baiget M. UGT1A1 gene variations and irinotecan treatment in patients with metastatic colorectal cancer. British Journal of Cancer. 2004;**91**(4):678-682. DOI: 10.1038/sj.bjc.6602042

[43] Caudle KE, Thorn CF, Klein TE, Swen JJ, McLeod HL, Diasio RB, Schwab M. Clinical Pharmacogenetics Implementation Consortium guidelines for dihydropyrimidine dehydrogenase genotype and fluoropyrimidine dosing. Clinical Pharmacology & Therapeutics. 2013;**94**(6):640-645. DOI: 10.1038/clpt.2013.172

[44] Hickey SE, Curry CJ, Toriello HV. ACMG practice guideline: Lack of evidence for MTHFR polymorphism testing. Genetics in Medicine. 2013;**15**(2):153-156. DOI: 10.1038/gim.2012.165

[45] Zhou SF, Di YM, Chan E, Du YM, Chow VD, Xue CC, Lai X, Wang JC, Li CG, Tian M, Duan W. Clinical pharmacogenetics and potential application in personalized medicine. Current Drug Metabolism. 2008;**9**(8):738-784. DOI: 10.2174/138920008786049302

[46] Tan BR, Thomas F, Myerson RJ, Zehnbauer B, Trinkaus K, Malyapa RS, Mutch MG, Abbey EE, Alyasiry A, Fleshman JW, McLeod HL. Thymidylate synthase genotype-directed neoadjuvant chemoradiation for patients with rectal adenocarcinoma. Journal of Clinical Oncology. 2011 Mar 1;**29**(7):875-883. DOI: 10.1200/JCO.2010.32.3212

[47] Lecomte T, Ferraz JM, Zinzindohoué F, Loriot MA, Tregouet DA, Landi B, Berger A, Cugnenc PH, Jian R, Beaune P, Laurent-Puig P. Thymidylate synthase gene polymorphism predicts toxicity in colorectal cancer patients receiving 5-fluorouracil-based chemotherapy. Clinical Cancer Research. 2004;**10**(17):5880-5888. DOI: 10.1158/1078-0432.CCR-04-0169

[48] Danenberg PV. Pharmacogenomics of thymidylate synthase in cancer treatment. Frontiers in Bioscience. 2004;**9**:2484-2494. DOI: 10.2741/1410

[49] Mandola MV, Stoehlmacher J, Zhang W, Groshen S, Yu MC, Iqbal S, Lenz HJ, Ladner RD. A 6 bp polymorphism in the thymidylate synthase gene causes message instability and is associated with decreased intratumoral TS mRNA levels. Pharmacogenetics. 2004;**14**(5):319-327. DOI: 10.1097/01.fpc.0000114730.08559.df

[50] Ulrich CM, Potter JD. Thymidylate synthase polymorphism and survival of colorectal cancer patients treated with 5-fluorouracil. British Journal of Cancer. 2002;**86**(8):1365. DOI: 10.1038/sj.bjc.6600229

[51] Rosmarin D, Palles C, Church D, Domingo E, Jones A, Johnstone E, Wang H, Love S, Julier P, Scudder C, Nicholson G, Gonzalez-Neira A, Martin M, Sargent D, Green E, McLeod H, Zanger UM, Schwab M, Braun M, Seymour M, Thompson L, Lacas B, Boige V, Ribelles N, Afzal S, Enghusen H, Jensen SA, Etienne-Grimaldi MC, Milano G, Wadelius M, Glimelius B, Garmo H, Gusella M, Lecomte T, Laurent-Puig P, Martinez-Balibrea E, Sharma R, Garcia-Foncillas J, Kleibl Z, Morel A, Pignon JP, Midgley R, Kerr D, Tomlinson I. Genetic markers of toxicity from capecitabine and other fluorouracil-based regimens: Investigation in the QUASAR2 study, systematic review, and meta-analysis. Journal of Clinical Oncology. 2014;**32**(10):1031-1039. DOI: 10.1200/JCO.2013.51.1857

[52] Hertz DL, Rae J. Pharmacogenetics of cancer drugs. Annual Review of Medicine. 2015;**66**:65-81. DOI: 10.1146/annurev-med-053013-053944

[53] Stanulla M, Schaeffeler E, Flohr T, Cario G, Schrauder A, Zimmermann M, Welte K, Ludwig WD, Bartram CR, Zanger UM, Eichelbaum M, Schrappe M, Schwab M. Thiopurine methyltransferase (TPMT) genotype and early treatment response to mercaptopurine in childhood acute lymphoblastic leukemia. Journal of the American Medical Association. 2005;**293**(12):1485-1489. DOI: 10.1001/jama.293.12.1485

[54] Luzzatto L, Seneca E. G6PD deficiency: A classic example of pharmacogenetics with on-going clinical implications. British Journal of Haematology. 2014;**164**(4):469-480. DOI: 10.1111/bjh.12665

[55] Manganelli G, Masullo U, Passarelli S, Filosa S. Glucose-6-phosphate dehydrogenase deficiency: Disadvantages and possible benefits. Cardiovascular & Haematological Disorders Drug Targets. 2013;**13**(1):73-82. DOI: 10.2174/1871529X11313010008

[56] Wei CY, Lee MT, Chen YT. Pharmacogenomics of adverse drug reactions: Implementing personalized medicine. Human Molecular Genetics. 2012;**21**(R1):R58–R65. DOI: 10.1093/hmg/dds341

[57] Bell GC, Crews KR, Wilkinson MR, Haidar CE, Hicks JK, Baker DK, Kornegay NM, Yang W, Cross SJ, Howard SC, Freimuth RR, Evans WE, Broeckel U, Relling MV, Hoffman JM. Development and use of active clinical decision support for preemptive pharmacogenomics. Journal of the American Medical Informatics Association. 2014;**21**(e1):e93–e99. DOI: 10.1136/amiajnl-2013-001993

[58] Swen JJ, Nijenhuis M, de Boer A, Grandia L, Maitland-van der Zee AH, Mulder H, Rongen GA, van Schaik RH, Schalekamp T, Touw DJ, van der Weide J, Wilffert B, Deneer VH, Guchelaar HJ. Pharmacogenetics: From bench to byte--an update of guidelines. Clinical Pharmacology & Therapeutics. 2011;**89**(5):662-673. DOI: 10.1038/clpt.2011.34

[59] Borges S, Desta Z, Jin Y, Faouzi A, Robarge JD, Philips S, Nguyen A, Stearns V, Hayes D, Rae JM, Skaar TC, Flockhart DA, Li L. Composite functional genetic and comedication CYP2D6 activity score in predicting tamoxifen drug exposure among breast cancer patients. The Journal of Clinical Pharmacology. 2010;**50**(4):450-458. DOI: 10.1177/0091270009359182

[60] Madlensky L, Natarajan L, Tchu S, Pu M, Mortimer J, Flatt SW, Nikoloff DM, Hillman G, Fontecha MR, Lawrence HJ, Parker BA, Wu AH, Pierce JP. Tamoxifen metabolite concentrations, CYP2D6 genotype, and breast cancer outcomes. Clinical Pharmacology & Therapeutics. 2011;**89**(5):718-725. DOI: 10.1038/clpt.2011.32

[61] Lorizio W, Wu AH, Beattie MS, Rugo H, Tchu S, Kerlikowske K, Ziv E. Clinical and biomarker predictors of side effects from tamoxifen. Breast Cancer Research and Treatment. 2012;**132**(3):1107-1118. DOI: 10.1007/s10549-011-1893-4

[62] Goossens N, Nakagawa S, Sun X, Hoshida Y. Cancer biomarker discovery and validation. Translational Cancer Research. 2015;**4**(3):256-269. DOI: 10.3978/j.issn.2218-676X.2015.06.04

Chapter 2

Genetic Polymorphisms in Aromatase (CYP19) Gene and Cancer

Arjumand S. Warsy, Fatimah Basil Almukaynizi,
Soad AlDaihan, Sophia Alam and Maha Daghastani

Additional information is available at the end of the chapter

http://dx.doi.org/10.5772/intechopen.69208

Abstract

Estrogens play an important role in the development and progression of several types of cancers. The synthesis of estrogens occurs in almost all tissues of the body in addition to the gonads. The enzyme aromatase (CYP19A1) encoded by *CYP19A1* gene is involved in the synthesis of estrogens. Genetic variations in *CYP19A1* gene influence both the structure-function relationship of the enzyme and the rate of its synthesis. Extensive studies have reported different types of polymorphisms in the *CYP19A1* gene and have shown that the polymorphisms, depending on their location in the gene, have different effects on the function and activity of the gene product. Association studies have been conducted and have led to the realization that interpopulation differences are widespread. Not only do polymorphic forms exert different effects on the development of different cancers, due possibly to the influence of other genetic variations, environmental, metabolic, and epigenetic factors, but also are important as they lead to the interindividual differences seen during treatment of the cancer state. This chapter covers important aspects of the aromatase function, the *CYP19A1* gene structure, polymorphisms identified in the gene, different cancers and associated polymorphisms, and the role of the polymorphic forms in affecting the treatment strategies.

Keywords: aromatase, aromatase inhibitors, cancer, CYP19A1, estrogens, polymorphism

1. Introduction

By the late 1990s, several epidemiological and clinical studies had shown that estrogens play an important role in the development and progression of several types of cancers, in particular breast, endometrial, prostrate, and colorectal cancer (CRC). A strong connection was shown to exist between initiation/promotion of cancer and excess of estrogens, as the latter increased mitotic activity. Initially, extensive studies linked the administration of exogenous hormones to the development of these cancers [1], and later it was shown that several estrogen-sensitive tissues act as intracrine organs, producing estrogens and hence elevating local hormone levels, which accelerated proliferation and growth of cancer cell [2].

There are four major naturally occurring estrogens, estrone (E1), estradiol (E2), estriol (E3), and estetrol (E4), which are produced only during pregnancy. Estradiol (E2) is an important estrogen, has the highest affinity to estrogen receptors, and is required for different physiological functions during all stages of life in both males and females [3]. Aromatase, due to its critical role in the synthesis of the different forms of estrogens from androgens [4], specifically estradiol from testosterone, estrone from androstenedione, and estriol from 16α-hydroxylated dehydroepiandrosterone, is incriminated as a major player in cancer biogenesis.

2. The enzyme "aromatase": a key player in estrogen synthesis

Aromatase (EC 1.14.14.1), also known as estrogen synthase, is the gene product of *CYP19A1* gene and is an important member of the cytochrome p450 superfamily, subfamily 19. It catalyzes a rate-limiting step during the aromatization of androgens to estrogens by three successive hydroxylations and eliminations of carbon at position 19 of the androgens (**Figure 1**) [5].

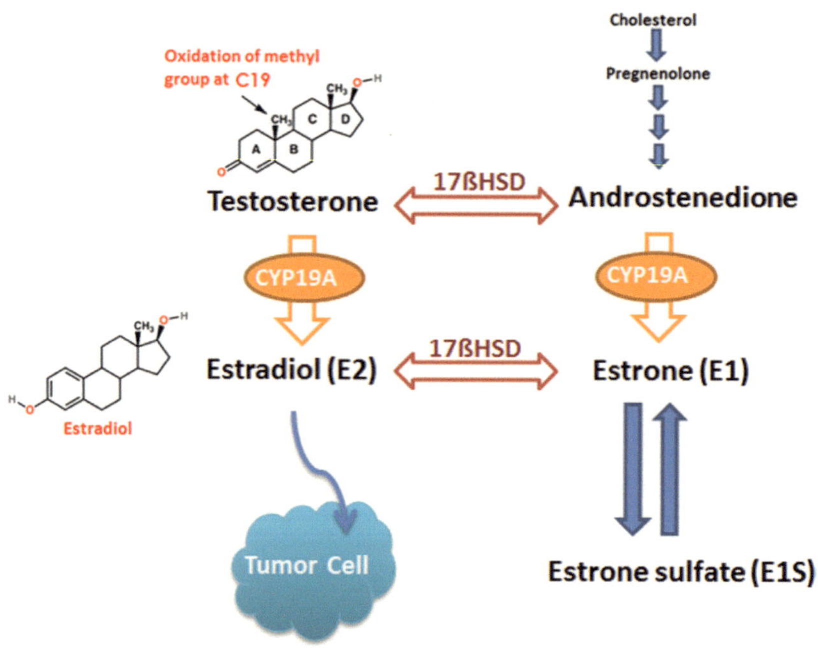

Figure 1. Role of aromatase in estrogen synthesis.

Several studies suggest that many tumors are dependent upon estrogens for their development and continued growth [6]. Blockage of any conversion in the pathway potentially leads to decreased estrogen production, but more specific suppression results from inhibition of the final step that is unique to estrogen biosynthesis, i.e., inhibition of aromatase. The key role of aromatase in estrogen biosynthesis has generated enormous interest in putative inhibitors of the enzyme and their use as therapy against endocrine-responsive tumors.

Initially, it was believed that the ovaries and placenta are the only site for the production of estrogens, which are involved in female reproductive functions. However, later studies conducted using many sophisticated and sensitive tests and equipment revealed that estrogens are also synthesized in the male gonadal tissues, i.e., the testis and epididymis, and in extra-gonadal tissues including liver, colon, prostate, brain, adrenal gland, skin, bone, hair follicles, adipose, and vascular tissues. This is due to the presence of aromatase, which is active in various tissues in both females and males, and hence estrogens are produced in gonads and in the extra-gonadal tissues [2, 7–9].

Aromatase is a dimer, a complex of two polypeptides; one is a specific cytochrome P450, which is the product of the *CYP19A1* gene. The other subunit is a flavoprotein, NADPH-cytochrome P450 reductase. This is ubiquitously present in most cells, and this wide distribution within the human body justifies its central role in different physiological processes [10].

2.1. Aromatase gene structure

The *CYP19A1* is located on chromosome 15 at q21.1 region and spans about 123 kb [11]. It has 10 exons and nine introns in all tissues where the coding region covers about 34 kb region, while the regulatory region is more than three times longer (approx. 95 kb) **(Figure 2)**. This is in the 5′ region of the gene and occurs as unique sequences, scattered upstream of the coding sequences. The regulatory region is unusually large and is composed of at least 10 tissue-specific promoters **(Figure 3)**. These promoters are used alternatively in different cell types. The regulation of each promoter depends on a distinct set of regulatory sequences in the DNA and specific transcription factors that bind to these sequences. The transcription factors bind the promoter, activating it and giving rise to splicing of an untranslated first exon onto this common junction immediately upstream of the translation start site in the coding region. The promoter region has the basic transcription elements, i.e., the TATA box, a CAAT box, and a GC box, and also contains different regulatory elements in different tissues [12].

This first exon (exon 1) occurs in multiple forms, which encode the 5′ untranslated region (UTR) of the *CYP19A* gene and are spliced out in a highly tissue-specific manner. Since the gene has multiple promoters, in each tissue the transcript is generated following tissue-specific splicing of alternative exons available for exon 1. For physiologic estrogen biosynthesis in the gonads, brain, vascular tissue, bone, adipose tissue, placenta, skin, and fetal liver, different partially tissue-specific promoters are used [13]. To date, nine different exon 1 subtypes have been reported, and each is expressed in a specific tissue as presented in **Table 1**. Exons 2–10 form the coding sequence of the gene and lie in a region, which is approximately 34 Kb in length. Exon 1, specific for the tissue, gets linked to exon 2 after splicing of the intervening sequences **(Figure 3)**. All transcripts have the same coding sequence generated from the sequences in exons 2–10 [12–14].

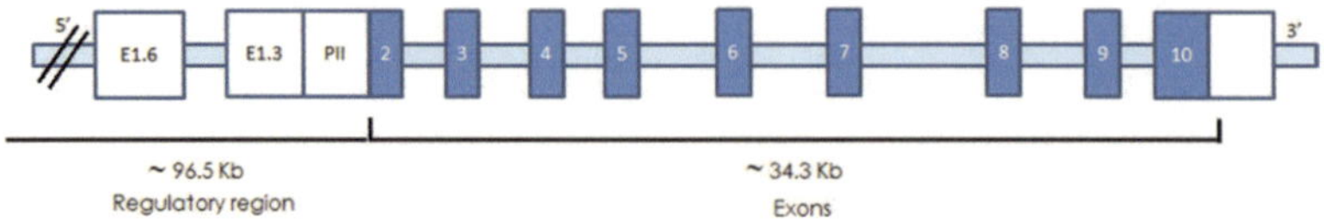

Figure 2. Structure of CYP19A gene.

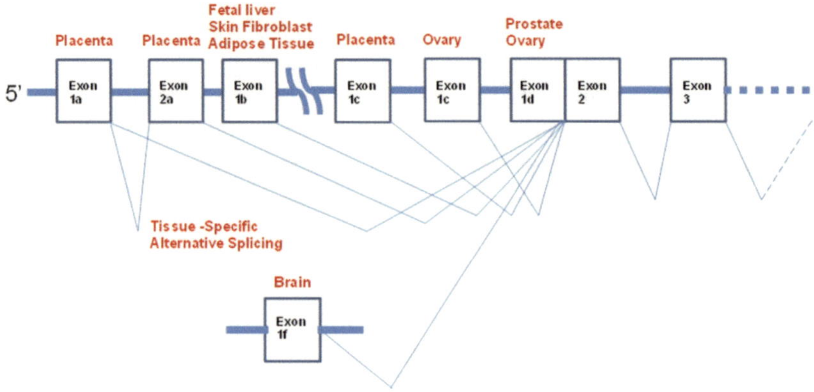

Figure 3. The 5′ gene region of the human *CYP19A1* gene. The 5′ untranslated region of the human aromatase gene is encoded by multiple exon 1. These are tissue specifically spliced and connected to exon 2 (modified from Ref. [4]). The lines linking exon 1 to exon 2 indicate that exon 1 is present as 5′ UTR in the tissue.

Exon 1 type	Expressed in (tissue)
I.1 (1a) and I.2 (1e)	—Placenta
I.3 (1c) and PII (1d)	—Ovary —Testis
I.4 (1b)	—Adipose tissue
I.5	—Fetal lung —Intestine
I.6	—Adipose —Bone tissues
I.7	—Adipose —Vascular endothelial tissues
1f	—Brain
II. I.3, I.7, and I.4	—Breast

Table 1. The multiple forms of exon 1 and the tissues in which each is expressed.

Investigations have shown the expression of aromatase gene in estrogen-dependent breast cancer (BC) tissues, endometrial carcinoma, and colorectal, gastric, liver, lung, ovarian, pancreatic, and prostatic cancers [2, 12]. The cell-specific expression of aromatase determines the presence or absence of aromatase activity in the tissue and hence the amount of available estrogens.

The transcriptional regulation of aromatase has been extensively investigated since the 1980s. Many mechanisms have been proposed to explain the underlying control of *CYP19A1* gene expression, in an attempt to elucidate the etiological role played by aromatase in cancer development and progression [15]. Several mechanisms at the transcriptional, posttranscriptional, and epigenetic levels have been unveiled. In addition to these mechanisms, extensive genetic variants of CYP19A1 gene have been identified that influence aromatase activity and may be regarded as prognostic factors for susceptibility to cancer development [16–18].

2.2. Genetic polymorphisms of the *CYP19A1* gene

The *CYP19A* gene seems to have acquired a number of variations in the coding, noncoding, and control sequences [17]. These variations result from different mutations, short tandem repeat (STR) polymorphisms, and single nucleotide polymorphisms (SNPs). The variations may influence expression of *CYP19A1* gene, activity of the enzyme, susceptibility to cancer development, and clinicopathological features of cancer, and some act as refractory and prognostic factors.

Frequencies at which the alleles occur in different populations differ considerably, and it is also shown that the differences in the plasma levels of several sex hormones may be due to the presence of different alleles, particularly in postmenopausal women. It is hypothesized that the genetic polymorphisms provide a probable explanation for differences in cancer risk among different ethnic groups. Hence, the presence of the different *CYP19A1* alleles may account partially for the racial differences in the frequency of the different types of cancer.

This section presents the polymorphisms identified in the *CYP19A1* gene and discusses their distribution in different populations, their association with different cancers, their influence on the development, prognosis, treatment strategies, and complications resulting from the treatment.

2.2.1. Short tandem repeat (STR) polymorphism

Short tandem repeats (STRs) were identified in the aromatase gene during the late 1990s, and some studies showed a higher incidence of cancers in individuals carrying different alleles of the *CYP19A1* gene. One of the most frequently reported STRs in *CYP19A1* is a tetranucleotide (TTTA) sequence, which occurs in different repeats ranging from 2 to 13.

Several studies conducted in different populations reported association between the tetranucleotide repeat sequence and cancer, while others failed to do so. Kristensen et al. [19] reported that a rare polymorphic A1 allele of *CYP19* repeat (TTTA)12 occurs at a significantly higher frequency in females suffering from breast cancer than controls (3.6 vs. 1.6%) and indicated that the carriers of the allele might have an increased risk of developing breast cancer (OR = 2.42; 95% CI = 1.03–5.80). Haiman et al. [20] showed that breast cancer cases had a statistically significant greater frequency of the (TTTA)10 repeat alleles (10 alleles; 2.3 vs. 0.7%; $p = 0.005$), but a nonsignificant increase in the frequency of the (TTTA)12 allele (12 alleles; 3.1 vs. 2.1%; $p = 0.11$). The 10 alleles were more frequent in patients with more advanced cancer disease, which were defined as four or more involved nodes or distant metastasis. A little later study on Japanese women reported similar results in breast cancer

(OR = 1.80; 95% CI = 0.97–3.36) risk [21]. Baxter et al. [22] also confirmed that breast cancer cases had a statistically significant positive association with the (TTTA)10 allele (1.5 vs. 0.2%; p = 0.028) and the (TTTA)8 allele (13.5 vs. 8.7%; p = 0.012), while the frequency of the (TTTA)12 allele was not statistically significant. A study by Miyoshi et al. [23] showed that the (TTTA)7 along with a trinucleotide deletion (−3bp) allele was increased significantly ($p < 0.05$) in breast cancer patients who were ER positive (OR = 1.72; 95% CI = 1.10–2.69), but not those who were ER negative. Among the Brazilian cancer patients, the (TTTA)10 allele associated positively with breast cancer development and the frequency of the allele was three times more compared to controls (p = 0.048) [24]. A study from China also showed a significantly higher frequency of (TTTA)10 allele in breast cancer cases (12.4%) than controls (8.2%) (p = 0.02) [25]. As presented in **Figure 4**, a recent study from Mexico showed significant differences in the repeat number in breast cancer patients compared to the normal controls.

Several studies were published from Russia, and it was shown by Artamonov et al. [26] that the allele (TTTA)8 was associated with BC (11.8 vs. 6.3%; p = 0.04). Risk of BC elevated if this allele was present with genotype A2/A2 of the tetranucleotide deletion (7.3 vs. 0%; $p < 0.01$). In Norwegian women [19], the association of breast cancer with the long allele (TTTA)12 was shown.

Kim et al. [28] reported that though there is no difference in the (TTTA)n genotype distribution between patients and controls, but there was a positive association between >(TTTA)10 and ER-negative tumors and between lower repeat polymorphism and ER-positive tumors (p = 0.019). A study on different ethnic groups (African-Americans, Japanese, Latinas, and non-Latina Whites) by Probst-Hensch et al. [29] reported contradictory results and showed no consistent association of (TTTA)n repeat polymorphism with breast cancer risk. This was in line with other studies from the USA [30] and Greece [31]. These studies show that the tetranucleotide polymorphism occurs in different populations, and the repeat variants show association with breast cancer in some and not others. Often, contradictory results are reported from the same population.

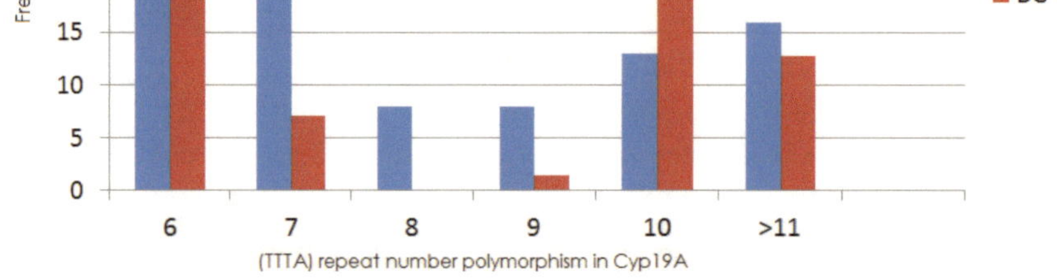

Figure 4. Frequency of TTTA repeat number polymorphism in breast cancer (BC) patients and normal (N) controls in a Mexican population (modified from Ref. [27]).

The (TTTA)n polymorphism has been reported to modify susceptibility to prostate cancer development in several studies in different populations. Most of the studies have shown that the longer alleles (TTTA)7 or more are associated with a higher risk of prostate cancer, and in some studies, it is shown that the association is also with cancer-specific survival [32, 33]. A study on the Japanese men reported that (TTTA)7 and (TTTA)8 alleles show association with the risk of prostate cancer [34]. It was also shown that when the patients were stratified according to the pathological grade or the clinical stage, there was no significant difference in the different genotypes. Tsuchiya et al. [35] regarded this polymorphism as a novel predictor of prostate cancer with bone metastasis. They showed that alleles longer than seven repeats (TTTA)7) were associated with worse cancer-specific survival. Tang et al. [36] further suggested that though these repeat polymorphism influence disease susceptibility, but the effect is modified by factors that alter hormone metabolism.

The (TTTA)n has also been investigated in endometrial cancer, and some studies have shown that the long alleles A6 and A7 occur at a higher frequency in the patients than the controls [37–39]. It was shown that the longer A6 and A7 alleles have higher intratumoral aromatase activity, thus predisposing to increased synthesis of estrogens and hence increasing the local estrogen concentration, which supports proliferation [40].

2.2.2. TCT insertion/deletion in intron 4

A TCT insertion/deletion (ins/del) polymorphism occurs in the intron 4 of the *CYP19A* gene, approximately 50 bp upstream to the (TTTA)n repeat. A few studies have linked breast cancer to the trinucleotide TCT deletion [31, 41]. In the British population, the TCT ins/del and a G-->T substitution in intron 4 were of rare occurrence (0.35 and 0.45, respectively), and both were in linkage disequilibrium with (TTTA)10 allele, which was reported to be linked to breast cancer susceptibility [41]. Similarly, in Korean breast cancer patients, 3-bp ins/del polymorphism showed a strong association with breast cancer risk [42], and other studies showed a stronger association with endometrial and prostate cancer risk [39, 43]. Coexisting (TTTA)n and 3-bp TCT deletion polymorphism show contradictory results in different studies [44, 45].

2.2.3. Single nucleotide polymorphisms

The presence of single nucleotide variations in the DNA sequence of *CYP19A1* gene was recognized in the earlier 1990s, and Ma et al. [46] reported 88 SNPs in 2005. To date several more SNPs have been identified, and several are of clinical interest, due to their predisposing or protective role in the development of cancer or other diseases. Some of these variations are rare, while others occur at a frequency of >1% and are polymorphic. Sourdaine et al. in 1994 [47] described several rare mutations in exons 3, 7, and 10 of the *CYP19A* gene in breast cancer patients. Kristensen et al. [48] reported a mutation in exon 10 (C > T) and showed that though the frequency of TT genotype was significantly higher in patients vs. controls ($p = 0.007$), particularly among those with stage III and IV diseases ($p = 0.004$) and with tumors larger than 5 cm ($p = 0.001$), it was a rare mutation. The T allele frequency was considerably higher in individuals who presented with more advanced disease and had larger (>5 cm) tumor size. The aromatase mRNA levels were high in the patient group and were associated with a switch to ovarian promoter from the one normally used, i.e., adipose promoter.

Single nucleotide polymorphism (SNP) association studies have been reported in several cancers and provide several interesting cues about the role of these variations. This section presents different types of cancer and the SNPs identified and studied.

3. CYP19A1 polymorphisms in different cancers

3.1. Variations in CYP19A1 gene and breast cancer

Breast cancer remains as the most frequently occurring cancer in all races and all ethnic groups (https://nccd.cdc.gov/uscs/toptencancers.aspx). Estrogens affect proliferation and growth of the cells in the breast. Thus, polymorphisms of the genes, which are involved in the estrogen biosynthesis and metabolism, have been regarded as factors affecting the risk of breast cancer. Research conducted since the early 1970s confirmed that the major risk and predisposing factor for breast cancer is increased exposure to estrogens and progesterone [49]. Obesity was also shown to be one of the factors since adipose tissues are an important source of endogenous estrogens [50]. Furthermore, local production of estrogens in the breast tissue was shown to play a major role in elevating hormone levels in the breast tissue, which in turn accelerates proliferation and growth of breast cells and subsequent progression to malignant transformation [51]. Genetic factors increase susceptibility to develop breast cancer, and in the 1990s, the identification of two breast cancer susceptibility genes, BRCA1 and BRCA2 [52], turned the attention of breast cancer research to the identification of possible genetic markers of breast cancer susceptibility. Extensive research has led to accumulation of knowledge about genetic variation in different genes, including the *CYP19A1* gene, due to its gene product, aromatase. **Table 2** summarizes some of the reports on SNPs in *CYP19A1* and shows that there are contradictions in different reports about the contribution of a SNP to breast cancer risk and there are population differences in the influence of the SNP on clinical presentation.

The rs10046 polymorphism is a C/T transition in the 3′ UTR of *CYP19A1* gene. It has been classified as a benign variant, which has recently been linked to aromatase deficiency (https://www.ncbi.nlm.nih.gov/clinvar/RCV000323501/). Recently, Farzaneh et al. [54] showed that there was a significant differences in allele and genotype frequencies for rs10046 in Iranian population with and without breast cancer (p-value = 0.01, OR (CI 95%) = 1.59 (1.1–2.3), p-value = 0.04, OR (CI 95%) = 1.7 (1.1–2.5), respectively). Zhang et al. [79] reported that among the ER+ Chinese women, the T allele of rs10046 was significantly associated with premenopausal breast cancer risk. Yoshimoto et al. [69] studied rs10046 polymorphism in Japanese women and reported that the C allele could be regarded as a risk predictor of breast cancer (p = 0.007). However, other studies on different populations failed to show any association. A study on Greenlandic Inuit women did not show any effect of rs10046 on the risk of breast cancer (%) [53]. Pineda et al. [72] showed that in a Spanish population the C allele may be linked to an increased risk of breast cancer. However, when they extended their findings to a meta-analysis, the association was lost. They concluded that it is possible that the effect of rs10046 is modified in the presence of other variants. Zins et al. [71], recently, showed that though rs10046 does not link to breast cancer risk, but the TT genotype affects the age of onset,

CYP19A1 SNP	Population/study location	Clinical implication	Reference
rs10046	Inuit women	Nonsignificant association with BC	[53]
rs10046	Iranian	Significant association with BC	[54]
rs762551 rs4646	Swedish	Predictive marker for early breast cancer events in AI-treated patients with ER-positive tumors	[8]
rs6493497	USA	Associated with decreased bone density with AI treatment	[10]
rs4646	China	AA is significantly associated with improved clinical outcome of hormone therapy; prolonged DFS	[55]
rs4646, rs10046, rs700518, rs749292 rs2289106, rs3759811, rs4775936	American	Significantly associated with decreases in triglycerides on letrozole treated	[12]
rs10046	Xinjiang Uigur women	TC genotype and an abortion can reduce the risk of the breast cancer	[56]
rs934635, rs60271534, rs700518	A meta-analysis	Treatment response	[57]
rs700518	Italy	Treatment response	[58]
rs4646, rs10046, rs936308	American	Were associated with bone AEs	[65]
rs4646	Chinese	Related to DFS in early breast cancer and that the prognosis index of the homozygous for the minor allele (AA) may depend on menopause status	[66]
rs700518, rs11856927	American ancestry, Hispanic Americans, and Mexico Whites	Significantly associated with increased breast cancer risk	[67]
rs4775936	UK	AI metabolism	[68]
rs10046	Japanese	Significant risk predictor	[69]
rs700519	India	Could be used as molecular markers to assess breast cancer	[70]
rs10046	Austrian population	Association with clinical characteristics	[71]
rs10046	Spain	Related to levels of circulating estradiol and to the estradiol/testosterone ratio	[72]
rs4646, rs1065779, rs1870050	Taiwan	Associated with poor survival of premenopausal women but does not affect survival of postmenopausal women	[73]
rs4646	American	May serve as a prognostic marker of the response to anastrozole in patients with MBC	[74]
rs10046, rs4646, rs2830, rs9926298, and rs9939609	China	Nonsignificant association with BC	[75]

CYP19A1 SNP	Population/study location	Clinical implication	Reference
rs700518, rs10459592, and rs4775936	Korea	Significantly associated with clinical efficacy	[76]
rs10046, rs4646, rs74929, rs727479	Italian	The aromatase enzyme function is not affected by polymorphisms of CYP19A1 gene in postmenopausal BC patients	[77]
rs4646, rs7167936	Swedish	Involved in both breast cancer risk and prognosis	[78]
Arg264Cys	Chinese	No association	[59]
Arg264Cys	Korean	Increased breast cancer risk	[60]
Arg264Cys	Chinese	No association	[61]
rs1008805	USA	G allele associates with breast cancer	[62]
rs2236722	Japanese	Trp more frequent in ER+	[63]
rs1870049, rs1004982, rs28566535, rs936306, rs11636639, rs767199, rs4775936, rs11575899, rs10046, rs4646	Chinese	No association	[64]

Table 2. Some of the SNP association studies reported in breast cancer.

where individuals carrying TT may develop breast cancer at an age younger than 50 years. It was also shown that the genotypes of rs10046 may influence the levels of estrogens and estrogen/testosterone ratio and also play a role in modulating the levels of other biochemical parameters [72].

The rs4646 polymorphism is an A/C transversion, located in the 3′ UTR of the *CYP19A1* gene. Some studies show it to be significantly associated with an increased risk of breast cancer. Among the Swedish breast cancer patients, rs4646 was strongly associated with the risk of breast cancer and the histological grade of the disease [78]. The A allele was associated with low histological grade and small tumor size ($p = 0.001$ and 0.015). Shao et al. [66] showed that AA is related to longer disease-free survival in Chinese breast cancer patient's population compared to the CC and CA genotype of the rs4646 genotype. Fasching et al. [80] showed that the rs4646 may influence disease-free intervals in breast cancer patients. They concluded that this variant may influence the prognosis of the disease but not through affecting estrogen levels.

Santa-Maria et al. [84] have recently reported that several SNPs influence the plasma lipid levels in patients treated with letrozole, where rs4646, rs10046, rs700518, rs749292, rs2289106, rs3759811, and rs4775936 decreased triglyceride levels and had a variable effect on the level of HDL-C.

A number of other SNPs have been investigated in breast cancer; some are associated with the risk of breast cancer, while others are not (**Table 2**). Some influence the clinical presentation of the disease, the prognosis, and the disease-free intervals, while still others modulate the effect of treatment and the associated complications.

http://dx.doi.org/10.5772/intechopen.69208

3.2. Variations in CYP19A1 gene and endometrial cancer

Endometrial cancer (EC) is one of the most frequently encountered gynecologic malignancies, and a strong association is shown to exist between excess of estrogens and initiation and promotion of endometrial cancer [81]. As early as 1975, it became evident that estrogen may act as a carcinogen when unopposed by an adequate amount of progesterone. Many studies demonstrated higher risk of endometrial cancer in females on hormone replacement therapy [82]. Since exposure to endogenous estrogens was regarded as an important determinant of risk of endometrial cancer, several studies were initiated to identify genetic variants and the role they play as risk factor for the development of endometrial cancer. One of the earliest studies was reported from Russia and implicated genetic variants of *CYP19A1* in the etiology of endometrial cancer [38]. Mikhailova et al. [83] investigated the C --> T transition (Arg264Cys) in exon 7 of CYP19A1 gene but did not find any association. G/A and T/C polymorphisms of *CYP19A1* were investigated, but no significant association was identified ($p > 0.05$) [85]. Tao et al. [86] investigated several SNPs (rs1065779, rs700519, rs28566535, rs752760, and rs1870050) in *CYP19A1* gene. The results showed that the rs1870050 in the promoter region associates inversely, where the genotypes CC and AC had a 0.81 (95% CI = 0.68–0.97) and 0.58 (95% CI = 0.42–0.80), respectively. Gulyaeva et al. [87] showed that the CT genotype of R264C polymorphism increases the risk of endometrial cancer significantly with an OR = 3.73, $p = 0.0004$. Setiawan et al. [88] showed the association of the A allele of rs749292 and rs727479 with increased risk of endometrial cancer and a 10–20% increase in circulating estrogen levels in postmenopausal women. In another study, the A allele of rs4775936 was significantly associated (OR (per allele) = 1.22; 95% CI = 1.01–1.47; p(trend) = 0.04), while the T allele of rs10046 was marginally associated with increased risk of endometrial cancer (OR (per allele) = 1.20; 95% CI = 0.99–1.45; p(trend) = 0.06) [89]. Recently, Thompson et al. [18] reported the results of a genome-wide study and showed that rs727479 was associated most significantly with endometrial cancer and elevation in circulating estrogen (E2). Further studies are required in different populations to confirm the association of genetic variants of CYP19A1 with endometrial cancer.

3.3. Variations in CYP19A1 gene and prostate cancer

Prostate cancer is among the most frequently encountered non-cutaneous malignancy in men. Extensive research has been carried out to identify the etiology and pathological mechanisms, but the mechanism of prostate cancer development is not fully clear. Several factors have been implicated in its etiology including environmental, dietary, hormonal, lifestyle, and genetic factors. Studies have confirmed that estrogens may be closely involved in predisposing to or even causing cancer [90]. Aromatase is shown to be altered in patients with prostate cancer, and its expression is elevated almost 30 times in the cancer tissue compared to the normal tissue [91, 92]. The mechanisms by which estrogens induce carcinogenesis in prostate tissue have been hypothesized in several studies and involve genotoxicity, after chronic inflammation, epigenotoxicity, hyperprolactinemia, and prostatic ER-mediated changes. The genetic factors in the patient are gaining considerable interest, and genetic polymorphisms are being regarded as prognostic predictors of metastatic prostate cancer [93].

A few studies have reported the influence of *rs700519* on prostate cancer risk. This SNP is a C > T transition in exon 7 of *CYP19A1* gene and results in the substitution of Arg at position 264 by Cys. No association was reported among Bulgarians [94], African Americans [95], and Japanese [96]. However, a study on North Indian population showed that the variant Cys was associated with statistically significant increased risk of prostate cancer (OR = 2.28; 95% CI = 1.20–4.35; p = 0.012) [97]. Another report on Japanese showed that when prostate cancer patients were stratified according to clinical stage and pathologic grade of cancer, the CT and TT genotypes were associated significantly with high-grade carcinoma (OR = 2.59; 95% CI = 1.47–4.46; p = 0.048) [98]. A study on Caucasians showed that the C/T mutation was associated with prostate cancer risk, with only borderline significance after age and BMI adjustment. Interestingly, when the effect of the C/T mutation was evaluated with a mutation in androgen receptor (AR), the significance of the association with prostate cancer risk increased considerably [99]. Mononen et al. [100] explored the association between 18 variants and prostate cancer risk and identified a novel SNP, T201M. This SNP showed association with prostate cancer (odds ratio (OR) = 2.04; 95% confidence interval (95% CI) = 1.03–4.03; p = 0.04). Onsory et al. [97] showed that Cys allele in exon 7 of *CYP19A1* was also associated with statistically significant increased risk of prostate cancer (OR = 2.28; 95% CI = 1.20–4.35; p = 0.012). Other studies also showed that CYP19A1 polymorphisms may influence prostate cancer risk and survival by modifying promoter activity, with subsequent effects on the sex hormone milieu [101].

A study recently reported on two populations of African ancestry failed to show any association between rs60271534 and prostate cancer risk [17]. Another SNP 1531 C > T was investigated in the Turkish prostate cancer patients, but no significant association was observed [102]. Lévesque et al. [103] reported a study in which results obtained in Caucasians and Taiwanese were compared. It was shown that rs12900487, rs4441215, and rs2470152 in *CYP19A1* gene do not follow Hardy-Weinberg equilibrium and did not differ in their frequency between the patient and control group. Two other SNPs rs1870050 and rs2446404 significantly increased the risk of prostate cancer in the Caucasian population, while in the Taiwanese, only rs1870050 was associated significantly in the Caucasians but not in the Taiwanese [103].

The effect of two or more coexisting SNPs in influencing predisposition to prostate cancer is shown in several studies, thereby implying that the SNPs may behave synergistically or have antagonistic effect and thus bringing further heterogeneity to SNP action [96]. Cussenot et al. [32] reported that the long allele (>175 bp) of the TTTA repeat of *CYP19A1*, when existing with V432L polymorphism of *CYP1B1*, increases the risk of prostate cancer significantly. This effect was more obvious in the younger patients. Huang et al. [42] working on a Taiwanese population reported that the risk of developing prostate cancer increased significantly (from OR = 1.59; 95% CI = 1.04–2.44; p = 0.044), when TCT del/del genotype of *CYP19A1* coexists with (TTTA)7. The coexisting ins allele and (TTTA)12 also in the *CYP19A1* reduced the risk of developing prostate cancer. More recently, Kachakova et al. [94] have shown that the 7/8 genotype of (TTTA)n repeat polymorphism in *CYP19A1*, when coexisting with the C allele of rs1056837 in *CYP1B1*, predisposes to prostate cancer, while the 8/9 and the 7/12 genotypes of (TTTA)n of *CYP19A1* when existing with the C allele of *CYP1B1* associate with lower risk of prostate cancer and a reduced risk for aggressive disease.

Interestingly, it was shown that some of the SNPs in *CYP19A1* gene have a significant effect on the level of circulating steroid hormones including LH, testosterone, estradiol, SHBG, and indices of insulin sensitivity. However, no association was reported between these polymorphisms and non-hormonal parameters including anthropometric parameters, blood pressure, lipids, hemoglobin, and prostate-specific antigen [104].

The plasma level of estrogens may also be altered by the presence of different SNPs in the *CYP19A1* gene. rs2470152, an intronic SNP, is significantly associated with the serum level of E2, while in individuals, the presence of rs2470152 results in the elevation of both E1 and E2 in men [105].

The presence of some SNPs also influences the effect of different nutritional and therapeutic agents used for protection from cancer. Sonoda et al. [106] report from Japan that the protective effect shown by isoflavones against prostate cancer is modified by the (TTTA) long repeat alleles and coexisting minor alleles of rs10046 in *CYP19A1*, even if the isoflavones are used at concentrations as high as 60 mg/day. On the other hand, homozygosity for the major allele of rs10046 in *CYP19A1* and also with coexisting short repeats of (TTTA) reduces the risk of prostate cancer development.

3.4. Variations in *CYP19A1* gene and colorectal cancer

It is well documented that estrogens play a role in the development and progression of colorectal cancer (CRC) [107–109]. The beneficial role played by estrogens in preventing CRC is obvious since males have a higher prevalence of CRC than premenopausal females, but the prevalence increases in menopausal females. Furthermore, females on hormone replacement therapy have a lower susceptibility to CRC [110]. However, it is shown that estrogens are locally produced in the colorectal tissue and result in a higher level of E2 and a lower level of E1. This imbalance in E2/E1 ratio may result in an increase in cell proliferation and concomitant decrease in apoptosis, thus increasing the risk of CRC [111–113]. Normally, in the colon, E2 is converted to E1 by 17β-HSD2 and 17β-HSD4. The E1 is antiproliferative, and the E2/E1 ratio keeps a check on the cell cycle. In colon cancer since this ratio is altered, proliferation is accelerated [111, 112]. A study on Chinese men showed that there were elevated E2 levels and the presence of CT/TT genotype of ESR2 receptor increased the risk of CRC to 2.3 (95% CI = 1.4–3.9), compared to those who had lower levels of E2 and the ESR2 genotype CC [114].

Polymorphisms are reported in *CYP19A1* gene, and some result in increased risk of CRC. Lin et al. [115] studied Caucasian patients of the European origin and genotyped the patients and controls for 13 different SNPs (rs4646, rs10046, rs2414096, rs727479, rs1008805, rs749292, rs93606, rs3751591, rs1004984, rs2445762, rs2446405, rs2740144, and rs32445765), distributed all over the *CYP19A1* gene. Only one SNP rs10046 showed a significant association with CRC risk. However, the significance was lost after correction for multiple comparisons. In a study from the USA, Slattery et al. [110] reported significant association of four SNPs (rs12591359, rs17523880, rs1961177, rs3751591) with increased risk of colon cancer and another four which increased the risk of rectal cancer [116]. However, after adjustment for multiple comparisons, only one SNP (rs12591359) showed significant association (OR = 1.44; 95% CI = 1.16–1.80). The AA genotype of this SNP was associated with an increased risk of cancer of the colon and decreased risk of the cancer of rectum. We genotyped Saudi CRC patients for six SNPs (rs4774585, rs936308, rs4775936, rs700518, rs28757184, and rs4646) in the *CYP19A1* gene but failed to see any association with CRC risk [117]. Lin et al. [116] studied haplotypes in the

CYP19A1 gene and identified one haplotype block, which associated with CRC, most likely reflecting association with the tagging SNP, rs1902584, in the block.

It has also been reported that aromatase also participates in metabolizing various compounds produced endogenously, including sex hormones, lipids, and other lipid derivatives. The rate of metabolism of these compounds depends on the amount and activity of the enzyme, which in turn may be altered by the alleles of the different SNPs. Metabolic end products produced may increase or decrease the risk of CRC and hence the interindividual differences in inherited metabolic susceptibility to CRC. Inflammatory response to different exogenous and endogenous factors may also have a role in CRC [110].

3.5. Variations in *CYP19A1* gene and ovarian cancer

Several clinical trials have provided evidence implicating hormone replacement therapy as a risk factor for development of ovarian cancer. However, the role played by estrogen in the etiology of ovarian cancer has yet to be unveiled. Polymorphisms in *CYP19A1* gene have been investigated in a few studies, to identify possible risk markers. Goodman et al. [118] conducted multiethnic (Japanese, Caucasian, Hawaiian, Filipino, and others) case-control study in Hawaii and investigated two SNPs (rs749292 and rs727479) in relation to ovarian cancer. They showed that the A allele of rs749292 was associated positively with ovarian cancer risk in a codominant model for all races combined, while the rs749479 did not show any association [118]. Both alleles increased the plasma estrogen levels by 10–20%. In an Australian population, no association was seen between rs10046 and ovarian cancer [119]. In a Polish population, several polymorphic loci were investigated, but no association was observed with any of the studied SNPs. More investigations are required to confirm association if any between the SNPs and ovarian cancer.

3.6. Variations in CYP19A1 gene and hepatocellular carcinoma

Worldwide, the prevalence of hepatocellular carcinoma (HCC) is high, classifying it as one of the most common malignancies. Studies have suggested that sex hormones, including androgen and estrogen, may be involved in HCC development and progression [120], pointing toward aromatase variants in HCC development. However, studies on *CYP19A1* polymorphism and the risk of HCC are few. Yuan et al. [121] failed to show any association between a non-synonymous SNP at codon 39 of the *CYP19A1* gene, which causes substitution of Trp by Arg and results in the synthesis of a nonfunctional aromatase. A positive association between A/C transversion and HCC risk was reported by Koh et al. [122]. This polymorphism occurs in the exon I.6 promoter of the *CYP19A1* gene and is located in a consensus sequence for a TFIID binding site. The C allele increases the expression of *CYP19A1* significantly, thereby increasing the synthesis of estrogens and androgens. Further studies are required to identify other risk markers for HCC in the *CYP19A1* gene.

3.7. Variations in *CYP19A1* gene and esophageal adenocarcinoma

Esophageal adenocarcinoma (EA) prevalence is on the rise in the young Western population. A strong gender bias is shown in epidemiological studies, with a sex ratio of 8:9.1. It is suggested that the estrogens may be a protecting factor in females, since estrogens have been shown to stimulate apoptosis and decrease the growth of the esophageal squamous cells [123]. It also decreases the expression of Ki-67 while increasing E-cadherin expression [124]. However, not many studies have explored the role of SNPs in *CYP19A1* gene and the risk of EA development. Wu et al. [125] studied the role of rs2445762 of *CYP19A1* and showed that there was a significant association between this SNP and an early onset of EA (≤55 vs. >55 years), all $p < 0.05$ after adjusting for covariates and false discovery rate.

Recently, a study by Lagergren et al. [126] pooled 14 studies from three continents (Australia, Europe, and North America) and investigated the effect of 60 SNPs in *CYP19A1* gene as a risk factor for EA. However, no significant association was identified for any of the SNPs in any of the populations. Further studies are required in different populations to identify possible association between *CYP19A1* polymorphisms and EA risk.

3.8. Variations in *CYP19A1* gene and gastric cancer

Gastric cancer is the fourth most common cause of cancer-related death in the world [http://www.who.int/mediacentre/factsheets/fs297/en/]. Studies have suggested that long exposure to estrogens, of ovarian or exogenous origin, may provide a protection against development of cancer [127, 128]. This finding has led to the implication of estrogen receptor defects in the development of gastric cancer [129]. There are very few reports on the association between CYP19A1 gene polymorphism and gastric cancer risk. Freedman et al. [130] investigated 58 SNPs in six genes (*COMT, CYP1B1, CYP17A1, CYP19A1, HSD17B1,* and *SHBG*) which are involved in the biosynthesis of estrogen and androgen. None of the *CYP19A1* gene showed any association with gastric cancer risk. More recently, Cho et al. [131] conducted a population-based genetic association study, in which they investigated the role of genes for proteins involved in the steroid hormone biosynthesis pathways. Of the 108 SNPs investigated in five genes (*CYP19A1, HSD3B1, HSD17B2, CYP17A1, HSD17B1*), 10 SNPs in *CYP19A1* were significantly associated with the risk of gastric cancer. They concluded that *CYP19A1* may be an important player in elevating the risk of gastric cancer and could be considered as a genetic marker for gastric cancer susceptibility ($p < 0.05$). Since the association is unclear, further studies on *CYP19A1* gene polymorphism and the risk of gastric cancer, in different populations, are warranted and may help in the identification of possible genetic marker.

3.9. Variations in *CYP19A1* gene and testicular germ cell tumor

In young men, testicular germ cell tumor (TGCT) is reported to be the most common cancer. It is hypothesized that an imbalance in the in utero level of androgens and estrogens may be the major predisposing factor in influencing TGCT risk. Kristiansen et al. [132] conducted an investigation on Norwegian-Swedish case-parent trios and genotyped 105 SNPs in 20 genes whose gene products were involved in the sex hormone pathways. Three SNPs (rs2414099, rs8025374, and rs3751592) showed a statistically significant association with TGCT risk in the case-parent analysis. For each of the studied SNP, the T alleles were associated with an elevated risk of TGCT (OR = 1.30, 1.30, and 1.21, respectively). No differences were identified in allelic effect estimates when the parental inherited genetic variation was correlated with the TGCT risk in the offspring. Furthermore, no differences were observed between the

Norwegian and the Swedish populations for each of the studied SNP. It was concluded that aromatase may be a factor playing a role in the etiology of TGCT. However, this statement needs confirmation from further population-based studies.

4. Effect of SNPs on prognosis and survival of breast cancer patients

Some of the SNPs in CYP19A1 gene have been linked to disease prognosis and survival. It was shown that rs28566535, rs730154, and rs936306 are significantly associated with plasma levels of estrone as well as with breast cancer survival [133, 134]. Long et al. [135] showed an association between genetic polymorphisms of the CYP19A1 gene and breast cancer survival. Udler et al. [136] presented preliminary evidence suggesting that germline variation in genes involved in steroid hormone metabolism may alter breast cancer prognosis.

5. Effect of SNPs on hormonal parameters

Variations related to the effect of SNPs on biochemical and hormonal parameters are also reported in a few studies. Huhtaniemi et al. [104] did not find any associations between *CYP19A1* polymorphism and non-hormonal variables including anthropometric parameters, blood pressure, cognition sexual hemoglobin, blood lipids, and hemoglobin. Kidokoro et al. [137] showed that SNPs in *CYP19A* gene alter the levels of estrogens. Eriksson et al. [105] presented data showing that rs2470152 is clearly associated with serum E2 and E1 levels in men. Other investigations show the association between SNPs rs10046 and rs11575899 and endogenous estrogen levels [138, 139].

Estrogen levels are influenced by the presence of different genotypes of a SNP, as reported in some studies but not in others. Thompson et al. [18] showed in a comprehensive study that the SNP rs727479 was associated most strongly with circulating E2 concentrations in postmenopausal healthy controls and its effect was stronger in obese females. Cai et al. [140] showed that rs1902584 in block 1 was associated with estradiol only in overweight postmenopausal women.

6. Influence of SNPs in CYP19A1 gene on treatment with aromatase inhibitors

The treatment strategies have been extensively investigated in breast cancer, due to the high prevalence and associated morbidity and motility. There are a number of options for the treatment of the different types of cancer, and generally a multidisciplinary approach is preferred. The options are dependent on the type of cancer, patients' history, and the characteristics of the tumor. Some of the more common treatment strategies are surgery, radiotherapy, chemotherapy, and hormonal therapy. The two common antiestrogen therapies are tamoxifen and aromatase inhibitors. The former is used generally for the treatment of ER+ breast cancer in premenopausal women, while the latter is under investigation for treatment of premenopausal breast cancer patients. In the postmenopausal women, the aromatase inhibitors (AIs) are reported to have a higher efficacy compared to tamoxifen in the postmenopausal group in relation to metastasis and prognosis in the presence of adjuvant treatment. However, ethnic differences and interindividual differences are frequently reported and are related to genetic variations.

As stated in the earlier part of this chapter, there are a significantly large number of SNPs in the CYP19A gene. Some of these have an influence on aromatase activity and hence influence the level of estrogens. Such mutations play a role in the effectiveness of the clinical efficacy related to treatment strategies.

Several studies have evaluated the effect of the genotype on the efficacy of the AI used for treatment of cancer. There are several contradictory reports, and the SNP may or may not associate with AI treatment complications. Those SNPs, which influence aromatase activity and are associated with elevated levels of estrogens, such as rs6493497 and rs7176005, seem to alter the effectiveness of AI [141]. On the other hand, it was shown that rs700518, rs10459592, and rs4775936 were significantly associated with higher clinical benefit rate with letrozole treatment [142]. Ferraldeschi et al. [68] investigated the effect of 56 SNPs on AI treatment and concluded that none of the variants independently were associated with improved AI efficacy and emphasized the significance of further studies on genetic biomarkers as prognostic factors in pharmacogenetic studies.

Table 3 lists a few SNPs and their influence on the outcome of AI treatment.

SNP	Effect on AI treatment	Reference
rs6493497	Almost 13-fold increase estradiol concentration in post-anastrozole. Alters effectiveness of AI treatment associated with decreased bone density in the exemestane-treated patients	[141]
rs7176005	Almost 11-fold increase estradiol concentration in post-anastrozole. Alters effectiveness of AI treatment	[141]
rs4646	Associated with poor response to the AI, letrozole ($p = 0.03$)	[134, 142]
rs700518	—GG genotype of rs700518 increases risk for significant loss of fat-free mass and increase in truncal fat with AI therapy —AA genotype of rs700518 is at risk for AI-associated bone loss	[142, 143]
rs700518	Significantly associated with higher clinical benefit rate with letrozole treatment	[142]
rs10459592		
rs4775936		
rs1062033	CC genotype in postmenopausal patients had lower spine and hip bone mineral density compared with the GG genotype. No correlation with AIs was established	[144]
rs60271534	Lower incidence of AI-associated arthralgia. But the effect was not definite as two different AIs were used	[145]
rs10046	Five-year disease-free survival was enhanced in premenopausal women on AI therapy	[146]
rs700519	Associated with lower aromatase activity, but no studies showed a significant correlation with AIs	[80]

AI, aromatase inhibitor.

Table 3. SNPs in CYP19A1 gene and their interaction with AI treatment.

7. Conclusions

Aromatase is an essential enzyme required for the synthesis of estrogens. The polymorphic forms of aromatase gene seem to contribute to the development of different forms of cancer, and several avenues await exploration. Population differences in the frequencies of different SNPs and the association with the different disease states need further detailed study. Association studies are required to confirm if there is a risk or protective effect of the SNP genotype. Studies on disease prognosis, in relation to the different genotypes of a SNP, are required. Finally, the influences of the SNP on treatment strategies are warranted. Individualized medicine is the dream of present-day clinicians. The role played by SNPs may contribute to achieve this dream.

Acknowledgements

We thankfully appreciate the support provided by the Central Laboratory during the preparation of this chapter.

Author details

Arjumand S. Warsy[1*], Fatimah Basil Almukaynizi[2], Soad AlDaihan[3], Sophia Alam[4] and Maha Daghastani[5]

*Address all correspondence to: aswarsy@gmail.com

1 Central Laboratory, Center for Science and Medical Studies for Girls, King Saud University, Riyadh, Saudi Arabia

2 Central Laboratory and Prince Naif for Health Research Center, King Saud University, Riyadh, Saudi Arabia

3 Department of Biochemistry, College of Science, King Saud University, Riyadh, Saudi Arabia

4 Dr.Hassan Clinic, Phelps Hospital, Northwell, Health, Sleepy Hollow, NY, USA

5 Department of Zoology, College of Science, King Saud University, Riyadh, Saudi Arabia

References

[1] Watanabe S, Kobayashi Y. Exogenous hormones and human cancer. Japanese Journal of Clinical Oncology. 1993;**23**(1):1-13

[2] Sasano H, Harada N. Intratumoral aromatase in human breast, endometrial, and ovarian malignancies. Endocrine Reviews. 1998;**19**:593-607

[3] Nelson LR, Bulun SE. Estrogen production and action. Journal of the American Academy of Dermatology. 2001;**45**(3):S116-S124

[4] Harada N. Structure, regulation and polymorphisms of the Aromatase gene in Larionov A, eds. Resistance to Aromatase Inhibitors in Breast Cancer, Resistance to Targeted Anti-Cancer Therapeutics 8, Switzerland: Springer International Publishing Switzerland; 2015

[5] Simpson ER, Davis SR. Minireview: Aromatase and the regulation of estrogen biosynthesis-Some new perspectives. Endocrinology. 2001;**142**(11):4589-4594

[6] Henderson BE, Ross R, and Bernstein L. Estrogens as a cause of human cancer: The Richard and Hinda Rosenthal Foundation award lecture. Cancer Research. 1988;**48**:246-253

[7] Simpson E, Rubin G, Clyne C, Robertson K, O'Donnell L, Davis S, Jones M. Local estrogen biosynthesis in males and females endocrine-related. Cancer. 1999;**6**:131-137

[8] Sasano H, Uzuki M, Sawai T, Nagura H, Matsunaga G, Kashimoto O, Harada N. Aromatase in human bone tissue. Journal of Bone and Mineral Research. 1997;**12**:1416-1423

[9] Harada N, Sasano H, Murakami H, Ohkuma T, Nagura H, Takagi Y. Localized expression of aromatase in human vascular tissues. Circulation Research. 1999;**84**:1285-1291

[10] Simpson, ER, Clyne, C, Rubin, G, Boon, WC, Robertson, K, Britt, K, Speed, C, and Jones, M. Aromatase-A brief overview. Annual Reviews of Physical Chemistry. 2002;**64**:93-127

[11] Chen SA, Besman MJ, Sparkes RS, Zollman S, Klisak I, Mohandas T, Hall PF, Shively JE. Human aromatase: cDNA cloning, southern blot analysis, and assignment of the gene to chromosome 15. DNA. 1988;**7**:27-38

[12] Harada N, Utsumi T, Takagi Y. Tissue-specific expression of the human aromatase cytochrome P450 gene by alternative use of multiple exons 1 and promoters, and switching of tissue-specific exons 1 in carcinogenesis. Proceedings of the National Academy of Sciences of the United States of America. 1993;**90**:11312-11316

[13] Shozu M, Zhao Y, Bulun SE, Simpson ER. Multiple splicing events involved in regulation of human aromatase expression by a novel promoter, I.6. Endocrinology. 1998;**139**:1610-1607

[14] Simpson ER, Mahendroo MS, Means GD, Kilgore MW, Hinshelwood MM, Graham-Lorence S, et al. Aromatase cytochrome P450, the enzyme responsible for estrogen biosynthesis. Endocrine Reviews. 1994;**15**:342-355

[15] McPhaul MJ, Herbst MA, Matsumine H, Young M, Lephart ED. Diverse mechanisms of control of aromatase gene expression. Journal of Steroid Biochemistry and Molecular Biology. 1993;**44**(4-6):341-346

[16] Chen S, Itoh T, Wu K, Zhou D, Yang C. Transcriptional regulation of aromatase expression in human breast tissue. Journal of Steroid Biochemistry and Molecular Biology. 2002;**83**:93-99

[17] Brureau L, Moningo D, Emeville E, Ferdinand S, Punga A, Lufuma S,et al, Polymorphisms of estrogen metabolism-related genes and prostate cancer risk in two populations of African ancestry. PLoS One. 2016;**11**(4):e0153609

[18] Thompson DJ, O'Mara TA, Glubb DM, Painter JN, Cheng T, Folkerd E, et al, CYP19A1 fine-mapping and Mendelian randomization: Estradiol is causal for endometrial cancer. Endocrine-Related Cancer. 2016;**23**(2):77-91

[19] Kristensen VN, Andersen TI, Lindblom A, Erikstein B, Magnus P, Børresen-Dale AL. A rare CYP19 (aromatase) variant may increase the risk of breast cancer. Pharmacogenetics. 1998;**8**(1):43-48

[20] Haiman CA, Hankinson SE, Spiegelman D, De Vivo I, Colditz GA, Willett WC, et al. A tetranucleotide repeat polymorphism in CYP19 and breast cancer risk. International Journal of Cancer. 2000;**87**(2):204-210

[21] Miyoshi Y, Iwao K, Ikeda N, Egawa C, Noguchi S. Breast cancer risk associated with polymorphism in CYP19 in Japanese women. International Journal of Cancer. 2000;**89**(4):325-328

[22] Baxter SW, Choong DY, Eccles DM, Campbell IG. Polymorphic variation in CYP19 and the risk of breast cancer. Carcinogenesis. 2001;**22**(2):347-349

[23] Miyoshi Y, Ando A, Hasegawa S, Ishitobi M, Yamamura J, Irahara N, et al. Association of genetic polymorphisms in CYP19 and CYP1A1 with the oestrogen receptor-positive breast cancer risk. European Journal of Cancer. 2003;**39**(17):2531-2537

[24] Ribeiro FS, de Amorim LM, de Almeida Simão T, Mendonça GA, de Moura Gallo CV, Pinto LF. CYP19 (TTTA)n polymorphism and breast cancer risk in Brazilian women. Toxicology Letters. 2006;**164**(1):90-95

[25] Hu MB, Xie W, Xiong B, Han DF, Li Y, Feng MH, et al. Study on the relationship between polymorphisms of genes (CYP17, CYP19 and SULT1A1) and susceptibility to breast cancer in Chinese women. Zhonghua Liu Xing Bing Xue Za Zhi. 2006;**27**(4):351-355

[26] Artamonov VV, Liubchenko LN, Shabanov MA, Babenko OV, Nemtsova MV, Zaletaev DV. Association of polymorphism of genetic markers of CYP19 and CYP17 with sporadic breast cancer. Molecular Biology (Mosk). 2003;**37**(6):975-982

[27] Murillo-Ortiz B, Martínez-Garza S, Suárez García D, Castillo Valenzuela RD, García Regalado JF, Cano Velázquez G Association between telomere length and CYP19 TTTA repetition polymorphism in healthy and breast cancer-diagnosed women. Breast Cancer (Dove Med Press). 2017;**9**:21-27

[28] Kim JY, Lee CS, Kim HO, Jo YH, Lee J, Jung MH,et al. The association between genetic polymorphisms in CYP19 and breast cancer risk in Korean women. Oncology Reports. 2009;**22**(3):487-492

[29] Probst-Hensch NM, Ingles SA, Diep AT, Haile RW, Stanczyk FZ, Kolonel LN, et al. Aromatase and breast cancer susceptibility. Endocrine-Related Cancer. 1999;**6**(2):165-173

[30] Thyagarajan B, Brott M, Mink P, Folsom AR, Anderson KE, Oetting WS, et al. CYP1B1 and CYP19 gene polymorphisms and breast cancer incidence: No association in the ARIC study. Cancer Letters. 2004;**207**(2):183-189

[31] Dialyna I, Tzanakakis G, Dolapsakis G, Tsatsakis A. A tetranucleotide repeat polymorphism in the CYP19 gene and breast cancer susceptibility in a Greek population exposed and not exposed to pesticides. Toxicology Letters. 2004;**151**(1):267-271

[32] Cussenot O, Azzouzi AR, Nicolaiew N, Fromont G, Mangin P, Cormier L, et al. Combination of polymorphisms from genes related to estrogen metabolism and risk of prostate cancers: The hidden face of estrogens. Journal of Clinical Oncology. 2007;**25**(24):3596-3602

[33] dos Santos RM, de Jesus CM, Trindade Filho JC, Trindade JC, de Camargo JL, Rainho CA, et al. PSA and androgen-related gene (AR, CYP17, and CYP19) polymorphisms and the risk of adenocarcinoma at prostate biopsy. DNA and Cell Biology. 2008;**27**(9):497-503

[34] Suzuki K, Nakazato H, Matsui H, Koike H, Okugi H, Ohtake N, et al. Association of the genetic polymorphism of the CYP19 intron 4[TTTA]n repeat with familial prostate cancer risk in a Japanese population. Anticancer Research. 2003;**23**(6D):4941-4946

[35] Tsuchiya N, Wang L, Suzuki H, Segawa T, Fukuda H, Narita S, et al. Impact of IGF-I and CYP19 gene polymorphisms on the survival of patients with metastatic prostate cancer. Journal of Clinical Oncology. 2006;**24**(13):1982-1989

[36] Tang L, Yao S, Till C, Goodman PJ, Tangen CM, Wu Y, et al, Repeat polymorphisms in estrogen metabolism genes and prostate cancer risk: Results from the prostate cancer prevention trial. Carcinogenesis. 2011;**32**(10):1500-1506

[37] Bershteĭn LM, Imianitov EN, Suspitsyn EN, Grigor'ev MIu, Sokolov EP, Togo AV, et al. A polymorphism study of the CYP19 gene in endometrial cancer patients. Voprosy Onkologii. 2000;**46**(3):302-305

[38] Berstein LM, Imyanitov EN, Suspitsin EN, Grigoriev MY, Sokolov EP, Togo A, et al. CYP19 gene polymorphism in endometrial cancer patients. Journal of Cancer Research and Clinical Oncology. 2001;**127**(2):135-138

[39] Olson SH, Bandera EV, Orlow I. Variants in estrogen biosynthesis genes, sex steroid hormone levels, and endometrial cancer: A HuGE review. American Journal of Epidemiology. 2007;**165**(3):235-245

[40] Berstein LM, Imyanitov EN, Kovalevskij AJ, Maximov SJ, Vasilyev DA, Buslov KG, et al. CYP17 and CYP19 genetic polymorphisms in endometrial cancer: Association with intratumoral aromatase activity. Cancer Letters. 2004;**207**(2):191-196

[41] Healey CS, Dunning AM, Durocher F, Teare D, Pharoah PD, Luben RN, et al. Polymorphisms in the human aromatase cytochrome P450 gene (CYP19) and breast cancer risk. Carcinogenesis. 2000;**21**(2):189-193

[42] Huang YC, Chen M, Lin MW, Chung MY, Chang YH, Huang WJ, et al. CYP19 TCT trinucleotide Del/Del genotype is a susceptibility marker for prostate cancer in a Taiwanese population. Urology. 2007;**69**(5):996-1000

[43] Olson SH, Orlow I, Bayuga S, Sima C, Bandera EV, Pulick K, et al. Variants in hormone biosynthesis genes and risk of endometrial cancer. Cancer Causes & Control. 2008;**19**(9):955-963

[44] Paynter RA, Hankinson SE, Colditz GA, Kraft P, Hunter DJ, De Vivo I. CYP19 (aromatase) haplotypes and endometrial cancer risk. International Journal of Cancer. 2005;**116**(2):267-274

[45] Suspitsin EN, Grigoriev MY, Togo AV, Kuligina ES, Belogubova EV, Pozharisski KM, Distinct prevalence of the CYP19 Delta3(TTTA)(7) allele in premenopausal versus postmenopausal breast cancer patients, but not in control individuals. European Journal of Cancer. 2002;**38**(14):1911-1916

[46] Ma CX, Adjei AA, Salavaggione OE, Coronel J, Pelleymounter L, Wang L, et al. Human aromatase: Gene resequencing and functional genomics. Cancer Research. 2005;**65**(23):11071-11082

[47] Sourdaine P, Parker MG, Telford J, Miller WR. Analysis of the aromatase cytochrome P450 gene in human breast cancers. Journal of Molecular Endocrinology. 1994;**13**(3):331-337

[48] Kristensen VN, Harada N, Yoshimura N, Haraldsen E, Lonning PE, Erikstein B, et al. Genetic variants of CYP19 (aromatase) and breast cancer risk. Oncogene. 2000;**19**(10):1329-1333

[49] Feigelson HS, Henderson BE. Estrogens and breast cancer. Carcinogenesis. 1996;**17**(11): 2279-2284

[50] Siiteri PK. Adipose tissue as a source of hormones. American Journal of Clinical Nutrition. 1987;**45**(1 Suppl):277-282

[51] O'Neill JS, Miller WR. Aromatase activity in breast adipose tissue from women with benign and malignant breast diseases. British Journal of Cancer. 1987;**56**(5):601-604

[52] Castilla LH, Couch FJ, Erdos MR, Hoskins KF, Calzone K, Garber JE, et al. Mutations in the BRCA1 gene in families with early-onset breast and ovarian cancer. Nature Genetics. 1994;**8**(4):387-391

[53] Ghisari M, Eiberg H, Long M, Bonefeld-Jørgensen EC. Polymorphisms in phase I and phase II genes and breast cancer risk and relations to persistent organic pollutant exposure: A case-control study in Inuit women. Environmental Health. 2014;**13**(1):19

[54] Farzaneh F, Noghabaei G, Barouti E, Pouresmaili F, Jamshidi J, Fazeli A, et al. Analysis of CYP17, CYP19 and CYP1A1 gene polymorphisms in Iranian women with breast cancer. Asian Pacific Journal of Cancer Prevention. 2016;**17**:(Spec No.):23-6

[55] Shao X, Cai J, Zheng Y, Wang J, Feng J, Huang Y, et al, S4646 polymorphism in CYP19A1 gene is associated with the efficacy of hormone therapy in early breast cancer. International Journal of Clinical and Experimental Pathology. 2015;**8**(5):5309-5317

[56] Yang L, Wang XY, Li YT, Wang HL, Wu T, Wang B, et al, CYP19 gene polymorphisms and the susceptibility to breast cancer in Xinjiang Uigur women. Genetics and Molecular Research. 2015;**14**(3):8473-8482

[57] Artigalás O, Vanni T, Hutz MH, Ashton-Prolla P, Schwartz IV.Influence of CYP19A1 polymorphisms on the treatment of breast cancer with aromatase inhibitors: A systematic review and meta-analysis. BMC Medicine. 2015;**13**:139

[58] Napoli N, Rastelli A, Ma C, Colleluori G, Vattikuti S, Armamento-Villareal R. Genetic polymorphism at Val80 (rs700518) of the CYP19A1 gene is associated with body composition changes in women on aromatase inhibitors for ER (+) breast cancer. Pharmacogenetics and Genomics. 2015;**25**(8):377-381

[59] Hu Z, Song CG, Lu JS, Luo JM, Shen ZZ, Huang W, et al. A multigenic study on breast cancer risk associated with genetic polymorphisms of ER Alpha, COMT and CYP19 gene in BRCA1/BRCA2 negative Shanghai women with early onset breast cancer or affected relatives. Journal of Cancer Research and Clinical Oncology. 2007;**133**(12):969-978

[60] Lee KM, Abel J, Ko Y, Harth V, Park WY, Seo JS, et al. Genetic polymorphisms of cytochrome P450 19 and 1B1, alcohol use, and breast cancer risk in Korean women. British Journal of Cancer. 2003;**88**(5):675-678

[61] Song CG, Hu Z, Yuan WT, Di GH, Shen ZZ, Huang W, et al. Effect of R264C polymorphism in CYP19A1 gene on BRCA1/2-negative hereditary breast cancer from Shanghai population of China. Zhonghua yi xue yi chuan xue za zhi= Zhonghua yixue yichuanxue zazhi= Chinese Journal of Medical Genetics. 2006;**23**(2):181-183

[62] Talbott KE, Gammon MD, Kibriya MG, Chen Y, Teitelbaum SL, Long CM, et al. A CYP19 (aromatase) polymorphism is associated with increased premenopausal breast cancer risk. Breast Cancer Research and Treatment. 2008;**111**(3):481-487

[63] Hamaguchi M, Nishio M, Toyama T, Sugiura H, Kondo N, Fujii Y, et al. Possible difference in frequencies of genetic polymorphisms of estrogen receptor alpha, estrogen metabolism and P53 genes between estrogen receptor-positive and -negative breast cancers. Japanese Journal of Clinical Oncology. 2008;**38**(11):734-742

[64] Chen C, Sakoda LC, Doherty JA, Loomis MM, Fish S, Ray RM, et al. Genetic variation in CYP19A1 and risk of breast cancer and fibrocystic breast conditions among women in Shanghai, China. Cancer Epidemiology Biomarkers Prevention. 2008;**17**(12): 3457-3466

[65] Leyland-Jones B, Gray KP, Abramovitz M, Bouzyk M, Young B, Long B, et al, CYP19A1 polymorphisms and clinical outcomes in postmenopausal women with hormone receptor-positive breast cancer in the BIG 1-98 trial. Breast Cancer Research and Treatment. 2015;**151**(2):373-384

[66] Shao X, Guo Y, Xu X, Zheng Y, Wang J, Chen Z, et al, The CYP19 RS4646 polymorphism IS related to the prognosis of stage I-II and operable stage III breast cancer. PLoS One. 2015;**10**(3):e0121535

[67] Boone SD, Baumgartner KB, Baumgartner RN, Connor AE, Pinkston CM, Rai SN, et al, Associations between CYP19A1 polymorphisms, Native American ancestry, and breast

cancer risk and mortality: The Breast Cancer Health Disparities Study. Cancer Causes & Control. 2014;**25**(11):1461-1471

[68] Ferraldeschi R, Arnedos M, Hadfield KD, A'Hern R, Drury S, Wardley A, et al, Polymorphisms of CYP19A1 and response to aromatase inhibitors in metastatic breast cancer patients. Breast Cancer Research and Treatment. 2012;**133**(3):1191-1198

[69] Yoshimoto N, Nishiyama T, Toyama T, Takahashi S, Shiraki N, Sugiura H, et al, Genetic and environmental predictors, endogenous hormones and growth factors, and risk of estrogen receptor-positive breast cancer in Japanese women. Cancer Science. 2011;**102**(11):2065-2072

[70] Chattopadhyay S, Siddiqui S, Akhtar MS, Najm MZ, Deo SV, Shukla NK, et al, Genetic polymorphisms of ESR1, ESR2, CYP17A1, and CYP19A1 and the risk of breast cancer: A case control study from North India. Tumour Biology. 2014;**35**(5):4517-4527

[71] Zins K, Mogg M, Schneeberger C, Abraham D, Schreiber M. Analysis of the rs10046 polymorphism of aromatase (CYP19) in premenopausal onset of human breast cancer. International Journal of Molecular Sciences. 2014;**15**(1):712-724

[72] Pineda B, García-Pérez MÁ, Cano A, Lluch A, Eroles P. Associations between aromatase CYP19 rs10046 polymorphism and breast cancer risk: From a case-control to a meta-analysis of 20,098 subjects. PLoS One. 2013;**8**(1):e53902

[73] Kuo SH, Yang SY, Lien HC, Lo C, Lin CH, Lu YS, et al, CYP19 genetic polymorphism haplotype AASA is associated with a poor prognosis in premenopausal women with lymph node-negative, hormone receptor-positive breast cancer. BioMed Research International. 2013;**2013**:562197

[74] Henry NL, Chan HP, Dantzer J, Goswami CP, Li L, Skaar TC, et al, Aromatase inhibitorinduced modulation of breast density: Clinical and genetic effects. British Journal of Cancer. 2013;**109**(9):2331-2339

[75] Liu L, Bai YX, Zhou JH, Sun XW, Sui H, Zhang WJ, et al, A polymorphism at the 3'-UTR region of the aromatase gene is associated with the efficacy of the aromatase inhibitor, anastrozole, in metastatic breast carcinoma. International Journal of Molecular Sciences. 2013;**14**(9):18973-18988

[76] Park IH, Lee YS, Lee KS, Kim SY, Hong SH, Jeong J, et al, Single nucleotide polymorphisms of CYP19A1 predict clinical outcomes and adverse events associated with letrozole in patients with metastatic breast cancer. Cancer Chemotherapy and Pharmacology. 2011;**68**(5):1263-1271

[77] Lunardi G, Piccioli P, Bruzzi P, Notaro R, Lastraioli S, Serra M, et al, Plasma estrone sulfate concentrations and genetic variation at the CYP19A1 locus in postmenopausal women with early breast cancer treated with letrozole. Breast Cancer Research and Treatment. 2013;**137**(1):167-174

[78] Darabi H, Czene K, Wedrén S, Li Y, Liu J, Hall P, et al. Genetic variation in the androgen estrogen conversion pathway in relation to breast cancer prognosticators. Breast Cancer Research and Treatment. 2011;**127**(2):503-509

[79] Zhang L, Gu L, Qian B, Hao X, Zhang W, Wei Q, et al. Association of genetic polymorphisms of ER-alpha and the estradiol-synthesizing enzyme genes CYP17 and CYP19 with breast cancer risk in Chinese women. Breast Cancer Research and Treatment. 2009;**114**(2):327-338

[80] Fasching PA, Loehberg CR, Strissel PL, Lux MP, Bani MR, Schrauder M,et al. Single nucleotide polymorphisms of the aromatase gene (CYP19A1), HER2/neu status, and prognosis in breast cancer patients. Breast Cancer Research and Treatment. 2008;**112**(1):89-98

[81] Ziel HK. Estrogen's role in endometrial cancer. Obstetrics and Gynecology. 1982 Oct;**60**(4):509-515

[82] Reich O, Regauer S, Tempfer C, Schneeberger C, Huber J. Polymorphism 1558 C > T in the aromatase gene (CYP19A1) in low-grade endometrial stromal sarcoma. European Journal of Gynaecological Oncology. 2011;**32**(6):626-627

[83] Mikhailova ON, Gulyaeva LF, Prudnikov AV, Gerasimov AV, Krasilnikov SE. 201. Estrogen-metabolizing gene polymorphisms in the assessment of female hormonedependent cancer risk. Pharmacogenomics Journal. 2006;**6**(3):189-193

[84] Santa-Maria CA, Blackford A, Nguyen AT, Skaar TC, Philips S, Oesterreich S, et al. Association of variants in candidate genes with lipid profiles in women with early breast cancer on adjuvant aromatase inhibitor therapy. Clinical Cancer Research. 2016;**22**(6):1395-1402

[85] Szyllo K, Smolarz B, Romanowicz-Makowska H, Lewy J, Kulig B. The T/C polymorphism of the CYP17 gene and G/A polymorphism of the CYP19 gene in endometrial cancer. Journal of Experimental & Clinical Cancer Research. 2006;**25**(3):411-416

[86] Tao MH, Cai Q, Zhang ZF, Xu WH, Kataoka N, Wen W, et al. Polymorphisms in the CYP19A1 (aromatase) gene and endometrial cancer risk in Chinese women. Cancer Epidemiology, Biomarkers & Prevention. 2007;**16**(5):943-949

[87] Gulyaeva LF, Mikhailova ON, PustyInyak VO, Kim IV, Gerasimov AV, Krasilnikov SE, et al. Comparative analysis of SNP in estrogen-metabolizing enzymes for ovarian, endometrial, and breast cancers in Novosibirsk, Russia. Advances in Experimental Medicine Biology. 2008;**617**:359-366

[88] Setiawan VW, Doherty JA, Shu XO, Akbari MR, Chen C, De Vivo I,et al. Two estrogen-related variants in CYP19A1 and endometrial cancer risk: A pooled analysis in the Epidemiology of Endometrial Cancer Consortium. Cancer Epidemiology, Biomarkers & Prevention. 2009; **18**(1):242-247

[89] Lundin E, Wirgin I, Lukanova A, Afanasyeva Y, Krogh V, Axelsson T, Selected polymorphisms in sex hormone-related genes, circulating sex hormones and risk of endometrial cancer. Cancer Epidemiology. 2012;**36**(5):445-452

[90] Barrett-Connor E, Garland C, McPhillips JB, Khaw KT, Wingard DL. A prospective, population based study of androstenedione, estrogens, and prostatic cancer. Cancer Research. 1990;**50**(1):169-173

[91] Ellem SJ, Schmitt JF, Pedersen JS, Frydenberg M, Risbridger GP. Local aromatase expression in human prostate is altered in malignancy. The Journal of Clinical Endocrinology and Metabolism. 2004;**89**:2431-2441

[92] Montgomery RB, Mostaghel EA, Vessella R, et al. Maintenance of intratumoral androgens in metastatic prostate cancer: A mechanism for castration-resistant tumor growth. Cancer Research 2008;**68**:4447-4454

[93] Nelles, JL Hu W, and Prins GS. Estrogen action and prostate cancer. Expert Review Endocrinology and Metabolism. 2011;**6**(3):437-451

[94] Kachakova D, Mitkova A, Popov E, Beltcheva O, Vlahova A, Dikov T, et al, Polymorphisms in androgen metabolism genes AR, CYP1B1, CYP19, and SRD5A2and prostate cancer risk and aggressiveness in Bulgarian patients. Turkish Journal of Medical Sciences. 2016;**46**(3):626-640

[95] Sarma AV, Dunn RL, Lange LA, Ray A, Wang Y, Lange EM, et al. Genetic polymorphisms in CYP17, CYP3A4, CYP19A1, SRD5A2, IGF-1, and IGFBP-3 and prostate cancer risk in African-American men: The Flint Men's Health Study. Prostate. 2008;**68**(3):296-305

[96] Fukatsu T, Hirokawa Y, Araki T, Hioki T, Murata T, Suzuki H, et al. Genetic polymorphisms of hormone-related genes and prostate cancer risk in the Japanese population. Anticancer Research. 2004;**24**(4):2431-2437

[97] Onsory K, Sobti RC, Al-Badran AI, Watanabe M, Shiraishi T, Krishan A, et al. Hormone receptor-related gene polymorphisms and prostate cancer risk in North Indian population. Molecular and Cellular Biochemistry. 2008;**314**(1-2):25-35

[98] Suzuki K, Nakazato H, Matsui H, Koike H, Okugi H, Kashiwagi B, et al. Genetic polymorphisms of estrogen receptor alpha, CYP19, catechol-O-methyltransferase are associated with familial prostate carcinoma risk in a Japanese population. Cancer. 2003;**98**(7):1411-1416

[99] Modugno F, Weissfeld JL, Trump DL, Zmuda JM, Shea P, Cauley JA, et al. Allelic variants of aromatase and the androgen and estrogen receptors: Toward a multigenic model of prostate cancer risk. Clinical Cancer Research. 2001;**7**(10):3092-3096

[100] Mononen N, Seppälä EH, Duggal P, Autio V, Ikonen T, Ellonen P, et al. Profiling genetic variation along the androgen biosynthesis and metabolism pathways implicates several single nucleotide polymorphisms and their combinations as prostate cancer risk factors. Cancer Research. 2006;**66**(2):743-747

[101] Kanda S, Tsuchiya N, Narita S, Inoue T, Huang M, Chiba S, et al. Effects of functional genetic polymorphisms in the CYP19A1 gene on prostate cancer risk and survival. International Journal of Cancer. 2015;**136**(1):74-82

[102] Ersekerci E, Sofikerim M, Taheri S, Demirtas A, Halis F. Genetic polymorphism in sex hormone metabolism and prostate cancer risk. Genetics and Molecular Research. 2015;**14**(3):7326-7334

[103] Lévesque É, Huang SP, Audet-Walsh É, Lacombe L, Bao BY, Fradet Y, et al, Molecular markers in key steroidogenic pathways, circulating steroid levels, and prostate cancer progression. Clinical Cancer Research. 2013;**19**(3):699-709

[104] Huhtaniemi IT, Pye SR, Holliday KL, Thomson W, O'Neill TW, Platt H, Payne D, et al. Effect of polymorphisms in selected genes involved in pituitary-testicular function on reproductive hormones and phenotype in aging men. Journal of Clinical Endocrinology and Metabolism. 2010;**95**(4):1898-1908

[105] Eriksson AL, Lorentzon M, Vandenput L, Labrie F, Lindersson M, Syvänen AC, et al. Genetic variations in sex steroid-related genes as predictors of serum estrogen levels in men. Journal of Clinical Endocrinology and Metabolism. 2009;**94**(3):1033-1041

[106] Sonoda T, Suzuki H, Mori M, Tsukamoto T, Yokomizo A, Naito S, et al. Polymorphisms in estrogen related genes may modify the protective effect of isoflavones against prostate cancer risk in Japanese men. European Journal of Cancer Prevention. 2010;**19**(2):131-137

[107] Nelson HD, Humphrey LL, Nygren P, et al. Postmenopausal hormone replacement therapy: Scientific review. JAMA 2002;**288**:872-881

[108] Nanda K, Bastian LA, Hasselblad V, Simel DL. Hormone replacement therapy and the risk of colorectal cancer: A meta-analysis. Obstetrics and Gynecology. 1999;**93**:880-888

[109] McMichael AJ, Potter JD. Reproduction, endogenous and exogenous sex hormones, and colon cancer: A review and hypothesis. Journal of the National Cancer Institute. 1980;**65**:1201-1207

[110] Slattery ML, Lundgreen A, Herrick JS, Kadlubar S, Caan BJ, Potter JD, and Roger K. Wolff Variation in the CYP19A1 gene and risk of colon and rectal cancer. Cancer Causes & Control. 2011;**22**(7):955-963

[111] English MA, Kane KF, Cruickshank N, Langman MJ, Stewart PM, Hewison M. Loss of estrogen inactivation in colonic cancer. Journal of Clinical Endocrinology and Metabolism. 1999;**84**:2080-2085

[112] English MA, Stewart PM, Hewison M. Estrogen metabolism and malignancy: Analysis of the expression and function of 17beta-hydroxysteroid dehydrogenases in colonic cancer. Molecular and Cellular Endocrinology. 2001;**171**:53-60

[113] Di Domenico M, Castoria G, Bilancio A, Migliaccio A, Auricchio F. Estradiol activation of human colon carcinoma-derived Caco-2 cell growth. Cancer Research. 1996;**56**:4516-4521

[114] Wu H, Xu L, Chen J, Hu J, Yu S, Hu G, et al. Association of estrogen receptor beta variants and serum levels of estradiol with risk of colorectal cancer: A case control study. BMC Cancer. 2012;**12**:276

[115] Lin J, Zee RY, Liu KY, Zhang SM, Lee IM, Manson JE, et al. Genetic variation in sex-steroid receptors and synthesizing enzymes and colorectal cancer risk in women. Cancer Causes & Control. 2010;**21**(6):897-908

[116] Lin JH, Manson JE, Kraft P, Cochrane BB, Gunter MJ, Chlebowski RT, et al, Estrogen and progesterone-related gene variants and colorectal cancer risk in women. BMC Medical Genetics. 2011;**12**:78

[117] Al-Mukaynizi FB, Alanazi M, Al-Daihan S, Parine NR, Almadi M, Aljebreen A, Azzam N, Alharbi O, Arafah M, Warsy A. CYP19A1 gene polymorphism and colorectal cancer etiology in Saudi population: Case-control study. OncoTargets and Therapy. 2017;**10**:1-9

[118] Goodman MT, Lurie G, Thompson PJ, McDuffie KE, Carney ME. Association of two common single-nucleotide polymorphisms in the CYP19A1 locus and ovarian cancer risk. Endocrine-Related Cancer. 2008;**15**(4):1055-1060

[119] Beesley J, Jordan SJ, Spurdle AB, Song H, Ramus SJ, Kjaer SK, et al. Association between single-nucleotide polymorphisms in hormone metabolism and DNA repair genes and epithelial ovarian cancer: Results from two Australian studies and an additional validation set. Cancer Epidemiology, Biomarkers & Prevention. 2007;**16**(12):2557-2565

[120] Di Maio M, Daniele B, Pignata S, Gallo C, De Maio E, Morabito A, et al. Is human hepatocellular carcinoma a hormone-responsive tumor? World Journal of Gastroenterology. 2008;**14**(11):1682-1689

[121] Yuan X, Zhou G, Zhai Y, Xie W, Cui Y, Cao J, et al. Lack of association between the functional polymorphisms in the estrogen-metabolizing genes and risk for hepatocellular carcinoma. Cancer Epidemiology, Biomarkers & Prevention. 2008;**17**(12):3621-3627

[122] Koh WP, Yuan JM, Wang R, Govindarajan S, Oppenheimer R, Zhang ZQ, et al. Aromatase (CYP19) promoter gene polymorphism and risk of nonviral hepatitis related hepatocellular carcinoma. Cancer. 2011;**117**(15):3383-3392

[123] Yang H, Sukocheva OA, Hussey DJ, Watson DI. Estrogen, male dominance and esophageal adenocarcinoma: Is there a link? World Journal of Gastroenterology. 2012;**18**(5):393-400

[124] Sukocheva OA, Wee C, Ansar A, Hussey DJ, Watson DI. Effect of estrogen on growth and apoptosis in esophageal adenocarcinoma cells. Diseases of the Esophagus. 2013;**26**(6):628-635

[125] Wu IC, Zhao Y, Zhai R, Liu G, Ter-Minassian M, Asomaning K, et al, Association between polymorphisms in cancer-related genes and early onset of esophageal adenocarcinoma. Neoplasia 2011;**13**:386-392

[126] Lagergren K, Ek WE, Levine D, Chow WH, Bernstein L, Casson AG, et al, Polymorphisms in genes of relevance for oestrogen and oxytocin pathways and risk of Barrett's oesophagus and oesophageal adenocarcinoma: A pooled analysis from the BEACON consortium. PLoS One. 2015;**10**(9):e0138738

[127] Camargo MC, Goto Y, Zabaleta J, Morgan DR, Correa P, Rabkin CS. Sex hormones, hormonal interventions, and gastric cancer risk: A meta-analysis. Cancer Epidemiology, Biomarkers & Prevention. 2012;**21**(1):20-38

[128] Lindblad M, Ye W, Rubio C, Lagergren J. Estrogen and risk of gastric cancer: A protective effect in a nationwide cohort study of patients with prostate cancer in Sweden. Cancer Epidemiology, Biomarkers & Prevention. 2004;**13**(12):2203-2207

[129] Wesołowska M, Pawlik P, Jagodziński PP. The clinicopathologic significance of estrogen receptors in human gastric carcinoma. Biomedicine & Pharmacotherapy. 2016;**83**:314-322

[130] Freedman ND, Ahn J, Hou L, Lissowska J, Zatonski W, Yeager M, et al. Polymorphisms in estrogen- and androgen-metabolizing genes and the risk of gastric cancer. Carcinogenesis. 2009;**30**(1):71-77

[131] Cho LY, Yang JJ, Ko KP, Ma SH, Shin A, Choi BY, et al, Genetic susceptibility factors on genes involved in the steroid hormone biosynthesis pathway and progesterone receptor for gastric cancer risk. PLoS One. 2012;**7**(10):e47603

[132] Kristiansen W, Andreassen KE, Karlsson R, Aschim EL, Bremnes RM, Dahl O, et al, Gene variations in sex hormone pathways and the risk of testicular germ cell tumour: A case-parent triad study in a Norwegian-Swedish population. Human Reproduction. 2012;**27**(5):1525-1535

[133] Huang CS, Kuo SH, Lien HC, Yang SY, You SL, Shen CY, et al. The CYP19 TTTA repeat polymorphism is related to the prognosis of premenopausal stage I-II and operable stage III breast cancers. The Oncologist. 2008;**13**(7):751-760

[134] Colomer R, Monzo M, Tusquets I, Rifa J, Baena JM, Barnadas A, et al. A single-nucleotide polymorphism in the aromatase gene is associated with the efficacy of the aromatase inhibitor letrozole in advanced breast carcinoma. Clinical Cancer Research. 2008;**14**(3):811-816

[135] Long JR, Kataoka N, Shu XO, Wen W, Gao YT, Cai Q, et al. Genetic polymorphisms of the CYP19A1 gene and breast cancer survival. Cancer Epidemiology, Biomarkers & Prevention. 2006;**15**(11):2115-2122

[136] Udler MS, Azzato EM, Healey CS, Ahmed S, Pooley KA, Greenberg D, et al. Common germline polymorphisms in COMT, CYP19A1, ESR1, PGR, SULT1E1 and STS and survival after a diagnosis of breast cancer. International Journal of Cancer. 2009;**125**(11):2687-2696

[137] Kidokoro K, Ino K, Hirose K, Kajiyama H, Hosono S, Suzuki T, et al. Association between CYP19A1 polymorphisms and sex hormones in postmenopausal Japanese women. Journal of Human Genetics. 2009;**54**(2):78-85

[138] Straume AH, Knappskog S, Lønning PE. Effect of CYP19 rs6493497 and rs7176005 haplotype status on in vivo aromatase transcription, plasma and tissue estrogen levels in postmenopausal women. Journal of Steroid Biochemistry and Molecular Biology. 2012;**128**(1-2):69-75

[139] Dunning AM, Dowsett M, Healey CS, Tee L, Luben RN, Folkerd E, et al. Polymorphisms associated with circulating sex hormone levels in postmenopausal women. Journal of the National Cancer Institute. 2004;**96**(12):936-945

[140] Cai H, Shu XO, Egan KM, Cai Q, Long JR, Gao YT, et al. Association of genetic polymorphisms in CYP19A1 and blood levels of sex hormones among postmenopausal Chinese women. Pharmacogenetics and Genomics. 2008;**18**(8):657-664

[141] Wang L, Ellsworth KA, Moon I, Pelleymounter LL, Eckloff BW, Martin YN, et al. Functional genetic polymorphisms in the aromatase gene CYP19 vary the response of breast cancer patients to neoadjuvant therapy with aromatase inhibitors. Cancer Research. 2010;**70**(1):319-328

[142] Garcia-Casado Z, Guerrero-Zotano A, Llombart-Cussac A, Calatrava A, Fernandez-Serra A, Ruiz-Simon A, et al. A polymorphism at the 3′-UTR region of the aromatase gene defines a subgroup of postmenopausal breast cancer patients with poor response to neoadjuvant letrozole. BMC Cancer 2010;**10**:36

[143] Napoli N, Rastelli A, Ma C, Colleluori G, Vattikuti S, Armamento-Villareal R. Genetic polymorphism at Val80 (rs700518) of the CYP19A1 gene is associated with body composition changes in women on aromatase inhibitors for ER (+) breast cancer. Pharmacogenet Genomics. 2015;**25**(8):377-388

[144] Napoli N, Rastelli A, Ma C, Yarramaneni J, Vattikutti S, Moskowitz G, et al. Genetic polymorphism at Val80 (rs700518) of the CYP19A1 gene is associated with aromatase inhibitor associated bone loss in women with ER + breast cancer. Bone. 2013;**55**(2):309-314

[145] Zarrabeitia MT, Hernandez JL, Valero C, A common polymorphism in the 5′-untranslated region of the aromatase gene influences bone mass and fracture risk. European Journal of Endocrinology. 2004;**150**:699-704

[146] Mao JJ, Su HI, Feng R, Association of functional polymorphisms in CYP19A1 with aromatase inhibitor associated arthralgia in breast cancer survivors. Breast Cancer Research 2011;**13**:R8

Single Nucleotide Polymorphisms and Colorectal Cancer Risk: The First Replication Study in a South American Population

Israel Gomy, Ligia Petrolini de Oliveira and
Benedito Mauro Rossi

Additional information is available at the end of the chapter

http://dx.doi.org/10.5772/intechopen.69994

Abstract

Colorectal cancer (CRC) heritability is determined by the complex interaction between inherited variants and environmental factors. CRC incidence rates have been increasing specially in developing countries, such as Brazil, where CRC is the third most frequent cancer in both genders. Genome-wide association studies (GWAS), based on thousands of cases and controls typed at thousands of single nucleotide polymorphisms (SNPs), have identified several variants that associate with gastrointestinal cancer risk. Less of half of the familial risk has been elucidated through GWAS that identified common SNPs in almost exclusively European populations. Replication studies in admixed heterogeneous populations are scarce and most failed to replicate all the imputed SNPs. Population stratification by ethnic subgroups with different allele frequencies and so with different patterns of linkage disequilibrium may cause expurious associations. Here, we show the first replication study of CRC inherited susceptibility in South America and aimed to identify known SNPs, which are associated with CRC risk in European populations.

Keywords: cancer susceptibility, cancer risk, colorectal cancer, single nucleotide polymorphism, South America

1. Introduction

1.1. Epidemiology

Colorectal cancer (CRC) is one of the most prevalent cancers in both genders worldwide, responsible for about 10% of all neoplasms, mainly in developed industrialized countries, such as Australia and New Zeland, North America, and Europe [1].

The variation in the CRC global incidence rates is progressively decreasing, and the increase of new cases in historically low incidence populations, such as Asian, seems to come along with a greater economic development and, consequently, a greater exposure to risk factors so-called "Western lifestyle." The highest incidence rates are in countries such as Australia, New Zealand, and in Western Europe, whereas the lowest incidence rates are in Africa and Southern Asia [2].

However, in developing countries such as Russia, Mexico, Chile, and Brazil, there is an increase of CRC incidence rates, possibly reflecting their population's lifestyles and the increased life expectancy, as well as the improved data records, the insufficient public health policies for CRC screening, and the lack of population awareness.

Data from international registries indicate that the overall 5-year survival rate is on average 55% in developed countries and 40% in developing countries and is higher in women than in men [3].

According to estimates from the National Cancer Institute for the 2016/2017 biennium, in Brazil, 34,280 individuals will develop CCR (17,620 women and 16,660 men), corresponding to the second most common malignancy in women and third most common malignancy in men [4].

The detection and early removal of premalignant lesions reduces CRC mortality as confirmed by several studies that have screened populations at general risk using the fecal occult blood test. In addition, the use of flexible sigmoidoscopy for screening has shown promising results in randomized trials in the United Kingdom [5] and the United States [6], where significant reductions in both incidence and mortality were observed. Improved survival was also observed with this approach in genetically determined high-risk groups [7]. Therefore, for those determined high-risk individuals could be offered a more intensive surveillance, with colonoscopy or flexible sigmoidoscopy periodically at shorter intervals. Colonoscopy is already offered to individuals at high risk due to personal or familial history of CRC, as well as for families with Lynch syndrome and intestinal polyposis syndromes, for which more assiduous surveillance is recommended [8]. Therefore, stratifying the general population into risk categories would allow the individualization of screening and prevention strategies.

1.2. Molecular pathogenesis

The classic adenoma-carcinoma sequence has revealed an intricate molecular pathogenesis of CRC, where tumor suppressor genes are inactivated, and proto-oncogenes are activated through several signaling pathways, such as *APC-B-cathenin*, *RAS-RAF*, *PIK3CA-PTEN*, and *TGF-B* [9].

Three main molecular mechanisms are involved in CRC pathogenesis: chromosomal instability, microsatellite instability, and serrated polyp pathway. The first one occurs in most sporadic cancers where the accumulation of mutations, rearrangements, and aneuploidy drives malignant transformation within decades [10]. The second one occurs in about 15% of sporadic CRC and in most hereditary CRC. In sporadic CRC, an epigenetic event—hypermethylation—occurs in CpG islands of MMR gene promoters, which silences them leading to a genetic instability in microsatellite regions of genome [11]. In Lynch syndrome, mutations in MMR genes lead to microsatellite instability and accelerate adenoma-carcinoma sequence

http://dx.doi.org/10.5772/intechopen.69994

more rapidly, the reason why Lynch syndrome families develop cancer in their 40's or even earlier. The most recently serrated polyp pathway involves molecular mechanisms other than the classic adenoma-carcinoma sequence but has not yet been fully elucidated [12].

1.3. Risk factors

Colorectal carcinoma is a multifactorial disease, where complex interactions between genetic and environmental factors determine individual risk. Among the latter are diets rich in red meat and animal fat and lower in fiber, smoking, alcohol consumption, obesity, sedentary lifestyle, and chronic inflammatory bowel disease [13]. In addition to age, gender, and previous history of polyps, familial history is considered the main risk factor, being the relative risk between siblings two to three times higher than in the general population [14].

Traditionally, CRC has been classified into sporadic and hereditary. The concept of familial CRC reflects one end of a risk spectrum determined by the contribution of genetic variants of susceptibility. Most are sporadic with no family history and known genetic susceptibility. Most of the CRC susceptibility genes were identified in families affected by inherited syndromes, which are caused by mutations with high penetrance. These syndromes account for about 6% of CRC cases and can be classified as syndromes with or without gastrointestinal polyposis [15]. Among the main syndromes with polyposis are familial adenomatous polyposis (FAP) caused by mutations in the *APC* gene; Peutz-Jeghers syndrome, attributable to mutations in the *STK11* gene; Juvenile polyposis, associated with the *BMPR1A* gene, and Cowden's syndrome, related to the *PTEN* gene. Among non-polyposis syndromes, the most prevalent is Lynch's syndrome, accounting for about 3% of all the cases with CRC, caused by mutations in the mismatch repair genes during DNA replication (*MLH1, MSH2, MSH6, PMS2,* and *EPCAM*) [16].

Most of the mutations identified in familial CRC are highly penetrant, that is, with a high chance of manifesting cancer throughout the life. However, there are families with CRC clusters that do not have mutations in genes associated with hereditary syndromes. This raises the hypothesis that there are other variants or mutations with low penetrance that make certain individuals more susceptible to the CRC development. Studies with brothers with and without CRC, as well as several association studies, have identified regions in the human genome in which single nucleotide polymorphisms (SNPs) variants are associated with CRC susceptibility [17].

Up to 25% of cases are familial CRC aggregations whose heritability has been partially uncovered by GWAS SNPs [18]. However, the large proportion of familial risk remains unexplained—so-called missing heritability.

1.4. Single nucleotide polymorphisms

Single nucleotide polymorphisms (SNPs) are variations of the human genome, where two or occasionally three alternative nucleotides are common in the population. In most cases, an SNP has two alternative forms, termed alleles, for example, A or G at a certain position in the genome.

There are 10 million SNPs estimated in the human genome, representing, along with other types of polymorphisms (such as copy number variations), about 90% of human genetic variation, including susceptibility to disease. Two individuals are 99.5% identical in their DNA sequences, and, every 1000 base pairs, there is one SNP [19].

Variants that have been deleterious during evolution are particularly rare due to natural selection. In turn, pathogenic variants that are deleterious in homozygosis may have become neutral or undergo a selection balance by conferring an advantage on asymptomatic heterozygotes. Therefore, alleles of frequent SNPs are not expected to have any significant phenotypic effect, either because natural selection would be in charge of eliminating it, - if it were detrimental by negative selection -, or fixing it, if beneficial by positive selection. Moreover, most SNPs are not located in either coding or regulatory sequences but in intergenic sequences [20].

1.5. Genome-wide association studies

Searching for population associations is an attractive option to identify disease susceptibility genes. Association studies are easier to conduct than linkage studies because they do not require multiple family cases segregating the phenotype. However, they depend on the linkage disequilibrium (LD)—the nonrandom association between alleles at different loci—with a susceptibility factor, which can only be identified by markers located in the same haplotype block (the set of alleles at a linked locus in a single chromosome) close to the factor [21].

SNPs are the markers of choice for studying LD for three reasons: (1) they are sufficiently abundant that they allow verifying very short chromosome segments; (2) compared to microsatellites, they have a lower mutation rate; (3) SNPs are easily large-scale genotyped on genome [20].

The structure of the human LD was investigated by the HapMap project, and the first result was a list of more than 3 million SNPs that captured most of the common genomic variation in some populations [22].

Genome-wide association studies (GWAS) are based on the LD principle at the population level, which is usually the result of a particular ancestral haplotype common in a population. Usually, loci that are physically close exhibit a stronger DL than those that are distant in a chromosome. The genomic distance at which LD decays determines how many genetic markers are required to "tag" a haplotype block, being the number of such markers much smaller than the total of segregating variants in the population. For example, the selection of about 500,000 common SNPs in the human genome is sufficient to "tag" the common variants in non-African population, even though the total SNPs are greater than 10 million [22]. These SNPs are called tagSNPs.

Although GWAS are not influenced by prior biological knowledge or genomic location of SNPs, they are influenced by LD between genotyped SNPs and non-genotyped causative variants. The strength of the statistical association between the alleles at the two loci in the genome depends, mainly, on their allelic frequencies. Thus, a rare variant—minor allele frequency (MAF) less than 0.01—will be low LD with a neighboring common variant, even though they are in the same recombination range. However, most of the SNPs selected in the SNP arrays are common (MAF higher than 0.05), and therefore, GWASs have the power to detect association of variants that are relatively common in the population [21]. On the other hand, it is suggested that the observed association between a common SNP and a complex trait may result from LD of the SNP with rare variants at the same locus. Since common alleles and causal rare variants are correlated in a low LD, the hypothesis of a "synthetic association" implies that the magnitude of the effect of the causative variants is much greater than that of the common genotyped SNPs by the GWAS. For example, if an SNP explains 0.1% of the phenotypic variance in the population, the causal variant would account for 5–10% [23].

1.6. GWAS and CRC

Most of the studies to identify low penetrance alleles for CRC susceptibility were based on a candidate gene approach, whose role in CRC pathogenesis was supposedly known. However, without the real understanding of the biology of predisposition, the choice of genes was problematic. Thus, until the advent of GWAS, few or no association studies based on this approach were able to identify alleles of susceptibility unequivocally associated with the CRC risk [17].

To date, seven GWAS and three meta-analyses have identified about 20 independent loci associated with CRC susceptibility [24–34].

The number of common variants contributing with more than 1% of the inherited risk is very low, and it is very unlikely that there will be other SNPs with similar effects (greater than 1.2) for alleles with frequencies greater than 20% in European populations. In fact, the GWAS identified on average 80% of the common SNPs in this population but only 12% of SNPs with a minor allele frequency (MAF) between 5 and 10% [17].

However, variants with this profile, if taken collectively, can confer substantial risks due to their multiplicity, and in the case of CRC, to date, explain about 10% of heritability [33]. In a model built on data from the Scottish GWAS, about 170 common independent variants would explain all the genetic variance of the CRC [35]. Therefore, most of the genetic susceptibility to CRC still needs to be defined the so-called "missing heritability". There are other possible causes of this unidentified portion: (1) the effect of rare variants; (2) failure to identify causal variants; and (3) allelic heterogeneity [36].

GWAS strategies to identify modest common risk alleles are not ideal for identifying rare variants (MAF below 1%) with potentially greater effects, as well as for capturing copy number variants and other structural variants, such as insertions, complex rearrangements, or expansions of microsatellite repeats, which may alter the risk of CRC. As efforts are made to scale up the GWAS meta-analyses, both in terms of sample size and coverage of SNPs, as well as to increase the number of SNPs considered for large-scale replication, it will be feasible to discover new variants. It is possible that a multiple loci approach based on haplotype markers identifies rare alleles. In addition, the use of exome sequencing may provide a more effective strategy for finding such variants [37].

2. Objectives

The overall objective of the present study was to replicate in individuals of the Brazilian population the 10 SNPs associated with CRC risk that are previously described in European populations. The specific objectives were to (1) calculate the allelic and genotype frequencies of the 10 SNPs in cases and controls; (2) analyze the association between the genotypes and alleles of the 10 SNPs and CRC risk; (3) calculate the magnitude of the effect on CRC risk; and (4) correlate the genotypes of the 10 SNPs with clinical-pathological characteristics and with familial history.

3. Research methods

3.1. Patient selection criteria

This is a retrospective study of case-control genetic association, whose sample comprised 727 cases and 740 controls, recruited from the Departments of Pelvic Surgery, Clinical Oncology, and Community Medicine at AC Camargo Cancer Center, in São Paulo, Brazil. All patients and controls authorized the present study by signing the informed consent form previously approved by the Research Ethics Committee of the institution under number 1231/09.

The inclusion criteria for cases were CRC diagnosis before age 75 years or with advanced colorectal adenoma (villous histology and/or greater than 1 cm and/or severe dysplasia) diagnosis before age 60 years, and controls were individuals without CRC who did not have first- or second-degree relatives with CRC. Controls were not matched with the cases in relation to the socioeconomic condition, ancestry, or self-referred ethnicity. The exclusion criteria were the presence of hereditary syndromes of predisposition to CRC, immunohistochemistry tests showing absence of proteins from DNA mismatch repair genes, the presence of high-penetrance germline mutations in susceptible genes to CRC, and appendix tumors and/or previous chronic inflammatory bowel disease.

3.2. SNP genotyping

After consent form was signed, 8 ml of peripheral blood was drawn to extract, purify, quantify, and amplify DNA. Quantitative PCRs for 10 tagSNPs (rs6983267, rs4939827, rs4779584, rs16892766, rs10795668, rs4444235, rs9929218, rs10411210, rs961253, and rs3802842) were performed using TaqMan® SNP Genotyping Assays and 7900HT Fast Real-Time PCR System (Thermo Scientific Fisher, CA, USA). Allelic discrimination analyses were made using the Sequence Detection Systems Automation Controller Software v2.3 and the auto-calling technique (Thermo Scientific Fisher, CA, USA).

As genotyping quality control, genotypes with the following criteria were excluded: (1) overall call <95%; (2) discordant duplicates; (3) Hardy-Weinberg imbalance ($p < 10^{-6}$ in cases and $p < 10^{-4}$ in controls); and (4) clusters of unsatisfactory genotypes in the X:Y axis inspection.

3.3. Statistics analysis

All tests were corrected for multiple analyses to avoid type I error. The allelic and genotypic frequencies of each SNP were calculated using the DeFinetti program [38], and the deviations of the genotype frequencies in cases and controls predicted by the Hardy-Weinberg equilibrium were calculated by the chi-square test with one degree of freedom or by Fisher's exact test, if the expected cell count was less than five.

Association analyses between the genotypes found in cases and controls for each SNP were performed with several types of genetic models, using the SNP and Variation Suite Version 7.6.10 program [39]. Multiple analyses were corrected by false discovery rate and Bonferroni.

4. Results

4.1. Clinical characteristics of cases and controls

Of the 727 cases included in this study, 51% were male, with a median age of diagnosis of 56.9 ± 10.1 SD years old; 30% fulfilled Bethesda criteria; 3% of tumors were high-risk adenomas; the most common site of CRC was the rectum and in about 10%, there was an extra-colonic second primary tumor; tubular adenocarcinomas moderately differentiated at clinical stage III was mostly diagnosed. The majority of patients was alive disease-free until data collection and about 30% of cases had no familial history of CRC, despite almost 20% did not know about affected relatives. Of the 740 controls included in this study, 52% were female, with a median age of 51.9 ± 12.3 SD years old. Cases and controls were age and sex matched ($p = 0.126$ and 0.193, respectively).

4.2. SNP genotyping and association tests

The genotypic frequencies of each SNP in cases and controls and their p-values are depicted in the following graphics:

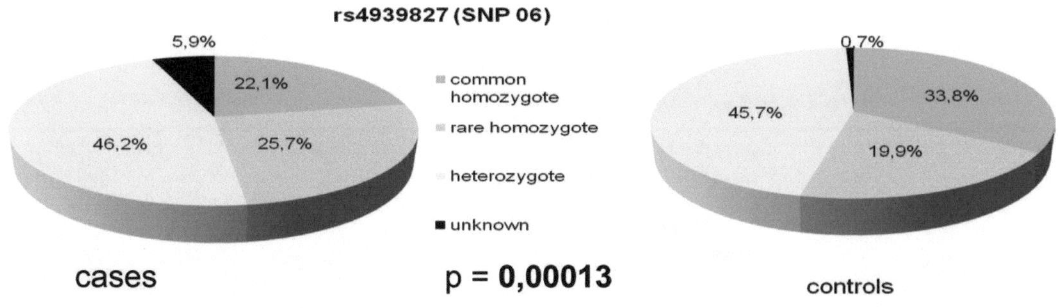

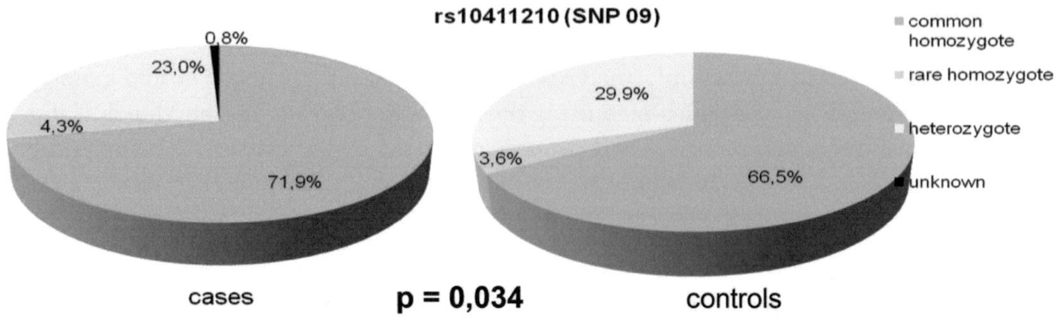
rs10411210 (SNP 09)
0,8%
23,0%
4,3%
71,9%
29,9%
3,6%
66,5%
common homozygote
rare homozygote
heterozygote
unknown
cases
p = 0,034
controls

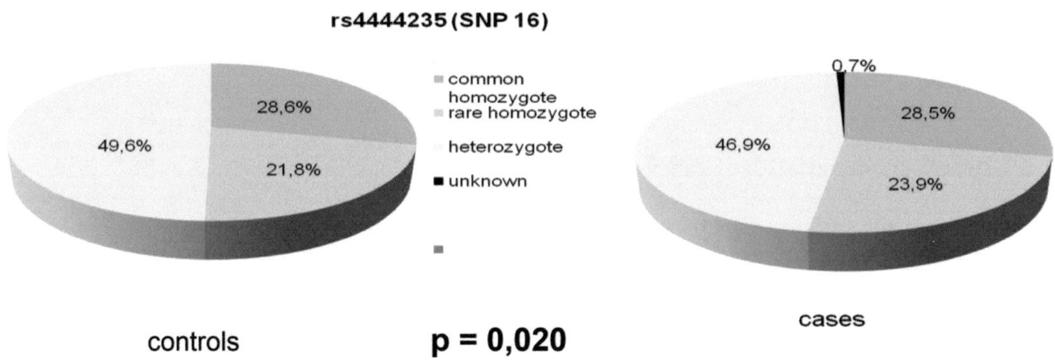
rs4444235 (SNP 16)
28,6%
49,6%
21,8%
common homozygote
rare homozygote
heterozygote
unknown
0,7%
28,5%
46,9%
23,9%
controls
p = 0,020
cases

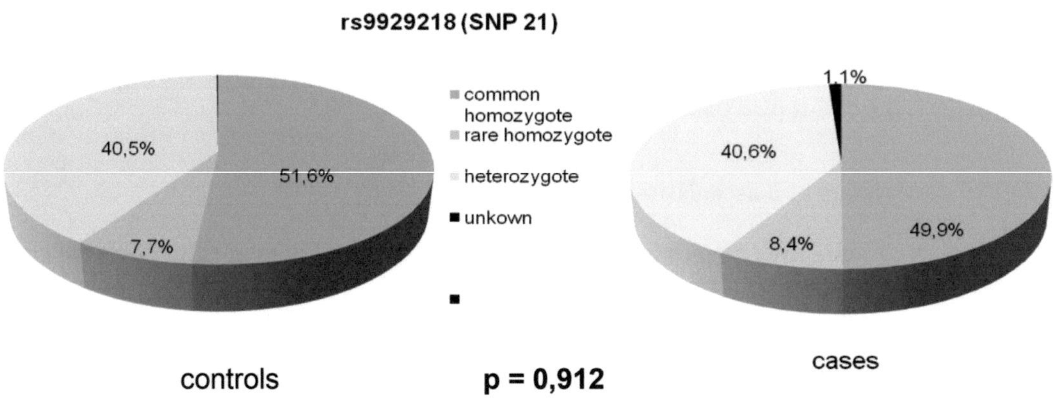
rs9929218 (SNP 21)
40,5%
51,6%
7,7%
common homozygote
rare homozygote
heterozygote
unkown
1,1%
40,6%
8,4%
49,9%
controls
p = 0,912
cases

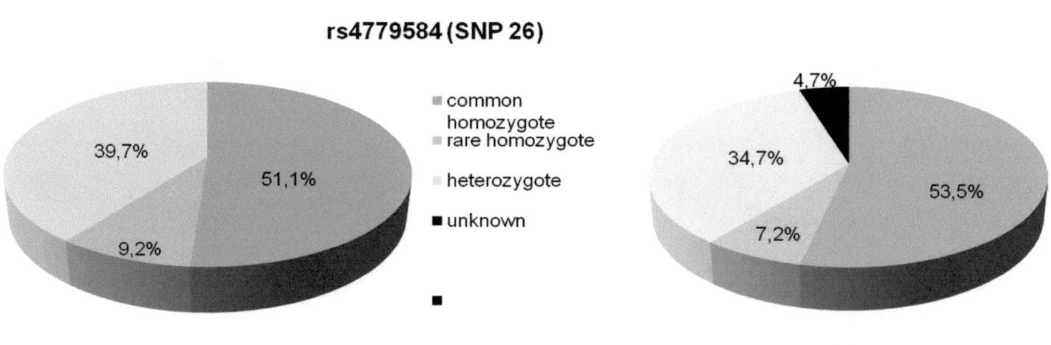
rs4779584 (SNP 26)
39,7%
51,1%
9,2%
common homozygote
rare homozygote
heterozygote
unknown
4,7%
34,7%
53,5%
7,2%
cases

http://dx.doi.org/10.5772/intechopen.69994

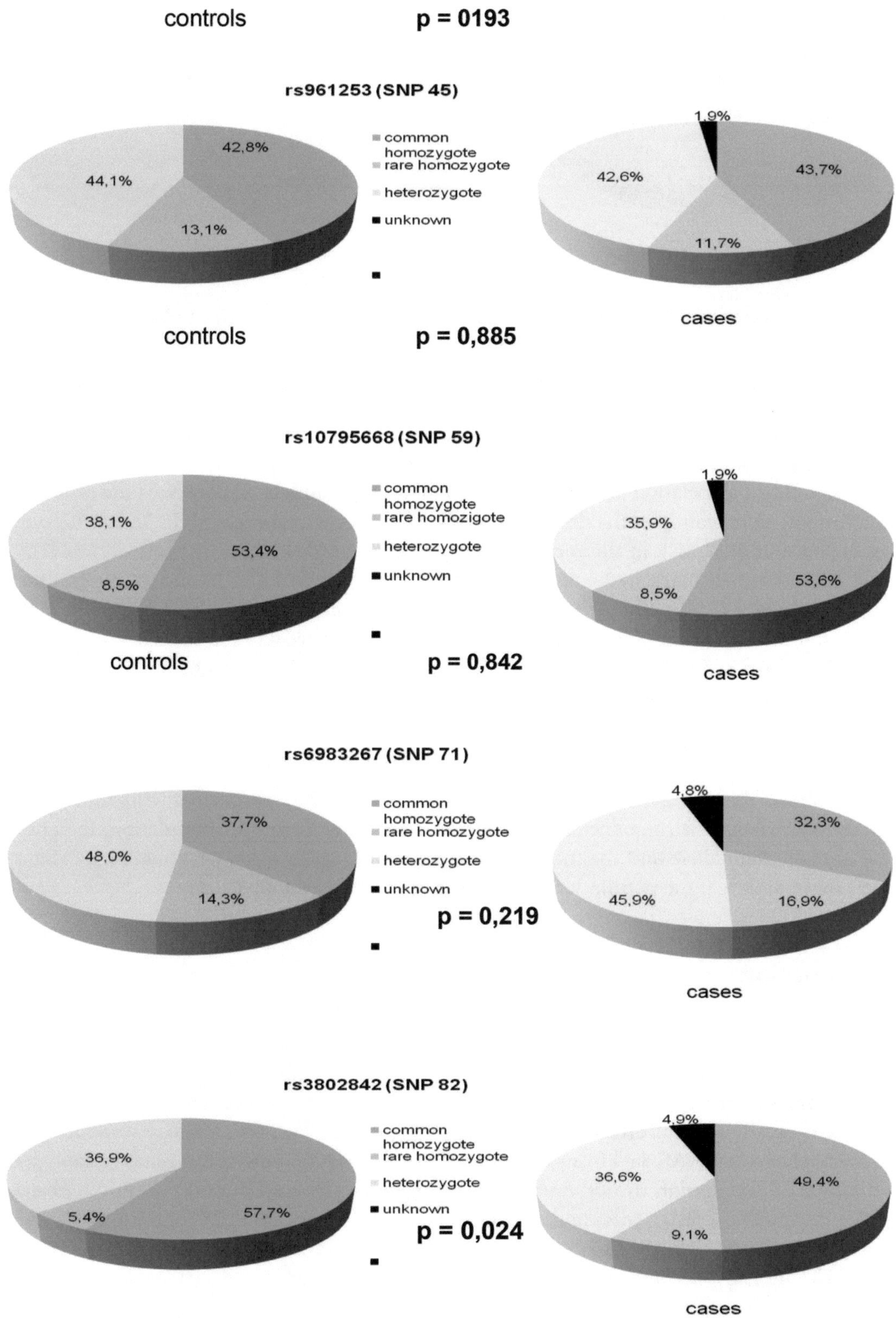

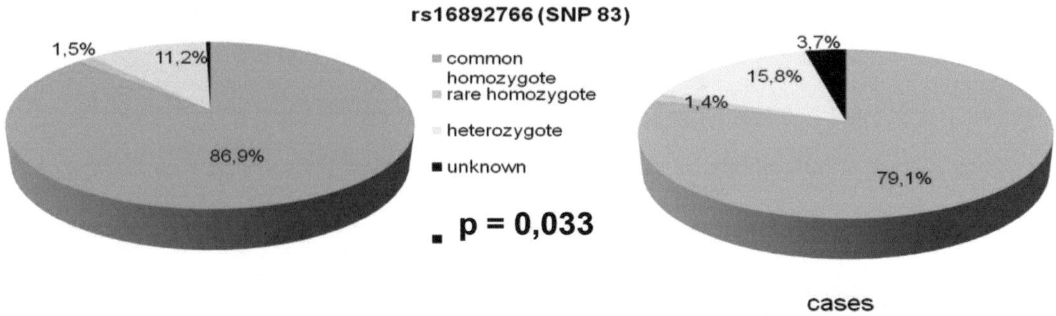

The allelic frequencies, the number of alleles, the genotyping rate, and the Hardy-Weinberg equilibrium (EHW) test are represented in **Table 1**.

The genetic association tests and their genetic models are shown in **Table 2**.

Of the 10 SNPs, 5 (06, 09 16, 82, and 83) were statistically significant ($p \leq 0.05$) associated with the risk of CRC and 2 (26 and 71) showed a trend to association ($p < 0.1$). SNP 06 showed the more significant association among all SNPs in all genetic models. SNP 09 was the only predictor of low risk, mainly in the dominant model (25% lower), whereas SNPs 16 and 82 were associated with high risk in the recessive model (45 and 85% higher, respectively). SNP 83 had higher risk principally in the dominant model (almost 50%). SNPs 26 and 71, on the other hand, obtained a marginally significant association only in the allelic and additive models, with a trend toward a higher risk with SNP 71 and lower risk with SNP 26. To sum up, of five SNPs associated with CRC risk, two (SNP 16 and 82) conferred higher risk among rare homozygotes than among heterozygotes and common homozygotes together through the recessive model and three (06, 09, and 83) showed higher risk among heterozygotes and rare homozygotes together than among common homozygotes through the dominant model.

Table 3 shows the five SNPs associated with CCR risk with their respective wild and variant alleles, their risk allele frequencies in comparison with the European population, the effect size of the variant allele and the their populational attributable risks, which is the incidence decrease of disease if the population was not exposed to the risk allele.

5. Discussion

In common diseases, such as CRC, it estimated that the most part of its genetic risk is due to the inherited multiple *loci* following polygenic model, each one with a common allelic frequency (MAF greater than 5%), whose effects show small sizes, between odds ratios 1.0 and 1.5. [17] Thus, to detect those small effects, it is necessary a big sample size. This strategy was validated by metanalyses of GWAS data from European populations with tens of thousands genotyped individuals through high throughput platforms, followed by validation by multiple phases with independent series of cases and controls. Even though only about 20 common SNPs with modest effects were identified so far, each one with a p value corrected by multiple tests ($<5.0 \times 10^{-8}$). In **Table 4**, GWAS data from European populations are compared to this study.

	EHW test		Allelic frequencies				Number of alleles				Frequencies		Genotyping rate		
	Cases	Controls	Cases		Controls		Cases		Controls				Cases	Controls	Global
SNP	p	p	*Major* allele	*Minor* allele	*Major* allele	*Minor* allele	*Major* allele	*Minor* allele	*Major* allele	*Minor* allele	*Major* allele	*Minor* allele	%	%	%
rs4939827 (SNP06)	0.7018	0.0978	0.48	0.52	0.57	0.43	658	710	838	632	0.53	0.47	94.1	99.3	96.7
rs10411210 (SNP09)	0.0007	0.7158	0.84	0.16	0.81	0.19	1213	229	1205	275	0.83	0.17	99.2	100.0	99.6
rs4444235 (SNP16)	0.1565	0.9411	0.48	0.52	0.53	0.47	689	755	791	689	0.51	0.49	99.3	100.0	99.7
rs9929218 (SNP21)	0.9279	0.9273	0.71	0.29	0.72	0.28	1021	417	1064	414	0.72	0.28	98.9	99.9	99.4
rs4779584 (SNP26)	0.2319	0.3270	0.74	0.26	0.71	0.29	1030	356	1050	430	0.73	0.27	95.3	100.0	97.7
rs961253 (SNP45)	0.5022	0.3750	0.66	0.34	0.65	0.35	946	480	960	520	0.66	0.34	98.1	100.0	99.0
rs10795668 (SNP59)	0.0576	0.2311	0.73	0.27	0.72	0.28	1041	385	1072	408	0.73	0.27	98.1	100.0	99.0
rs6983267 (SNP71)	0.8151	0.7557	0.58	0.42	0.62	0.38	804	580	913	567	0.60	0.40	95.2	100.0	97.6
rs3802842 (SNP82)	0.1146	0.7613	0.71	0.29	0.76	0.24	984	398	1127	353	0.74	0.26	95.0	100.0	97.5
rs16892766 (SNP83)	0.1287	0.0005	0.9	0.10	0.93	0.07	1265	135	1369	105	0.92	0.08	96.3	99.6	98.0

Table 1. Allelic frequencies, number of alleles, genotyping rate and Hardy-Weinberg equilibrium (EHW) test.

Models SNP	Risk allele (minor)	RAF	Allelic OR [95% CI]	p	Dominant OR [95% CI]	p	Recessive OR [95% CI]	p	Additive OR [95% CI]	p
rs4939827 (SNP 06)	C	0.47	1.43 [1.23–1.66]	2.12×10^{-5}	1.67 [1.33–2.11]	0.0001	1.51 [1.18–1.93]	0.011	1.54 [1.20–1.98]	3.49×10^{-5}
rs10411210 (SNP 09)	T	0.17	0.83 [0.68–1.00]	0.080	0.75 [0.60–0.94]	0.040	1.19 [0.70–2.01]	0.749	0.71 [0.56–0.90]	0.083
rs4444235 (SNP16)	C	0.49	1.26 [1.09–1.45]	0.011	1.26 [1.00–1.60]	0.097	1.45 [1.14–1.83]	0.012	1.38 [1.07–1.78]	0.012
rs3802842 (SNP 21)	A	0.26	1.29 [1.09–1.53]	0.010	1.26 [1.02–1.56]	0.072	1.85 [1.23–2.78]	0.009	1.69 [1.1 –2.60]	0.011
rs16892766 (SNP 26)	C	0.08	1.39 [1.07–1.82]	0.038	1.49 [1.11–1.99]	0.035	0.96 [0.40–2.27]	0.920	1.55 [1.14–2.10]	0.049
rs6983267 (SNP 45)	T	0.40	1.16 [1.00–1.35]	0.086	1.18 [0.95–1.46]	0.2	1.29 [0.97–1.72]	0.188	1.23 [0.91–1.66]	0.082
rs4779584 (SNP 59)	T	0.27	0.84 [0.72–1.00]	0.089	0.82 [0.66–1.00]	0.092	0.80 [0.55–1.17]	0.498	0.83 [0.67–1.04]	0.097
rs9929218 (SNP 71)	A	0.28	1.05 [0.89–1.23]	0.629	1.05 [0.85–1.29]	0.645	1.11 [0.76–1.62]	0.737	1.03 [0.83–1.28]	0.628
rs961253 (SNP 82)	A	0.34	0.94 [0.80–1.09]	0.515	0.93 [0.76–1.15]	0.623	0.90 [0.66–1.22]	0.824	0.95 [0.76–1.18]	0.524
rs10795668 (SNP 83)	A	0.27	0.97 [0.83–1.14]	0.739	0.95 [0.77–1.17]	0.682	1.02 [0.71–1.48]	1	0.94 [0.75–1.17]	0.739

RAF, risk allele frequency.

Table 2. Genetic association tests and genetic models.

SNP	**Wild allele***	**Risk allele**	**Risk allele frequencies(RAF)**	**Minor allele frequency (Europeans)***	**Effect size**	**Populational attributable risk** (%)**
rs4939827 (SNP 06)	*T (major)*	*C (minor)*	0.47	0.47	43% higher	16.8
rs10411210 (SNP 09)	*C (major)*	*T (minor)*	0.17	0.10	25% lower	–
rs4444235 (SNP 16)	*T (major)*	*C (minor)*	0.49	0.48	26% higher	11.3
rs3802842 (SNP 82)	*C (minor)*	*C (minor)*	0.26	0.27	29% higher	7.0
rs16892766 (SNP 83)	*A (major)*	*C (minor)*	0.08	0.09	39% higher	3.0

* From 1000 genomes.
** (RAF(OR – 1))/(1 + RAF(OR – 1)).

Table 3. The five SNPs associated with CCR risk.

SNP	**Risk allele**	**RAF**	**Effect size (odds ratio)**	**PAR (%)**	**Sample size (total)**	**References**
rs4939827 (SNP 06)	*C (major)*	0.52	1.18	8.6	15,362	Broderick et al. [27]
rs10411210 (SNP 09)	*T (minor)* *C (major)*	0.10 0.90	0.87 1.15	– 11.9	41,259	Houlston et al. [31]
rs4444235 (SNP 16)	*C (minor)*	0.46	1.11	4.8	41,259	Houlston et al. [31]
rs9929218 (SNP 21)	*G (major)*	0.71	1.10	6.6	41,259	Houlston et al. [31]
rs4779584 (SNP 26)	*T (minor)*	0.18	1.26	4.5	14,663	Jaeger et al. [28]
rs961253 (SNP 45)	*A (minor)*	0.36	1.12	4.0	41,259	Houlston et al. [31]
rs10795668 (SNP 59)	*G (major)*	0.67	1.12	7.4	37,371	Tomlinson et al. [30]
rs6983267 (SNP 71)	*G (major)*	0.51	1.21	9.7	14,470	Tomlinson et al. [25]
rs3802842 (SNP 82)	*C (minor)*	0.29	1.12	3.4	27,794	Tenesa et al. [29]
rs16892766 (SNP 83)	*C (minor)*	0.07	1.25	1.7	37,371	Tomlinson et al. [30]

RAF, risk allele frequency; PAR, populational attributable risk.

Table 4. GWAS data from European populations compared to this data.

In this study, there was an association with CRC risk in half of SNPs (06, 09 16, 82 and 83), whose risk alleles revealed similar frequencies as to European GWAS, except SNP 06. Effect sizes were modest as well as European GWAS. SNP 06 was the variant that resulted the greatest effect with the most statistically significant association ($p_{trend} = 3.49 \times 10^{-5}$), which conferred the highest populational risk, whereas in European GWAS, the risk augmented up to 23%, representing 8.6% of the populational risk [35]. In the original study, the same SNP also showed the greatest association ($p_{trend} = 1.0 \times 10^{-12}$) [27]. SNP 09 (rs10411210) was associated with a low risk in a dose-dependent way [31]. In this study, however, this effect was detected only in the dominant model. It is noteworthy that in European studies the *major* allele *(C)* confers 15% higher risk, responsible for 12% of the populational risk [35]. In the present study, there was a trend to a higher risk but not statistically significant ($p = 0.08$). Moreover, SNP 16 was associated with a higher risk in this study than from European GWAS, as well as the populational attributable risk [35]. Likewise, SNPs 82 and 83 also increased more the CRC risk and populational risk in the present study than from European GWAS [35].

In the present study, the populational stratification by ancestry was not investigated. However, the Brazilian population, although greatly admixed, has a high prevalence of individuals from European ancestry, whose the great majority is located in the South (79.5%) and Southeast (74.2%) [40].

6. Conclusion

This study partially replicated European GWAS in Brazilian Southeastern population with a predominantly European genetic background. Small sample size and lack of stratification by ancestry are prone to type I and II errors, respectively. Further studies in admixed populations would certainly aid to uncover the missing heritability of CRC and help to build the genetic architecture of CRC susceptibility.

Author details

Israel Gomy[1]*, Ligia Petrolini de Oliveira[2] and Benedito Mauro Rossi[3]

*Address all correspondence to: isgomy@gmail.com

1 Universidade Federal do Paraná, Curitiba, Brazil

2 Universidade Federal do ABC, Santo André, Brazil

3 Hospital Sírio Libanês, São Paulo, Brazil

References

[1] Ferlay J, Shin HR, Bray F, Forman D, Mathers C, Parkin DM. Estimates of worldwide burden of cancer in 2008: GLOBOCAN 2008. International Journal of Cancer. 2010;**127**: 2893-2917. DOI: 10.1002/ijc.25516

[2] Edwards BK, Ward E, Kohler BA, et al. Annual report to the nation on the status of cancer, 1975-2006, featuring colorectal cancer trends and impact of interventions (risk factors, screening, and treatment) to reduce future rates. Cancer. 2010;**116**:544-573. DOI: 10.1002/cncr.24760

[3] Center MM, Jemal A, Ward E. International trends in colorectal cancer incidence rates. Cancer Epidemiology Biomarkers & Prevention. 2009;**18**:1688-1694. DOI: 10.1158/1055-9965.EPI-09-0090

[4] Ministério da Saúde. Estimativa 2016: Incidência de Câncer no Brasil. Instituto Nacional de Câncer José Alencar Gomes da Silva, Coordenação de Prevenção e Vigilância. Rio de Janeiro: INCA; 2015

[5] Atkin WS, Edwards R, Kralj-Hans I, et al. Once-only flexible sigmoidoscopy screening in prevention of colorectal cancer: A multicentre randomised controlled trial. Lancet. 2010;**375**:1624-1633. DOI: 10.1016/S0140-6736(10)60551-X

[6] Schoen RE, Pinsky PF, Weissfeld JL, et al. Colorectal-cancer incidence and mortality with screening flexible sigmoidoscopy. The New England Journal of Medicine. 2012;**366**: 2345-2357. DOI: 10.1056/NEJMoa1114635

[7] de Jong AE, Hendriks YM, Kleibeuker JH, et al. Decrease in mortality in Lynch syndrome families because of surveillance. Gastroenterology. 2006;**130**:665-671. DOI: 10.1053/j.gastro.2005.11.032

[8] Levin B, Lieberman DA, McFarland B, et al. Screening and surveillance for the early detection of colorectal cancer and adenomatous polyps, 2008: A joint guideline from the American Cancer Society, the US Multi-Society Task Force on Colorectal Cancer, and the American College of Radiology. Gastroenterology. 2008;**134**:1570-1595. DOI: 10.1053/j.gastro.2008.02.002

[9] Vogelstein B, Fearon ER, Hamilton SR, et al. Genetic alterations during colorectal-tumor development. The New England Journal of Medicine. 1988;**319**:525-532. DOI: 10.1056/NEJM198809013190901

[10] Lengauer C, Kinzler KW, Vogelstein B. Genetic instabilities in human cancers. Nature. 1998;**396**:643-649. DOI: 10.1038/25292

[11] Cunningham JM, Christensen ER, Tester DJ, et al. Hypermethylation of the hMLH1 promoter in colon cancer with microsatellite instability. Cancer Research. 1998;**58**:3455-3460

[12] Noffsinger AE. Serrated polyps and colorectal cancer: New pathway to malignancy. Annual Review of Pathology. 2009;**4**:343-364. DOI: 10.1146/annurev.pathol.4.110807.092317

[13] Cunningham D, Atkin W, Lenz HJ, et al. Colorectal cancer. Lancet. 2010;**375**:1030-1047. DOI: 10.1016/S0140-6736(10)60353-4

[14] Cannon-Albright LA, Skolnick MH, Bishop DT, Lee RG, Burt RW. Common inheritance of susceptibility to colonic adenomatous polyps and associated colorectal cancers. The New England Journal of Medicine. 1988;**319**:533-537. DOI: 10.1056/NEJM198809013190902

[15] Aaltonen L, Johns L, Jarvinen H, Mecklin JP, Houlston R. Explaining the familial colorectal cancer risk associated with mismatch repair (MMR)-deficient and MMR-stable tumors. Clinical Cancer Research. 2007;**13**:356-361. DOI: 10.1158/1078-0432.CCR-06-1256

[16] Aaltonen LA, Salovaara R, Kristo P, et al. Incidence of hereditary nonpolyposis colorectal cancer and the feasibility of molecular screening for the disease. The New England Journal of Medicine. 1998;**338**:1481-1487. DOI: 10.1056/NEJM199805213382101

[17] Tomlinson IP, Dunlop M, Campbell H, et al. COGENT (COlorectal cancer GENeTics): An international consortium to study the role of polymorphic variation on the risk of colorectal cancer. British Journal of Cancer. 2010;**102**:447-454. DOI: 10.1038/sj.bjc.6605338

[18] St John DJ, McDermott FT, Hopper JL, Debney EA, Johnson WR, Hughes ES. Cancer risk in relatives of patients with common colorectal cancer. Annals of Internal Medicine. 1993;**118**:785-790. DOI: 10.7326/0003-4819-118-10-199305150-00005

[19] Sachidanandam R, Weissman D, Schmidt SC, et al. A map of human genome sequence variation containing 1.42 million single nucleotide polymorphisms. Nature. 2001;**409**:928-933. DOI: 10.1038/35057149

[20] Strachan T, Read A. Human genetic variability and its consequences. In Human Molecular Genetics. 4th ed. New York: Garland Science; 2011. pp. 405-440

[21] Visscher PM, Brown MA, McCarthy MI, Yang J. Five years of GWAS discovery. American Journal of Human Genetics. 2012;**90**:7-24. DOI: 10.1016/j.ajhg.2011.11.029

[22] International HapMap Consortium. A haplotype map of the human genome. Nature. 2005;**437**:1299-1320. DOI: 10.1038/nature04226

[23] Dickson SP, Wang K, Krantz I, et al. Rare variants create synthetic genome-wide associations. PLoS Biology. 2010;**8**:e1000294. DOI: 10.1371/journal.pbio.1000294

[24] Zanke BW, Greenwood CM, Rangrej J, et al. Genome-wide association scan identifies a colorectal cancer susceptibility locus on chromosome 8q24. Nature Genetics. 2007;**39**:989-994. DOI: 10.1038/ng2089

[25] Tomlinson I, Webb E, Carvajal-Carmona L, et al. A genome-wide association scan of tag SNPs identifies a susceptibility variant for colorectal cancer at 8q24.21. Nature Genetics. 2007;**39**:984-988. DOI: 10.1038/ng2085

[26] Haiman CA, Le Marchand L, Yamamato J, et al. A common genetic risk factor for colorectal and prostate cancer. Nature Genetics. 2007;**39**:954-956. DOI: 10.1038/ng2098

[27] Broderick P, Carvajal-Carmona L, Pittman AM, et al. A genome-wide association study shows that common alleles of SMAD7 influence colorectal cancer risk. Nature Genetics. 2007;**39**:1315-1317. DOI: 10.1038/ng.2007.18

[28] Jaeger E, Webb E, Howarth K, et al. Common genetic variants at the CRAC1 (HMPS) locus on chromosome 15q13.3 influence colorectal cancer risk. Nature Genetics. 2008;**40**:26-28. DOI: 10.1038/ng.2007.41

[29] Tenesa A, Farrington SM, Prendergast JG, et al. Genome-wide association scan identifies a colorectal cancer susceptibility locus on 11q23 and replicates risk loci at 8q24 and 18q21. Nature Genetics. 2008;**40**:631-637. DOI: 10.1038/ng.133

[30] Tomlinson IP, Webb E, Carvajal-Carmona L, et al. A genome-wide association study identifies colorectal cancer susceptibility loci on chromosomes 10p14 and 8q23.3. Nature Genetics. 2008;**40**:623-630. DOI: 10.1038/ng.111

[31] Houlston RS, Webb E, Broderick P, et al. Meta-analysis of genome-wide association data identifies four new susceptibility loci for colorectal cancer. Nature Genetics. 2008;**40**:1426-1435. DOI: 10.1038/ng.262

[32] Houlston RS, Cheadle J, Dobbins SE, et al. Meta-analysis of three genome-wide association studies identifies susceptibility loci for colorectal cancer at 1q41, 3q26.2, 12q13.13 and 20q13.33. Nature Genetics. 2010;**42**:973-977. DOI: 10.1038/ng.670

[33] Dunlop MG, Dobbins SE, Farrington SM, et al. Common variation near CDKN1A, POLD3 and SHROOM2 influences colorectal cancer risk. Nature Genetics. 2012;**44**:770-776. DOI: 10.1038/ng.2293

[34] Peters U, Hutter CM, Hsu L, et al. Meta-analysis of new genome-wide association studies of colorectal cancer risk. Human Genetics. 2012;**131**:217-234. DOI: 10.1007/s00439-011-1055-0

[35] Tenesa A, Dunlop MG. New insights into the aetiology of colorectal cancer from genome-wide association studies. Nature Reviews Genetics. 2009;**10**:353-358. DOI: 10.1038/nrg2574

[36] Ehret GB, Lamparter D, Hoggart CJ, et al. A Multi-SNP locus-association method reveals a substantial fraction of the missing heritability. American Journal of Human Genetics. 2012;**91**:863-871. DOI: 10.1016/j.ajhg.2012.09.013

[37] Fletcher O, Houlston RS. Architecture of inherited susceptibility to common cancer. Nature Reviews Cancer. 2010;**10**:353-361. DOI: 10.1038/nrc2840

[38] DeFinetti program [Internet]. Available from: http://ihg2.helmholtz-muenchen.de/cgi-bin/hw/hwa2.pl [Accessed: 30 January 2013]

[39] SNP & Variation Suite™ (Version 7.6.10) [Software]. Bozeman, MT: Golden Helix, Inc. Available from: http://www.goldenhelix.com [Accessed: 30 January 2013]

[40] Pena SD, Di Pietro G, Fuchshuber-Moraes M, et al. The genomic ancestry of individuals from different geographical regions of Brazil is more uniform than expected. PLoS One. 2011;**6**:e17063. DOI: 10.1371/journal.pone.0017063

Chapter 4

Osteopontin (OPN) Gene Polymorphisms and Autoimmune Diseases

Beata Kaleta

Additional information is available at the end of the chapter

http://dx.doi.org/10.5772/intechopen.69528

Abstract

Osteopontin (OPN) is a pleiotropic protein, important in bone remodeling and immune system signaling. OPN is synthesized in a variety of cells and tissues. It can be found not only in bone cells but also in immune cells (B and T lymphocytes, natural killer (NK) cells, natural killer T (NKT) cells, macrophages, neutrophils, and dendritic cells). OPN regulates T-helper 1/T-helper 2 (Th1/Th2) balance, stimulates B cells to antibodies production, regulates macrophages and neutrophils function, and activates dendritic cells. A number of factors, including hormones, cytokines, and polymorphisms of promoter region of *OPN* gene, regulate protein expression. OPN and variants of the *OPN* gene have been associated with the pathogenesis of multiple disorders, including systemic lupus erythematosus, multiple sclerosis, rheumatoid arthritis, systemic sclerosis, inflammatory bowel diseases, asthma, type 1 diabetes, and many other. However, some studies gave different or inconclusive results. Thus, the role of *OPN* polymorphic variants in autoimmune diseases needs to be better defined and explored as a diagnostic and therapeutic target to monitor and treat immune-mediated conditions.

Keywords: asthma, autoimmune, gene, immunomodulation, inflammatory bowel diseases, multiple sclerosis, osteopontin, polymorphism, rheumatoid arthritis, sarcoidosis, systemic lupus erythematosus, systemic sclerosis, type 1 diabetes

1. Introduction

There are more than 200 genetic loci that have been associated with one or more disorders. Today, at least 90 autoimmune diseases have been identified [1]. The etiology of autoimmune diseases is not fully elucidated; however, the causes are likely based on a combination of environmental and genetic factors, which lead to immunological abnormalities [2, 3]. Recent genome-wide association studies (GWAS) and single-nucleotide polymorphism (SNP) arrays have allowed the identification of several genetic variants associated with immune-mediated disorders. Genetic polymorphisms can influence the susceptibility, clinical manifestations, as well as response to therapy [4, 5].

A wide spectrum of inflammatory and immune mediators is currently under investigation in the context of autoimmune diseases. One of them is osteopontin (OPN), also known as early T lymphocyte activation-1 (Eta-1) or secreted phosphoprotein 1 (SPP-1). OPN is a member of the small integrin-binding ligand N-linked glycoprotein (SIBLING) family proteins [6, 7]. OPN was identified in 1986 as a major sialoprotein of bone [8], where is involved in many biological processes, such as biomineralization and remodeling [9]. OPN is synthesized in a variety of cells and tissues. It can be found in bone cells, immune cells (B and T lymphocytes, natural killer (NK) cells, natural killer T (NKT) cells, macrophages, neutrophils, dendritic cells), breast epithelial cells, neurons, Kupffer cells, hepatic macrophages, hepatic stellate cells (HSCs), lung cells, adipocytes, and many other [10]. OPN is a pleiotropic protein and its functions are linked to various physiological processes and pathological conditions. OPN, secreted by osteoblasts, osteoclasts, and osteocytes, is important in mineralization and bone resorption [9]. Recently, this protein was found to be relevant in regulation of immunity and inflammation, angiogenesis, oncogenesis, cancer progression, and apoptosis [10–12]. OPN interacts with most cells using two binding domains. Signaling via integrins ($\alpha v\beta 1$, $\alpha v\beta 3$, $\alpha v\beta 5$, $\alpha v\beta 6$, $\alpha 8\beta 1$, $\alpha 5\beta 1$, $\alpha 9\beta 1$, $\alpha 4\beta 1$, and $\alpha 4\beta 7$) modulates the phosphorylation of kinases, which are involved in nuclear factor-kappa B (NF-κB) activation and regulation of cytokines production [13–16]. Moreover, OPN is an extracellular ligand for CD44 receptors. Signaling through CD44 modulates T cell chemotaxis, fibroblast adhesion, and interleukin (IL)-10 gene expression in macrophages [17]. OPN expression and function are influenced by post-translational modifications (phosphorylation, O-linked glycosylation, sialylation, tyrosine sulfation), hormones (calcitriol, retinoid acid, steroids), pro-inflammatory cytokines, growth and differentiation factors (epidermal growth factor, platelet-derived growth factor, transforming growth factor beta), and genetic polymorphisms of its promoter [18].

2. Osteopontin gene—structure and polymorphism

The human OPN gene (*OPN*) is mapped on the long arm of chromosome 4 (4q21-4q25). *OPN* contains seven exons (protein-coding regions) and six introns. The gene spans ~9 kb. The open reading frame (ORF) consists of 942 nucleotides from the start codon (in exon 2) to the stop codon (in exon 7) [19]. The 5′-untranslated (5′-UTR) region, of 67 bases, contains exon 1, which starts with transcription start site AGC (also referred to as the GCC box). The 3′-UTR region, of 415 bases, consists of the last part of exon 7 and includes three polyadenylation signals (AATAA). Exons 2–7 contain coding sequences: signal peptide and two first amino acids (exon 2), two Ser-Ser-Glu-Glu phosphorylation sequences (exons 3 and 5), two trans-glutaminase-reactive glutamine residues (exon 4), and aspartic acid-rich sequence (exon 6). Exon 7 encodes about half of the protein and contains the RGD motif and the central thrombin cleavage site [20].

OPN is highly polymorphic. Several polymorphisms in the human OPN gene have been identified. Single-nucleotide polymorphisms (SNPs) have been proposed as a tool for identifying genes associated with multiple autoimmune disorders. Polymorphisms in a human *OPN* have been reported to exhibit functional implications and have been evaluated in several conditions. Genetic association studies have suggested that some *OPN* SNPs may serve as a potential marker to predict immune-mediated diseases in some populations.

3. Osteopontin gene polymorphism and autoimmune diseases

3.1. Systemic lupus erythematosus

Systemic lupus erythematosus (SLE) is a chronic multisystemic autoimmune disease. SLE is caused by environmental, hormonal, and genetic factors, which lead to immunological dysfunction [21, 22]. Deregulation of B and T lymphocytes activation leads to abnormalities in cytokine expression and production of autoantibodies, which form complexes with antigens. Complexes are deposited in organs and cause inflammation and tissue damage [23, 24]. Deregulation in cytokine expression is also a cause of tissue injury [25]. OPN promotes activation of T lymphocytes and regulates the T-helper 1/T-helper 2 (Th1/Th2) balance. OPN upregulates IL-12 production and downregulates IL-10 [26]. Recent findings revealed that OPN enhances interferon (IFN)-α expression through the interferon regulatory factor 7 (IRF7) activation upon toll-like receptor (TLR)9 stimulation in plasmacytoid dendritic cells (pDCs) [27] and stimulates antibodies production by B lymphocytes [26, 28]. In addition, it has been demonstrated that OPN enhances IL-17 producing Th17 cell responses [29, 30]. Thus, OPN plays an important role in regulating inflammation and immunity. Therefore, several studies have been performed to assess the association of OPN and predisposition to SLE.

In the literature, there are reports suggesting that OPN participates in the pathogenesis of SLE. It has been demonstrated that serum OPN level is elevated in SLE patients [31–36]. Moreover, OPN level correlates positively with disease activity index [33–35]. Polymorphic *OPN* alleles have been implicated in the mouse model of lupus [37]. The association between OPN gene polymorphisms and SLE susceptibility in humans has also been investigated.

In 2002, a study of Forton et al. [38] showed that polymorphic T allele of the polymorphism at position 707 in exon 7 (707C/T, rs1126616) is associated with opportunistic infections and renal insufficiency but is protective for avascular necrosis in Caucasian SLE patients. This was the first demonstration of a phenotypic association with an *OPN* polymorphism.

In a study of D'Alfonso et al. [39], a total of 13 SNPs in OPN gene were identified (six in the 5′ flanking region, one in intron 3, three in exons 6, 7 and three in the 3′-UTR). Two polymorphisms: −156G/GG (rs7687316, in promoter) and +1239A/C (rs9138, in 3′-UTR) were significantly associated with SLE. The −156G and +1239C alleles were more frequent in SLE patients than in the control group. In addition, significant association was seen between lymphadenopathy and −156 genotypes. Significantly increased OPN serum level was detected in healthy individuals carrying +1239C.

In 2007, Xu et al. [40] demonstrated that SNP at position 9250 in exon 7 of the *OPN* gene (9250C/T) exists in the Chinese Han ethnic population and is associated with SLE. The frequency of TT genotype was lower and the frequency of TC genotype was higher in SLE patients than in controls. When authors separated patients and controls into women and men, significant differences of frequencies were noted in TT genotype, TC genotype and allele in women, but not in men. Moreover, the TT genotype was lower in SLE patients with lupus nephritis (LN) [41].

In a large study of SLE patients, Han et al. [42] reported that minor alleles of rs1126616 and rs9138 (T and C, respectively) were correlated with higher risk of SLE in European-American and African-American populations (in males, not in females). In addition, haplotype analysis identified rs1126616T-rs1126772A-rs9138C which demonstrated association with SLE in general, especially in males. It was the first description of a gender-specific human lupus genetic association.

In another study, Trivedi et al. [43] genotyped the rs11730582, rs28357094, rs6532040, and rs9138 SNPs in the *OPN* gene in SLE patients. The group proved that photosensitivity was associated with the risk allele rs9138C. In addition, the study demonstrated that the C allele of rs11730582 polymorphism is associated with thrombocytopenia and hemolytic anemia.

Kariuki et al. [44] revealed an association of the rs9138C allele with higher levels of OPN and INF-α in male SLE patients. Moreover, two SNPs, rs11730582 and rs28357094, were associated with the presence of anti-ribonucleoprotein (anti-RNP) autoantibodies.

Salimi and colleagues [36] genotyped the rs1126616 SNP in SLE patients and age, gender, and ethnically matched controls. There was no association between the polymorphism and SLE susceptibility. However, the frequency of CT and TT genotypes was higher in SLE patients with LN than in those without LN. In addition, no correlation between OPN serum levels and rs1126616 polymorphism has been found.

In conclusion, a number of studies demonstrated that some *OPN* polymorphic variants are associated with SLE susceptibility and/or clinical manifestations of the disease in humans. However, some studies gave different or inconclusive results. Reasons for such divergences may be low statistical power or clinical variety. Only few studies evaluated the correlation coefficient between *OPN* polymorphisms and SLE. Moreover, limited clinical data were provided.

3.2. Multiple sclerosis

Multiple sclerosis (MS) is an autoimmune disease affecting the central nervous system (CNS) with the basic pathological hallmark of inflammatory demyelination in the white matter and cortex, implying a disturbance of the symbiotic relationship of the axon and myelin sheath [45]. Infiltrating $CD4^+$ Th1 cells, which produce IFN-γ, and $CD4^+$ Th17, which produce IL-17, has been shown to be involved in pathogenesis of MS. In addition, activated monocytes and B cells are present in the CNS, which results in degradation of the myelin sheath surrounding nerves [45, 46]. For MS development, both genetic predisposition and environmental factors are responsible [47]. OPN, a pleiotropic cytokine, plays an important role in immune-mediated disorders. OPN may influence development of MS through enhancing the pro-inflammatory Th1 and Th17 cell responses and inhibiting the anti-inflammatory Th2 cell responses [11, 29].

In the literature, there are reports suggesting that OPN participates in the pathogenesis of MS. OPN was identified as one of the disease-specific markers in plaques from brains of patients with MS [48]. In addition, it has been demonstrated that this protein is expressed higher in blood and CNS in MS patients than in healthy controls [49]. Moreover, OPN level correlated positively with disease activity and relapse rate [50–53]. However, there are studies which showed that higher OPN serum level in MS patients is not associated with disease severity [54, 55].

A large body of data indicates that *OPN* gene variants have an impact on MS pathogenesis and progression.

In a study of Niino et al. [56], three SNPs in the *OPN* gene (8090 in a coding region of exon 6, 9250 in a coding region of exon 7, and 9583 in the 3′-UTR region of exon 7) were analyzed in Japanese MS patients and healthy controls. It has been demonstrated that the CC genotype at the 8090th position was more prevalent in MS than in the control group. For the 9583rd position polymorphism, patients with GG genotype showed a later disease onset than GA and AA genotypes. However, there were no significant correlations between *OPN* variants and disease progression. These results suggest that the 8090th polymorphism might be associated with susceptibility to MS, whereas the 9583rd polymorphism with age of onset of MS.

In another study, Caillier and colleagues [57] investigated whether four SNPs (327T/C, 795C/T, 1128A/G, and 1284A/C) in the *OPN* gene were correlated with susceptibility to MS or clinical manifestations in a group of MS patients. As a result of the strong disequilibrium observed between SNPs within the OPN locus, only two SNPs were selected to study potential genotype-phenotype correlations: 1284A/C and 327T/C. No evidence of genetic association between the *OPN* polymorphisms and MS susceptibility has been observed. However, a modest trend for association with disease course was detected in patients carrying at least one wild-type 1284A allele. Patients with this allele/genotype were less likely to have a mild disease course and were at increased risk for a secondary progressive clinical type.

Similar to study of Caillier et al., no evidence of association between *OPN* variants and MS susceptibility and severity was observed in a study of Hensiek et al. [58].

Chiocchetti et al. [59, 60] identified four SNPs in the *OPN* gene: +282T/C(rs4754), +750C/T (rs11226616), +1083A/G (rs1126772), and +1239A/C(rs9138) in 3′ UTR, which form three haplotypes: A (282T-750C-1083A-1239A), B (282C-750T-1083A-1239C), and C (282C-750T-1083G-1239C). The group demonstrated that haplotype A homozygotes showed lower risk of developing MS and lower OPN serum levels than haplotype B or C carriers. In the next study, analysis was extended to a gene polymorphism at the 5′ end on the −156G/GG SNP and replicated previous findings at the 3′ end on the +1239A/C SNP. It has been demonstrated that +1239A/C SNP was associated with MS development. +1239A and −156/GG homozygosity was associated with slower disease progression. Moreover, patients homozygous for +1239A showed lower relapse rate than those carrying +1239C [61].

Most of the results indicate that OPN and its gene SNPs might be a good marker for the susceptibility to and severity of MS. Despite this, further studies are needed to improve our understanding of the *OPN* gene role in disease pathogenesis.

3.3. Rheumatoid arthritis

Rheumatoid arthritis (RA) is a chronic inflammatory disease that affects joints, connective tissues, muscle, tendons, and fibrous tissue [62]. In RA, immune cells (monocytes, macrophages, B cells, $CD4^+$ and $CD8^+$ T cells, neutrophils) infiltrate the synovial fluid. Activation of T cells leads to the production of pro-inflammatory cytokines. Humoral adaptive immunity is also integral to RA. B cells are activated through interactions with T cells and through soluble cytokines that enhance their proliferation and differentiation. Mature B cells (plasma cells) are a source of autoantibodies (known as rheumatoid factors and anti-citrullinated peptide antibodies, ACPA). Synovial macrophages produce pro-inflammatory cytokines, including tumor necrosis factor (TNF), IL-1, IL-6, IL-8, and granulocyte-macrophage colony-stimulating factor (GMCSF). Neutrophils in the synovial fluid are in an activated state, releasing oxygen-derived free radicals that promote joints damage [63]. Gene-environment interactions appear as the most plausible underlying cause of RA.

A wide spectrum of immune mediators is currently under investigation in the context of RA pathogenesis and progression. One of them is OPN. This protein has been found to be elevated in plasma and synovial fluid of RA patients as well as in peripheral blood mononuclear cells (PBMCs) and synovial fluid mononuclear cells [64–66]. High OPN level has been correlated with serum C-reactive protein (CRP) level and inflammation markers [67]. It has been demonstrated that OPN concentration is higher during disease progression. Moreover, OPN correlates with bone resorption markers [68]. To support the role of OPN in RA, several studies have been conducted to investigate the role of *OPN* gene variants in disease pathogenesis and progression.

In 2005, Urcelay et al. [69] studied the association of four *OPN* SNPs (327T/C in the coding region of exon 6, 795C/T in the coding region of exon 7, 1128A/G, and 1284A/C in the 3′-UTR) and predisposition to RA in a Spanish population. Analysis of the haplotypes defined by these SNPs did not identify association with RA.

In another study, Xu and colleagues [66] investigated whether genetic polymorphisms of the *OPN* gene were associated with susceptibility to RA in Chinese Han nationality. Analysis revealed a total of 14 SNPs. Finally, six SNPs were selected for analysis (two newly identified SNPs in the promoter region: −631G/T and −458T/C and four in exons: rs4754, rs1126616, rs1126772, rs9138). Similarly to a study of Urcelay et al., prevalence of OPN genotype and allele frequencies did not differ significantly between RA patients and healthy controls.

For the first time, the association between *OPN* gene polymorphism and RA susceptibility was demonstrated in a study of Ceccarelli et al. [70] in an Italian cohort. A statistically significant association between RA and OPN −156G/GG (rs7687316) was found. There was no association of +1239A/C (rs9138) polymorphism and RA.

In 2013, Gazal et al. [71] evaluated the contribution of the OPN rs11439060 (−156-/G) and rs9138 (1239A/C) SNPs in a large cohort of RA patients and controls. The group reported a significant contribution of the combination of the rs11439060 and rs9138 frequent alleles to risk of RA, especially in ACPA-negative patients. In the next study of this group, it has been demonstrated that rs9138 variants contribute to joint damage progression in ACPA-negative patients [72].

OPN is relatively a newly identified RA susceptibility gene. Data about the role of *OPN* variants in disease pathogenesis are very scanty and contradictory. Therefore, more studies are necessary for further elucidation of *OPN* polymorphism role in RA.

3.4. Systemic sclerosis

Systemic sclerosis (SSc) is an immune-mediated connective tissue disorder, characterized by an overproduction of collagen, immune dysfunction, and blood vessel damage [73]. Multiple organ damage is a consequence of this disease [74]. Immunological abnormalities of innate and adaptive immune system, including mononuclear cell infiltration of affected tissues, deregulation of cytokines (transforming growth factor beta [TGFβ], TNFα, IL-6, IL-10, IL-17, IL-4, IL-13) and chemokines (CCL18, CCL19, CXCL13, CCL2, CCL3, CXCL4, CCR1, CCR2, CCR3) synthesis, and autoantibodies production, have long been recognized in SSc [75].

Despite intense research, the pathogenesis of SSc is only partly understood, but it likely involves an interaction between environmental factors in a genetic predisposing background [76].

OPN, plays an important role during both acute and chronic inflammation. In the literature, there are reports suggesting that this protein participates in the pathogenesis of SSc. OPN has a chemotactic and pro-fibrotic properties [77, 78]. Moreover, enhances the pro-inflammatory Th1 cell response, which is believed to be crucial in SSc pathogenesis. It has been demonstrated that mice with OPN overexpression have higher levels of anti-DNA autoantibodies, as well as increased gamma globulins [26]. This protein has been found to be elevated in plasma in SSc patients [79–81]. In addition, high OPN level was found to be correlated with serum CRP level [79].

The association between *OPN* gene polymorphisms and SSc susceptibility in humans has been investigated in a study of Barizzone et al. [82]. The group analyzed the association of two *OPN* SNPs: −156G/GG and +1239A/C and serum level of OPN in Italian SSc patients and controls. In SSc patients, there was a significantly increased frequency of the alleles −156G and +1239C, compared with controls. Moreover, OPN serum levels were significantly higher in SSc patients. However, no association between OPN levels and +1239 or −156 genotypes was observed.

These few data suggest that *OPN* genetic variations may have a role in SSc susceptibility, but further studies are needed to confirm these findings.

3.5. Inflammatory bowel diseases

Inflammatory bowel diseases (IBDs), especially Crohn's disease (CD) and ulcerative colitis (UC), are idiopathic, multifactorial disorders, characterized by chronic intestinal inflammation [83]. CD is a transmural and segmental inflammatory disease. It may affect any part of the gastrointestinal tract, from the mouth to the anus, but is located usually in the terminal ileum.

It is characterized by the formation of ulcers, fistulas, stenosis, and intestinal granulomas, with periods of aggravation and remission. UC can affect only the mucosa of the colon and the rectum [84]. The etiology of IBDs is not fully elucidated. However, available evidence suggests that an abnormal immune response against the microorganisms of the intestinal flora is responsible for the disease in genetically susceptible individuals [85]. CD is characterized as a Th1 directed disease, with elevated $CD4^+$ T-cell synthesis of IFN-γ and high TNF-α and IL-12 production by activated macrophages. UC is associated with incorrect Th2 response mediated by NKT cells, which secrete IL-13 [86].

In the literature, there are reports suggesting that OPN, as an immunomodulator, participates in the pathogenesis of IBDs in animal models and in humans. It has been demonstrated that serum OPN level is elevated in IBD patients and correlates with disease activity [87–91]. However, some studies in humans and in animal models of colitis gave opposite results, suggesting a dual or protective function of OPN in intestinal inflammation [86, 91–99].

The association between *OPN* gene polymorphisms and IBD susceptibility in humans has also been investigated. In a study of Glas et al. [100], 9 *OPN* SNPs (rs2728127, rs2853744, rs11730582, rs11739060, rs28357094, rs4754=p.Asp80Asp, rs1126616=p.Ala236Ala, rs1126772, and rs9138) were analyzed in a large group of Caucasian individuals (841 patients with CD, 473 patients with UC, and 1505 healthy unrelated controls). For rs4754, rs1126616, rs1126772, and rs9138, significantly different distributions between male and female CD patients were observed (rs4754 was protective in male patients). None of the other investigated *OPN* SNPs was associated with CD or UC susceptibility. However, several haplotypes demonstrated significant associations with CD susceptibility. The strongest association was found for a haplotype rs2728127-rs2853744-rs11730582-rs11439060-rs28357094-rs112661-rs1126772-rs9138. Moreover, no correlation was found between SNPs and IL-22 serum levels. The results argue against a major role for *OPN* gene polymorphism in the IBDs susceptibility. However, further analysis is required to clarify the role of *OPN* variants in the pathogenesis of the disease.

3.6. Type 1 diabetes

Type 1 diabetes (T1D) is a chronic, immune-mediated metabolic disorder of childhood and adolescence. T1D develops as a result of an autoimmune process, leading to β-cell destruction [101]. Activated NK cells, DCs, macrophages, and T-cells are attracted to the islets, which is followed by production of pro-inflammatory cytokines and free radicals, causing β-cell dysfunction and apoptosis [101, 102].

OPN plays an essential role in the regulation of immune cell response. It has been demonstrated that OPN induces adipose tissue inflammation, upregulates pro-inflammatory cytokines, and stimulates B lymphocytes to antibodies production. Consequently, OPN promotes the destruction of pancreatic β-cell and development of T1D [10, 103]. Therefore, several studies have been performed to assess the association of OPN and predisposition to T1D. This protein has been found to be elevated in pediatric and adult patients with T1D [104–106]. Moreover, OPN has correlated with some clinical and biochemical parameters in T1D patients, including higher body mass index (BMI), systolic blood pressure (SBP), diastolic blood pressure (DBP), lower high-density lipoprotein (HDL), and microalbuminuria [104, 107]. In addition, OPN has been found to be an independent predictor of diabetic retinopathy and nephropathy [107].

The *OPN* encoding gene can be considered as a candidate for genetic susceptibility to T1D. Several studies have been conducted to investigate the role of *OPN* polymorphisms in disease pathogenesis. In 2009, Marciano et al. [108] genotyped T1D patients and controls for three OPN SNPs: −156G/GG, −66T/G (in promoter) and biallelic ins/del variant TG/TGTG at +245 in the first intron. It has been demonstrated that the G allele at −66 SNP had higher frequency in controls than in patients. The association has been confirmed in females but not in males.

In another study, Chiocchietti and colleagues [109] evaluated the role of +1239A/C SNP in a 3′-UTR of *OPN* gene in an Italian T1D patients and controls. The analysis revealed that C allele carriers displayed higher risk of T1D than A allele carriers. The group suggested that this SNP is associated with T1D development.

In 2013, a study of Karamizadeh et al. [105] showed that rs1126772 SNP is not associated with T1D children, although serum OPN levels were significantly higher in diabetic patients than in controls.

The results from these studies are inconclusive; thus, more research is necessary for further elucidation of *OPN* polymorphism role in T1D.

3.7. Asthma

Asthma is the most common chronic lung disease. It is characterized by airway inflammation and respiratory symptoms, such as wheeze, shortness of breath, chest tightness, and cough [110]. Multiple immune cells are involved in the inflammatory response in asthma. Th2 cells, which produce Il-4, IL-5, and IL-13, are responsible for eosinophils accumulation in the lungs of asthmatic patients. Th17 cells release IL-17 and recruit neutrophils, which attract eosinophils indirectly. Th1 and regulatory T (Treg) lymphocytes are also involved in the development of asthma. An elevation of Th17 cells, the absence of Treg cells, and an imbalance in Treg/Th17 are associated with the disease [110–112].

Asthma is thought to be caused by a combination of genetic and environmental factors. A wide spectrum of immune mediators is currently under investigation in the context of this disorder. OPN plays an important role during inflammation and regulates function of immune cells. In the literature, there are reports suggesting that this protein participates in the pathogenesis of asthma. Several studies have demonstrated that OPN level is increased in asthmatic patients and is associated with disease phenotypes [113–116]. In addition, the chromosomal region of 4q24 (where *OPN* gene is mapped) has been associated with atopy in asthmatic patients [117]. These studies suggest that *OPN* gene may be a candidate gene for asthma susceptibility.

The case-control study of Tanino et al. [118] investigated the association of *OPN* variants with serum immunoglobulin E (IgE) levels, atopy, and asthma in a Japanese population. The group genotyped three promoters and two exon polymorphisms at *OPN* gene: −1687A/G; −381T/C;

−94 deletion/G; 5891C/T; and 7052T/C. Association analyses demonstrated that homozygotes for the 5891T allele and 7052C allele were significantly associated with increased levels of total IgE in non-asthmatic subjects. However, these variants were not associated with asthma and atopy.

Different results have been obtained in a study of Arjomandi and colleagues [119]. To determine whether SNPs in *OPN* gene are associated with risk of asthma, six SNPs (rs6812524, rs7435825, rs1126616, rs4660, rs1126772, and rs9138) have been genotyped in the Latino Americans population of 294 Mexican and 365 Puerto Rican parent-child asthma trios. Haplotype analysis identified rs1126616C-rs1126772A-rs9138A to be associated with an increased risk and severity of asthma in Puerto Rican subjects with elevated IgE. However, there was no association between the SNPs and asthma outcomes in Mexicans.

Only these two studies have been conducted to investigate the role of *OPN* gene variants in asthma pathogenesis and progression; therefore, further investigation in this field is indispensable.

3.8. Sarcoidosis

Sarcoidosis is a chronic inflammatory condition characterized by the formation of non-caseating epithelioid granulomata at various sites in the body (lungs, thorax, skin, eyes, liver, heart, and nervous and musculoskeletal system) [120]. The cause of the disease is still unknown, but several immune aberrations are thought to play a role in its pathogenesis. Studies have revealed an increase of B-cell activity with elevated plasma levels of immunoglobulins and immune-complexes in patients. In addition, inflammation in sarcoidosis is dependent on persistent stimulation by $CD4^+$ Th1 cells [120, 121]. Sarcoidosis is thought to be caused by a combination of genetic and environmental factors, but the exact etiology remains unclear. In the literature, there are reports suggesting that OPN participates in the pathogenesis of sarcoidosis. High levels of this protein have been found to be increased in serum and granulomas from patients with sarcoidosis [122–124]. Moreover, it has been demonstrated that OPN induced the chemotaxis of T cells and acted as an adhesion factor for activated T cells [123].

The *OPN* encoding gene can be considered as a candidate for susceptibility to sarcoidosis. Two studies have been conducted to investigate the role of *OPN* polymorphisms in disease pathogenesis. In 2004, Akahoshi et al. [125] investigated the 2514C/T SNP in Japanese patients with sarcoidosis and in healthy controls. The group did not find any significant association between genotypes/alleles and disease pathogenesis.

In another study, Maver and colleagues [126] genotyped three *OPN* SNPs: rs11730582, rs11728697, and rs4754 in Slovenian patients and healthy subjects. The analysis revealed a significant difference in genotype frequencies at rs4754 SNP in patients and controls. However, these results failed to reach significance after correction for multiple testing. In addition, analysis demonstrated that frequency of rs11730582T-rs11728697T-rs4754T haplotype was decreased in the group of patients compared to controls. It has been suggested that TTT haplotype of *OPN* gene is a protective factor in sarcoidosis.

These scanty studies have yielded conflicting and inconclusive results. Thus, further analyses are required to understand the role of OPN and its gene polymorphism in sarcoidosis.

4. Conclusions and future perspectives

OPN is highly expressed by various cell types, including cells of the immune system. This pleiotropic protein regulates both, innate and adaptive immune response. A large number of publications suggest that OPN participates in the pathogenesis of multiple autoimmune conditions. Moreover, there are reports suggesting the role of *OPN* gene polymorphism in the pathogenesis and/or clinical manifestations of immune-mediated diseases. However, some investigations failed to demonstrate any associations of *OPN* SNPs with autoimmune conditions. The main causes for these differences include ethnic, environmental and still unknown factors. Moreover, some studies do not meet the current rigorous standards for non-biased large-cohort trials. Future research should focus on selecting the best study groups to investigate the role of *OPN* variants in diseases pathogenesis and progression. Studies of *OPN* polymorphisms must take into account the gene-environment, gene-gene interactions, and ethnic factors.

The role of *OPN* polymorphic variants in autoimmune diseases needs to be better defined and explored as a diagnostic and therapeutic target to monitor and treat immune-mediated conditions. Advances in understanding specific SNPs in *OPN* may be helpful to create genetic profiles for predisposition to autoimmune diseases in order to adopt prevention strategies from childhood to adulthood.

Author details

Beata Kaleta

Address all correspondence to: kaletabeata1@gmail.com

Department of Clinical Immunology, Transplantation Institute, Medical University of Warsaw, Warsaw, Poland

References

[1] Ercolini A, Miller SD. The role of infections in autoimmune disease. Clinical and Experimental Immunology. 2009;**155**:1-15. DOI: 10.1111/j.1365-2249.2008.03834.x

[2] Campbell AW. Autoimmunity and the gut. Autoimmune Diseases. 2014;**2014**:152428. DOI: 10.1155/2014/152428

[3] Davidson A, Diamond B. Autoimmune diseases. The New England Journal of Medicine. 2001;**345**:340-350. DOI: 10.1056/NEJM200108023450506

[4] Costenbader KH, Gay S, Alarcón-Riquelme ME, Iaccarino L, Doria A. Genes, epigenetic regulation and environmental factors: Which is the most relevant in developing autoimmune diseases? Autoimmunity Reviews. 2012;**11**:604-609. DOI: 10.1016/j.autrev.2011.10.022

[5] Cho JH, Feldman M. Heterogeneity of autoimmune diseases: Pathophysiologic insights from genetics and implications for new therapies. Nature Medicine. 2015;**21**:730-738. DOI: 10.1038/nm.3897

[6] Fisher LW, Torchia DA, Fohr B, Young MF, Fedarko NS. Flexible structures of SIBLING proteins, bone sialoprotein, and osteopontin. Biochemical and Biophysical Research Communications. 2001;**280**:460-465. DOI: 10.1006/bbrc.2000.4146

[7] Ramaiah SK, Rittling S. Pathophysiological role of osteopontin in hepatic inflammation, toxicity, and cancer. Toxicological Sciences. 2008;**103**:4-13. DOI: 10.1093/toxsci/kfm246

[8] Oldberg A, Franzén A, Heinegård D. Cloning and sequence analysis of rat bone sialoprotein (osteopontin) cDNA reveals an Arg-Gly-Asp cell-binding sequence. Proceedings of the National Academy of Sciences of the United States of America. 1986;**83**:8819-8823

[9] Kruger TE, Miller AH, Godwin AK, Wang J. Bone sialoprotein and osteopontin in bone metastasis of osteotropic cancers. Critical Reviews in Oncology/Hematology. 2014;**89**:330-341. DOI: 10.1016/j.critrevonc.2013.08.013

[10] Denhardt DT, Guo X. Osteopontin: A protein with diverse functions. FASEB Journal. 1993;**7**:1475-1482

[11] Cantor H. The role of Eta-1/osteopontin in the pathogenesis of immunological disorders. Annals of the New York Academy of Sciences. 1995;**760**:143-150

[12] Cao DX, Li ZJ, Jiang XO, Lum YL, Khin E, Lee NP, Wu GH, Luk JM. Osteopontin as potential biomarker and therapeutic target in gastric and liver cancers. World Journal of Gastroenterology. 2012;**18**:3923-3930. DOI: 10.3748/wjg.v18.i30.3923

[13] Hu DD, Lin EC, Kovach NL, Hoyer JR, Smith JW. A biochemical characterization of the binding of osteopontin to integrins alpha v beta 1 and alpha v beta 5. The Journal of Biological Chemistry. 1995;**270**:26232-26238

[14] Green PM, Ludbrook SB, Miller DD, Horgan CM, Barry ST. Structural elements of the osteopontin SVVYGLR motif important for the interaction with alpha(4) integrins. FEBS Letters. 2001;**503**:75-79

[15] Yokosaki Y, Tanaka K, Higashikawa F, Yamashita K, Eboshida A. Distinct structural requirements for binding of the integrins alphavbeta6, alphavbeta3, alphavbeta5, alpha5beta1 and alpha9beta1 to osteopontin. Matrix Biology: Journal of the International Society for Matrix Biology. 2005;**24**:418-427. DOI: 10.1016/j.matbio.2005.05.005

[16] Urtasun R, Lopategi A, George J, Leung TM, Lu Y, Wang X, Ge X, Fiel MI, Nieto N. Osteopontin, an oxidant stress sensitive cytokine, up-regulates collagen-I via integrin $\alpha(V)\beta(3)$ engagement and PI3K/pAkt/NFκB signaling. Hepatology. 2012;**55**:594-608. DOI: 10.1002/hep.24701

[17] Weber GF, Ashkar S, Glimcher MJ, Cantor H. Receptor-ligand interaction between CD44 and osteopontin (Eta-1). Science. 1996;**271**:509-512

[18] Subraman V, Thiyagarajan M, Malathi N, Rajan ST. OPN -Revisited. Journal of Clinical and Diagnostic Research. 2015;**6**:ZE10-ZE13. DOI: 10.7860/JCDR/2015/12872.6111

[19] Hijiya N, Setoguchi M, Matsuura K, Higuchi Y, Akizuki S, Yamamoto S. Cloning and characterization of the human osteopontin gene and its promoter. The Biochemical Journal. 1994;**303**:255-262

[20] Rodrigues LR, Teixeira JA, Schmitt FL, Paulsson M, Lindmark-Mänsson H. The role of osteopontin in tumor progression and metastasis in breast cancer. Cancer Epidemiology, Biomarkers and Prevention. 2007;**16**:1087-1097. DOI: 10.1158/1055-9965.EPI-06-1008

[21] Kotzin BL. Systemic lupus erythematosus. Cell. 1996;**85**:303-306

[22] Mills JA. Systemic lupus erythematosus. The New England Journal of Medicine. 1994;**330**:1871-1879

[23] Giles BM, Boackle SA. Linking complement and anti-dsDNA antibodies in the pathogenesis of systemic lupus erythematosus. Immunology Research. 2013;**55**:10-21. DOI: 10.1007/s12026-012-8345-z

[24] Marks SD, Tullus K. Autoantibodies in systemic lupus erythematosus. Pediatric Nephrology. 2012;**27**:1855-1868. DOI: 10.1007/s00467-011-2078-4

[25] Yap DY, Lai KN. The role of cytokines in the pathogenesis of systemic lupus erythematosus - From bench to bedside. Nephrology. 2013;**18**:243-255. DOI: 10.1111/nep.12047

[26] Ashkar S, Weber GF, Panoutsakopoulou V, Sanchirico ME, Jansson M, Zawaideh S, Rittling SR, Denhardt DT, Glimcher MJ, Cantor H. Eta-1 (osteopontin): An early component of type-1 (cell-mediated) immunity. Science. 2000;**287**:860-864

[27] Shinohara ML, Lu L, Bu J, Werneck MB, Kobayashi KS, Glimcher LH, Cantor H. Osteopontin expression is essential for interferon-alpha production by plasmacytoid dendritic cells. Nature Immunology. 2006;**7**:498-506. DOI: 10.1038/ni1327

[28] Lampe MA, Patarca R, Iregui MV, Cantor H. Polyclonal B cell activation by the Eta-1 cytokine and the development of systemic autoimmune disease. Journal of Immunology. 1991;**147**:2902-2906

[29] Murugaiyan G, Mittal A, Weiner HL. Increased osteopontin expression in dendritic cells amplifies IL-17 production by CD4+ T cells in experimental autoimmune encephalomyelitis and in multiple sclerosis. Journal of Immunology. 2008;**181**:7480-7488

[30] Shinohara ML, Kim JH, Garcia VA, Cantor H. Engagement of the type I interferon receptor on dendritic cells inhibits T helper 17 cell development: Role of intracellular osteopontin. Immunity. 2008;**29**:68-78. DOI: 10.1016/j.immuni.2008.05.008

[31] Katagiri Y, Mori K, Hara T, Tanaka K, Murakami M, Uede T. Functional analysis of the osteopontin molecule. Annals of the New York Academy of Sciences. 1995;**760**:371-374

[32] Lou B, Lv J, Zheng M. The relationship between osteopontin plasma concentration and disease activity in systemic lupus erythematosus. Chinese Journal of Dermatology. 2006;**39**:320-321

[33] Wong CK, Lit LC, Tam LS, Li EK, Lam CW. Elevation of plasma osteopontin concentration is correlated with disease activity in patients with systemic lupus erythematosus. Rheumatology (Oxford). 2005;**44**:602-606. DOI: 10.1093/rheumatology/keh558

[34] Rullo OJ, Woo JM, Parsa MF, Hoftman AD, Maranian P, Elashoff DA, Niewold TB, Grossman JM, Hahn BH, McMahon M, McCurdy DK, Tsao BP. Plasma levels of osteopontin identify patients at risk for organ damage in systemic lupus erythematosus. Arthritis Research & Therapy. 2013;**15**:R18. DOI: 10.1186/ar4150

[35] Afify MF, Mohamed GB, El-Maboud MA, Abdel-Latif EA. Plasma concentration of osteopontin (OPN) in children with systemic lupus erythematosus: Relationship with disease activity. The Open Autoimmunity Journal. 2009;**1**:59-63. DOI: 10.2174/1876894600901010059

[36] Salimi S, Noora M, Nabizadeh S, Rezaei M, Shahraki H, Milad MK, Naghavi A, Farajian-Mashhadi F, Zakeri Z, Sandoughi M. Association of the osteopontin rs1126616 polymorphism and a higher serum osteopontin level with lupus nephritis. Biomedical Reports. 2016;**4**:355-360. DOI: 10.3892/br.2016.589

[37] Miyazaki T, Ono M, Qu WM, Zhang MC, Mori S, Nakatsuru S, Nakamura Y, Sawasaki T, Endo Y, Nose M. Implication of allelic polymorphism of osteopontin in the development of lupus nephritis in MRL/lpr mice. European Journal of Immunology. 2005;**35**:1510-1520. DOI: 10.1002/eji.200425672

[38] Forton AC, Petri MA, Goldman D, Sullivan KE. An osteopontin (SPP1) polymorphism is associated with systemic lupus erythematosus. Human Mutation. 2002;**19**:459. DOI: 10.1002/humu.9025

[39] D'Alfonso S, Barizzone N, Giordano M, Chiocchetti A, Magnani C, Castelli L, Indelicato M, Giacopelli F, Marchini M, Scorza R, Danieli MG, Cappelli M, Migliaresi S, Bigliardo B, Sabbadini MG, Baldissera E, Galeazzi M, Sebastiani GD, Minisola G, Ravazzolo R, Dianzani U, Momigliano-Richiardi P. Two single-nucleotide polymorphisms in the 5' and 3' ends of the osteopontin gene contribute to susceptibility to systemic lupus erythematosus. Arthritis and Rheumatism. 2005;**52**:539-547. DOI: 10.1002/art.20808

[40] Xu AP, Bai J, Lü J, Liang YY, Li JG, Lai DY, Wan X, Huang HH. Osteopontin gene polymorphism in association with systemic lupus erythematosus in Chinese patients. Chinese Medical Journal. 2007a;**120**:2124-2128

[41] Xu AP, Liang YY, Lü J, Li JG, Wang Z. Association of osteopontin gene polymorphism with lupus nephritis in Chinese Han population. Journal of Southern Medical University. 2007b;**27**:1348-1351. Chinese

[42] Han S, Guthridge JM, Harley IT, Sestak AL, Kim-Howard X, Kaufman KM, Namjou B, Deshmukh H, Bruner G, Espinoza LR, Gilkeson GS, Harley JB, James JA, Nath SK. Osteopontin and systemic lupus erythematosus association: A probable gene-gender interaction. PLoS One. 2008;**3**:e0001757. DOI: 10.1371/journal.pone.0001757

[43] Trivedi T, Franek BS, Green SL, Kariuki SN, Kumabe M, Mikolaitis RA, Jolly M, Utset TO, Niewold TB. Osteopontin alleles are associated with clinical characteristics in systemic lupus erythematosus. Journal of Biomedicine and Biotechnology. 2011;**2011**:802581. DOI: 10.1155/2011/802581

[44] Kariuki SN, Moore JG, Kirou KA, Crow MK, Utset TO, Niewold TB. Age- and gender-specific modulation of serum osteopontin and interferon-alpha by osteopontin genotype in systemic lupus erythematosus. Genes and Immunity. 2009;**10**:487-494. DOI: 10.1038/gene.2009.15

[45] Trapp BD, Nave KA. Multiple sclerosis: An immune or neurodegenerative disorder? Annual Review of Neuroscience. 2008;**31**:247-269. DOI: 10.1146/annurev.neuro.30.051606.094313

[46] Trager N, Butler JT, Haque A, Ray SK, Beeson C, Banik NL. The involvement of calpain in CD4+ T helper cell bias in multiple sclerosis. Journal of Clinical and Cellular Immunology. 2013;**4**:1000153. DOI: 10.4172/2155-9899.1000153

[47] Nylander A, Hafler DA. Multiple sclerosis. The Journal of Clinical Investigation. 2012;**122**:1180-1188. DOI: 10.1172/JCI58649

[48] Chabas D, Baranzini SE, Mitchell D, Bernard CC, Rittling SR, Denhardt DT, Sobel RA, Lock C, Karpuj M, Pedotti R, Heller R, Oksenberg JR, Steinman L. The influence of the proinflammatory cytokine, osteopontin, on autoimmune demyelinating disease. Science. 2001;**294**:1731-1735. DOI: 10.1126/science.1062960

[49] Sinclair C, Mirakhur M, Kirk J, Farrell M, McQuaid S. Up-regulation of osteopontin and alphaBeta-crystallin in the normal-appearing white matter of multiple sclerosis: An immunohistochemical study utilizing tissue microarrays. Neuropathology and Applied Neurobiology. 2005;**31**:292-303. DOI: 10.1111/j.1365-2990.2004.00638.x

[50] Comabella M, Pericot I, Goertsches R, Nos C, Castillo M, Blas Navarro J, Río J, Montalban X. Plasma osteopontin levels in multiple sclerosis. Journal of Neuroimmunology. 2005;**158**:231-239. DOI: 10.1016/j.jneuroim.2004.09.004

[51] Szalardy L, Zadori D, Simu M, Bencsik K, Vecsei L, Klivenyi P. Evaluating biomarkers of neuronal degeneration and neuroinflammation in CSF of patients with multiple sclerosis-osteopontin as a potential marker of clinical severity. Journal of Neurological Science. 2013;**331**:38-42. DOI: 10.1016/j.jns.2013.04.024

[52] Vogt MH, Floris S, Killestein J, Knol DL, Smits M, Barkhof F, Polman CH, Nagelkerken L. Osteopontin levels and increased disease activity in relapsing-remitting multiple

sclerosis patients. Journal of Neuroimmunology. 2004;**155**:155-160. DOI: 10.1016/j.jneuroim.2004.06.007

[53] Wen SR, Liu GJ, Feng RN, Gong FC, Zhong H, Duan SR, Bi S. Increased levels of IL-23 and osteopontin in serum and cerebrospinal fluid of multiple sclerosis patients. Journal of Neuroimmunology. 2012;**244**:94-96. DOI: 10.1016/j.jneuroim.2011.12.004

[54] Kivisäkk P, Healy BC, Francois K, Gandhi R, Gholipour T, Egorova S, Sevdalinova V, Quintana F, Chitnis T, Weiner HL, Khoury SJ. Evaluation of circulating osteopontin levels in an unselected cohort of patients with multiple sclerosis: Relevance for biomarker development. Multiple Sclerosis. 2014;**20**:438-444. DOI: 10.1177/1352458513503052

[55] Runia TF, van Meurs M, Nasserinejad K, Hintzen RQ. No evidence for an association of osteopontin plasma levels with disease activity in multiple sclerosis. Multiple Sclerosis. 2014;**20**:1670-1671. DOI: 10.1177/1352458514528765

[56] Niino M, Kikuchi S, Fukazawa T, Yabe I, Tashiro K. Genetic polymorphisms of osteopontin in association with multiple sclerosis in Japanese patients. Journal of Neuroimmunology. 2003;**136**:125-129

[57] Caillier S, Barcellos LF, Baranzini SE, Swerdlin A, Lincoln RR, Steinman L, Martin E, Haines JL, Pericak-Vance M, Hauser SL, Oksenberg JR. Osteopontin polymorphisms and disease course in multiple sclerosis. Genes and Immunity. 2003;**4**:312-315. DOI: 10.1038/sj.gene.6363952

[58] Hensiek AE, Roxburgh R, Meranian M, Seaman S, Yeo T, Compston DA, Sawcer SJ. Osteopontin gene and clinical severity of multiple sclerosis. Journal of Neurology. 2003;**250**:943-947. DOI: 10.1007/s00415-003-1120-2

[59] Chiocchetti A, Indelicato M, Bensi T, Mesturini R, Giordano M, Sametti S, Castelli L, Bottarel F, Mazzarino MC, Garbarini L, Giacopelli F, Valesini G, Santoro C, Dianzani I, Ramenghi U, Dianzani U. High levels of osteopontin associated with polymorphisms in its gene are a risk factor for development of autoimmunity/lymphoproliferation. Blood. 2004;**103**:1376-1382. DOI: 10.1182/blood-2003-05-1748

[60] Chiocchetti A, Comi C, Indelicato M, Castelli L, Mesturini R, Bensi T, Mazzarino MC, Giordano M, D'Alfonso S, Momigliano-Richiardi P, Liguori M, Zorzon M, Amoroso A, Trojano M, Monaco F, Leone M, Magnani C, Dianzani U. Osteopontin gene haplotypes correlate with multiple sclerosis development and progression. Journal of Neuroimmunology. 2005;**163**:172-178. DOI: 10.1016/j.jneuroim.2005.02.020

[61] Comi C, Cappellano G, Chiocchetti A, Orilieri E, Buttini S, Ghezzi L, Galimberti D, Guerini F, Barizzone N, Perla F, Leone M, D'Alfonso S, Caputo D, Scarpini E, Cantello R, Dianzani U. The impact of osteopontin gene variations on multiple sclerosis development and progression. Clinical and Developmental Immunology. 2012;**2012**:212893. DOI: 10.1155/2012/212893

[62] Carmona L, Cross M, Williams B, Lassere M, March L. Rheumatoid arthritis. Best Practice and Research: Clinical Rheumatology. 2010;**24**:733-745. DOI: 10.1016/j.berh.2010.10.001

[63] McInnes IB, Schett G. The pathogenesis of rheumatoid arthritis. The New England Journal of Medicine. 2011;**365**:2205-2219. DOI: 10.1056/NEJMra1004965

[64] Petrow PK, Hummel KM, Schedel J, Franz JK, Klein CL, Müller-Ladner U, Kriegsmann J, Chang PL, Prince CW, Gay RE, Gay S. Expression of osteopontin messenger RNA and protein in rheumatoid arthritis: Effects of osteopontin on the release of collagenase 1 from articular chondrocytes and synovial fibroblasts. Arthritis and Rheumatism. 2000;**43**:1597-1605. DOI: 10.1002/1529-0131(200007)43:7<1597::AID-ANR25>3.0.CO;2-0

[65] Shio K, Kobayashi H, Asano T, Saito R, Iwadate H, Watanabe H, Sakuma H, Segawa T, Maeda M, Ohira H. Thrombin-cleaved osteopontin is increased in urine of patients with rheumatoid arthritis. The Journal of Rheumatology. 2010;**37**:704-710. DOI: 10.3899/jrheum.090582

[66] Xu G, Sun W, He D, Wang L, Zheng W, Nie H, Ni L, Zhang D, Li N, Zhang J. Overexpression of osteopontin in rheumatoid synovial mononuclear cells is associated with joint inflammation, not with genetic polymorphism. The Journal of Rheumatology. 2005;**32**:410-416

[67] Zheng W, Li R, Pan H, He D, Xu R, Guo TB, Guo Y, Zhang JZ. Role of osteopontin in induction of monocyte chemoattractant protein 1 and macrophage inflammatory protein 1beta through the NF-kappaB and MAPK pathways in rheumatoid arthritis. Arthritis and Rheumatism. 2009;**60**:1957-1965. DOI: 10.1002/art.24625

[68] Iwadate H, Kobayashi H, Kanno T, Asano T, Saito R, Sato S, Suzuki E, Watanabe H, Ohira H. Plasma osteopontin is correlated with bone resorption markers in rheumatoid arthritis patients. International Journal of Rheumatoid Diseases. 2014;**17**:50-56. DOI: 10.1111/1756-185X.12115

[69] Urcelay E, Martínez A, Mas-Fontao A, Peris-Pertusa A, Pascual-Salcedo D, Balsa A, Fernández-Arquero M, de la Concha E. Osteopontin gene polymorphisms in Spanish patients with rheumatoid arthritis. The Journal of Rheumatology. 2005;**32**:405-409

[70] Ceccarelli F, D'Alfonso S, Perricone C, Carlomagno Y, Alessandri C, Croia C, Barizzone N, Montecucco C, Galeazzi M, Sebastiani GD, Minisola G, Fiocco U, Valesini. The role of eight polymorphisms in three candidate genes in determining the susceptibility, phenotype, and response to anti-TNF therapy in patients with rheumatoid arthritis. Clinical and Experimental Rheumatology. 2012;**30**:939-942

[71] Gazal S, Sacre K, Allanore Y, Teruel M, Goodall AH, Tohma S, Alfredsson L, Okada Y, Xie G, Constantin A, Balsa A, Kawasaki A, Nicaise P, Amos C, Rodriguez-Rodriguez L, Chiocchia G, Boileau C, Zhang J, Vittecoq O, Barnetche T, Gonzalez Gay MA, Furukawa H, Cantagrel A, Le Loët X, Sumida T, Hurtado-Nedelec M, Richez C, Chollet-Martin S, Schaeverbeke T, Combe B, Khoryati L, Coustet B, El-Benna J, Siminovitch K, Plenge R, Padyukov L, Martin J, Tsuchiya N, Dieudé P. Identification of secreted phosphoprotein 1 gene as a new rheumatoid arthritis susceptibility gene. Annals of the Rheumatic Diseases. 2015;**74**:e19. DOI: 10.1136/annrheumdis-2013-204581

[72] Juge PA, van Steenbergen HW, Constantin A, Tobon GJ, Schaeverbeke T, Gazal S, Combe B, Devauchelle-Pensec V, Nigon D, van der Helm-van Mil AH, Dieude P. SPP1

rs9138 variant contributes to the severity of radiological damage in anti-citrullinated protein autoantibody-negative rheumatoid arthritis. Annals of the Rheumatic Diseases. 2014;**73**:1840-1843. DOI: 10.1136/annrheumdis-2014-205539

[73] Ferri C, Sebastiani M, Lo Monaco A, Iudici M, Giuggioli D, Furini F, Manfredi A, Cuomo G, Spinella A, Colaci M, Govoni M, Valentini G. Systemic sclerosis evolution of disease pathomorphosis and survival. Our experience on Italian patients' population and review of the literature. Autoimmunity Reviews. 2014;**13**:1026-1034. DOI: 10.1016/j.autrev.2014.08.029

[74] Chizzolini C, Brembilla NC, Montanari E, Truchetet ME. Fibrosis and immune dysregulation in systemic sclerosis. Autoimmunity Reviews. 2011;**10**:276-281. DOI: 10.1016/j.autrev.2010.09.016

[75] Fuschiotti P. Current perspectives on the immunopathogenesis of systemic sclerosis. Immunotargets and Therapy. 2016;**5**:21-35. DOI: 10.2147/ITT.S82037

[76] Geyer M, Müller-Ladner U. The pathogenesis of systemic sclerosis revisited. Clinical Reviews in Allergy & Immunology. 2011;**40**:92-103. DOI: 10.1007/s12016-009-8193-3

[77] Collins AR, Schnee J, Wang W, Kim S, Fishbein MC, Bruemmer D, Law RE, Nicholas S, Ross RS, Hsueh WA. Osteopontin modulates angiotensin II-induced fibrosis in the intact murine heart. Journal of the American College of Cardiology. 2004;**43**:1698-1705. DOI: 10.1016/j.jacc.2003.11.058

[78] Wolak T, Kim H, Ren Y, Kim J, Vaziri ND, Nicholas SB. Osteopontin modulates angiotensin II-induced inflammation, oxidative stress, and fibrosis of the kidney. Kidney International. 2009;**76**:32-43. DOI: 10.1038/ki.2009.90

[79] Lorenzen JM, Krämer R, Meier M, Werfel T, Wichmann K, Hoeper MM, Riemekasten G, Becker MO, Haller H, Witte T. Osteopontin in the development of systemic sclerosis—Relation to disease activity and organ manifestation. Rheumatology (Oxford). 2010;**49**:1989-1991. DOI: 10.1093/rheumatology/keq223

[80] Corallo C, Volpi N, Franci D, Montella A, Biagioli M, Mariotti G, D'Onofrio F, Gonnelli S, Nuti R, Giordano N. Is osteopontin involved in cutaneous fibroblast activation? Its hypothetical role in scleroderma pathogenesis. International Journal of Immunopathology and Pharmacology. 2014;**27**:97-102

[81] Wu M, Schneider DJ, Mayes MD, Assassi S, Arnett FC, Tan FK, Blackburn MR, Agarwal SK. Osteopontin in systemic sclerosis and its role in dermal fibrosis. The Journal of Investigative Dermatology. 2012;**132**:1605-1614. DOI: 10.1038/jid.2012.32

[82] Barizzone N, Marchini M, Cappiello F, Chiocchetti A, Orilieri E, Ferrante D, Corrado L, Mellone S, Scorza R, Dianzani U, D'Alfonso S. Association of osteopontin regulatory polymorphisms with systemic sclerosis. Human Immunology. 2011;**72**:930-934. DOI: 10.1016/j.humimm.2011.06.009

[83] Baumgart DC, Sandborn WJ. Inflammatory bowel disease: Clinical aspects and established and evolving therapies. Lancet. 2007;**369**:1641-1657. DOI: 10.1016/S0140-6736(07)60751-X

[84] Sands BE. From symptom to diagnosis: Clinical distinctions among various forms of intestinal inflammation. Gastroenterology. 2004;**126**:1518-1532. DOI: 10.1053/j.gastro.2004.02.072

[85] Silva FA, Rodrigues BL, Ayrizono ML, Leal RF. The immunological basis of inflammatory bowel disease. Gastroenterology Research and Practice. 2016;**2016**:2097274. DOI: 10.1155/2016/2097274

[86] Heilmann K, Hoffmann U, Witte E, Loddenkemper C, Sina C, Schreiber S, Hayford C, Holzlöhner P, Wolk K, Tchatchou E, Moos V, Zeitz M, Sabat R, Günthert U, Wittig BM. Osteopontin as two-sided mediator of intestinal inflammation. Journal of Cellular and Molecular Medicine. 2009;**13**:1162-1174. DOI: 10.1111/j.1582-4934.2008.00428.x

[87] Gassler N, Autschbach F, Gauer S, Bohn J, Sido B, Otto HF, Geiger H, Obermüller N. Expression of osteopontin (Eta-1) in Crohn disease of the terminal ileum. Scandinavian Journal of Gastroenterology. 2002;**37**:1286-1295

[88] Masuda H, Takahashi Y, Asai S, Takayama T. Distinct gene expression of osteopontin in patients with ulcerative colitis. The Journal of Surgical Research. 2003;**111**:85-90

[89] Sato T, Nakai T, Tamura N, Okamoto S, Matsuoka K, Sakuraba A, Fukushima T, Uede T, Hibi T. Osteopontin/Eta-1 upregulated in Crohn's disease regulates the Th1 immune response. Gut. 2005;**54**:1254-1262. DOI: 10.1136/gut.2004.048298

[90] Mishima R, Takeshima F, Sawai T, Ohba K, Ohnita K, Isomoto H, Omagari K, Mizuta Y, Ozono Y, Kohno S. High plasma osteopontin levels in patients with inflammatory bowel disease. Journal of Clinical Gastroenterology. 2007;**41**:167-172. DOI: 10.1097/MCG.0b013e31802d6268

[91] Komine-Aizawa S, Masuda H, Mazaki T, Shiono M, Hayakawa S, Takayama T. Plasma osteopontin predicts inflammatory bowel disease activities. International Surgery. 2015;**100**:38-43. DOI: 10.9738/INTSURG-D-13-00160.1

[92] Agnholt J, Kelsen J, Schack L, Hvas CL, Dahlerup JF, Sørensen ES. Osteopontin, a protein with cytokine-like properties, is associated with inflammation in Crohn's disease. Scandinavian Journal of Immunology. 2007;**65**:453-460. DOI: 10.1111/j.1365-3083.2007.01908.x

[93] Tang R, Yang G, Zhang S, Wu C, Chen M. Opposite effects of interferon regulatory factor 1 and osteopontin on the apoptosis of epithelial cells induced by TNF-α in inflammatory bowel disease. Inflammatory Bowel Disease. 2014;**20**:1950-1961. DOI: 10.1097/MIB.0000000000000192

[94] Chen F, Liu H, Shen Q, Yuan S, Xu L, Cai X, Lian J, Chen SY. Osteopontin: Participation in inflammation or mucosal protection in inflammatory bowel diseases? Digestive Diseases and Sciences. 2013;**58**:1569-1580. DOI: 10.1007/s10620-012-2556-y

[95] Zhong J, Eckhardt ER, Oz HS, Bruemmer D, de Villiers WJ. Osteopontin deficiency protects mice from Dextran sodium sulfate-induced colitis. Inflammatory Bowel Diseases. 2006;**12**:790-796

[96] da Silva AP, Pollett A, Rittling SR, Denhardt DT, Sodek J, Zohar R. Exacerbated tissue destruction in DSS-induced acute colitis of OPN-null mice is associated with downregulation of TNF-alpha expression and non-programmed cell death. Journal of Cellular Physiology. 2006;**208**:629-639

[97] da Silva AP, Ellen RP, Sørensen ES, Goldberg HA, Zohar R, Sodek J. Osteopontin attenuation of dextran sulfate sodium-induced colitis in mice. Laboratory Investigation. 2009;**89**:1169-1181. DOI: 10.1038/labinvest.2009.80

[98] Toyonaga T, Nakase H, Ueno S, Matsuura M, Yoshino T, Honzawa Y, Itou A, Namba K, Minami N, Yamada S, Koshikawa Y, Uede T, Chiba T, Okazaki K. Osteopontin deficiency accelerates spontaneous colitis in mice with disrupted gut microbiota and macrophage phagocytic activity. PLoS One. 2015;**10**:e0135552. DOI: 10.1371/journal.pone.0135552

[99] Kanwar JR, Kanwar RK, Stathopoulos S, Haggarty NW, MacGibbon AK, Palmano KP, Roy K, Rowan A, Krissansen GW. Comparative activities of milk components in reversing chronic colitis. Journal of Dairy Science. 2016;**99**:2488-2501. DOI: 10.3168/jds.2015-10122

[100] Glas J, Seiderer J, Bayrle C, Wetzke M, Fries C, Tillack C, Olszak T, Beigel F, Steib C, Friedrich M, Diegelmann J, Czamara D, Brand S. The role of osteopontin (OPN/SPP1) haplotypes in the susceptibility to Crohn's disease. PLoS One. 2011;**6**:e29309. DOI: 10.1371/journal.pone.0029309

[101] Schranz DB, Lernmark A. Immunology in diabetes: An update. Diabetes/Metabolism Reviews. 1998;**14**:3-29

[102] Daneman D. Type 1 diabetes. Lancet. 2006;**367**:847-858. DOI: 10.1016/S0140-6736(06)68341-4

[103] Ahlqvist E, Osmark P, Kuulasmaa T, Pilgaard K, Omar B, Brons C, Kotova O, Zetterqvist AV, Stancakova A, Jonsson A, Hansson O, Kuusisto J, Kieffer TJ, Tuomi T, Isomaa B, Madsbad S, Gomez MF, Poulsen P, Laakso M, Degerman E, Pihlajamaki J, Wierup N, Vaag A, Groop L, Lyssenko V. Link between GIP and osteopontin in adipose tissue and insulin resistance. Diabetes. 2013;**62**:2088-2094. DOI: 10.2337/db12-0976

[104] Talat MA, Sherief LM, El-Saadany HF, Rass AA, Saleh RM, Sakr MM. The role of osteopontin in the pathogenesis and complications of type 1 diabetes mellitus in children. Journal of Clinical Research in Pediatric Endocrinology. 2016;**8**:399-404. DOI: 10.4274/jcrpe.3082

[105] Karamizadeh Z, Kamali Sarvestani E, Saki F, Karamifar H, Amirhakimi GH, Namavar Shooshtarian MH, Ashkani-Esfahani S. Investigation of osteopontin levels and genomic variation of osteopontin and its receptors in Type 1 diabetes mellitus. Journal of Endocrinological Investigation. 2013;**36**:1090-1093. DOI: 10.3275/9098

[106] Barchetta I, Alessandri C, Bertoccini L, Cimini FA, Taverniti L, Di Franco M, Fraioli A, Baroni MG, Cavallo MG. Increased circulating osteopontin levels in adult patients with type 1 diabetes mellitus and association with dysmetabolic profile. European Journal of Endocrinology. 2016;**174**:187-192. DOI: 10.1530/EJE-15-0791

[107] Gordin D, Forsblom C, Panduru NM, Thomas MC, Bjerre M, Soro-Paavonen A, Tolonen N, Sandholm N, Flyvbjerg A, Harjutsalo V, Groop PH; FinnDiane Study Group. Osteopontin is a strong predictor of incipient diabetic nephropathy, cardiovascular disease, and all-cause mortality in patients with type 1 diabetes. Diabetes Care. 2014;**37**:2593-2600. DOI: 10.2337/dc14-0065

[108] Marciano R, D'Annunzio G, Minuto N, Pasquali L, Santamaria A, Di Duca M, Ravazzolo R, Lorini R. Association of alleles at polymorphic sites in the Osteopontin encoding gene in young type 1 diabetic patients. Clinical Immunology. 2009;**131**:84-91. DOI: 10.1016/j.clim.2008.11.004

[109] Chiocchetti A, Orilieri E, Cappellano G, Barizzone N, D'Alfonso S, D'Annunzio G, Lorini R, Ravazzolo R, Cadario F, Martinetti M, Calcaterra V, Cerutti F, Bruno G, Larizza D, Dianzani U. The osteopontin gene +1239A/C single nucleotide polymorphism is associated with type 1 diabetes mellitus in the Italian population. International Journal of Immunopathology and Pharmacology. 2010;**23**:263-269

[110] Lloyd CM, Hessel EM. Functions of T cells in asthma: More than just T(H)2 cells. Nature Reviews. Immunology. 2010;**10**:838-848. DOI: 10.1038/nri2870

[111] Dunican EM, Fahy JV. The role of Type 2 inflammation in the pathogenesis of asthma exacerbations. Annals of the American Thoracic Society. 2015;12(Suppl 2):S144-S149. DOI:10.1513/AnnalsATS.201506-377AW

[112] Kay AB. The role of T lymphocytes in asthma. Chemical Immunology and Allergy. 2006;**91**:59-75. DOI: 10.1159/000090230

[113] Xanthou G, Alissafi T, Semitekolou M, Simoes DC, Economidou E, Gaga M, Lambrecht BN, Lloyd CM, Panoutsakopoulou V. Osteopontin has a crucial role in allergic airway disease through regulation of dendritic cell subsets. Nature Medicine. 2007;**13**:570-578. DOI: 10.1038/nm1580

[114] Samitas K, Zervas E, Xanthou G, Panoutsakopoulou V, Gaga M. Osteopontin is increased in the bronchoalveolar lavage fluid and bronchial tissue of smoking asthmatics. Cytokine. 2013;**61**:713-715. DOI: 10.1016/j.cyto.2012.12.028

[115] Takahashi A, Kurokawa M, Konno S, Ito K, Kon S, Ashino S, Nishimura T, Uede T, Hizawa N, Huang SK, Nishimura M. Osteopontin is involved in migration of eosinophils in asthma. Clinical and Experimental Allergy. 2009;**39**:1152-1159. DOI: 10.1111/j.1365-2222.2009.03249.x

[116] Yang AM, Huang R, Jin SJ. ORMDL3 polymorphisms and their relationship with OPN and TGF-β1 levels in children with asthma in Hunan, China: An analysis of 98 cases. Chinese Journal of Contemporary Pediatrics. 2016;**18**:324-328. Chinese

[117] Haagerup A, Bjerke T, Schøitz PO, Binderup HG, Dahl R, Kruse TA. Allergic rhinitis—A total genome-scan for susceptibility genes suggests a locus on chromosome 4q24-q27. European Journal of Human Genetics. 2001;**9**:945-952. DOI: 10.1038/sj.ejhg.5200753

[118] Tanino Y, Hizawa N, Konno S, Fukui Y, Takahashi D, Maeda Y, Huang SK, Nishimura M. Sequence variants of the secreted phosphoprotein 1 gene are associated with total serum immunoglobulin E levels in a Japanese population. Clinical and Experimental Allergy. 2006;**36**:219-225. DOI: 10.1111/j.1365-2222.2006.02414.x

[119] Arjomandi M, Galanter JM, Choudhry S, Eng C, Hu D, Beckman K, Chapela R, Rodríguez-Santana JR, Rodríguez-Cintrón W, Ford J, Avila PC, Burchard EG. Polymorphism in osteopontin gene (SPP1) is associated with asthma and related phenotypes in a Puerto Rican population. Pediatric Allergy, Immunology, and Pulmonology. 2011;**24**:207-214. DOI: 10.1089/ped.2011.0095

[120] Valeyre D, Prasse A, Nunes H, Uzunhan Y, Brillet PY, Müller-Quernheim J. Sarcoidosis. Lancet. 2014;**383**:1155-1167. DOI: 10.1016/S0140-6736(13)60680-7

[121] James DG, Neville E, Siltzbach LE. A worldwide review of sarcoidosis. Annals of the New York Academy of Sciences. 1976;**278**:321-334

[122] Carlson I, Tognazzi K, Manseau EJ, Dvorak HF, Brown LF. Osteopontin is strongly expressed by histiocytes in granulomas of diverse etiology. Laboratory Investigation. 1997;**77**:103-108

[123] O'Regan AW, Chupp GL, Lowry JA, Goetschkes M, Mulligan N, Berman JS. Osteopontin is associated with T cells in sarcoid granulomas and has T cell adhesive and cytokine-like properties in vitro. Journal of Immunology. 1999;**162**:1024-1031

[124] Maeda K, Takahashi K, Takahashi F, Tamura N, Maeda M, Kon S, Uede T, Fukuchi Y. Distinct roles of osteopontin fragments in the development of the pulmonary involvement in sarcoidosis. Lung. 2001;**179**:279-291. DOI: 10.1007/s004080000068

[125] Akahoshi M, Ishihara M, Remus N, Uno K, Miyake K, Hirota T, Nakashima K, Matsuda A, Kanda M, Enomoto T, Ohno S, Nakashima H, Casanova JL, Hopkin JM, Tamari M, Mao XQ, Shirakawa T. Association between IFNA genotype and the risk of sarcoidosis. Human Genetics. 2004;**114**:503-509. DOI: 10.1007/s00439-004-1099-5

[126] Maver A, Medica I, Salobir B, Tercelj M, Peterlin B. Genetic variation in osteopontin gene is associated with susceptibility to sarcoidosis in Slovenian population. Disease Markers. 2009;**27**:295-302. DOI: 10.3233/DMA-2009-0675

Chapter 5

Genetic Single Nucleotide Polymorphisms (GSNPs) in the DNA Repair Genes and Hepatocellular Carcinoma Related to Aflatoxin B1 among Guangxiese Population

Xue-Ming Wu, Zhi-Feng Xi, Jun Lu, Xing-Zhizi Wang, Tian-Qi Zhang, Xiao-Ying Huang, Jin-Guang Yao, Chao Wang, Zhong-Heng Wei, Chun-Ying Luo, Bing-Chen Huang, Qun-Qing Xu, Wen-Pei Yang, Qiang Xia and Xi-Dai Long

Additional information is available at the end of the chapter

http://dx.doi.org/10.5772/intechopen.69530

Abstract

Aflatoxin B1 (AFB1) is an important environmental carcinogen for the development of hepatocellular carcinoma (HCC). HCC is a complex disease likely resulting from genetic single nucleotide polymorphisms (GSNPs) of multiple interacting genes and gene-environment interactions. Recent efforts have been made to analyze the associations between risk of this malignancy and GSNPs in genes involved in the repair of DNA damage induced by AFB1. Here, we reviewed the results of published case-control studies that have examined the effects of common alleles of all susceptible DNA repair genes, including XRCC1, XRCC3, XRCC4, XRCC7, XPC, and XPD, on risk of AFB1-related HCC among Guangxi population. Statistically significant differences in genotype frequencies found in case-control comparisons were rs25487, rs80309960, rs861539, rs7003908, rs28383151, rs3734091, rs13181, and rs2228001 polymorphism. The overall effects of these GNSPs were moderate in terms of relative risk, with ORs ranging from 2 to 10. Furthermore, some evidence of the interaction of GSNPs in DNA repair genes and AFB1 exposure modulate risk of this cancer was also found, although the results require confirmation with larger sample size studies.

Keywords: genetic single nucleotide polymorphism, hepatocellular carcinoma, DNA repair, DNA damage, aflatoxin B1, Guangxiese population

1. Introduction

In China, hepatocellular carcinoma (HCC) is the fourth most common malignant tumors and accounts for about 50% of the world's HCC cases [1, 2]. This malignancy occurs more often in some hot and humid areas such as Guangxi area, mainly because of high aflatoxin B1(AFB1) exposure [3, 4]. However, accumulating epidemiological evidence has shown that although many people are exposed to this risk factor, only a relatively small proportion of people with chronic AFB1 exposure develop HCC [3, 4]. This suggests that an individual susceptibility related to genetic factors including genetic single nucleotide polymorphisms (GSNPs) in DNA repair genes might be correlated with HCC tumorigenesis [3–5]. In past several decade years, evidence has been accumulated to support the hypothesis that GSNPs in DNA repair genes may be of importance in determining individual susceptibility to AFB1-related HCC [6–8]. Here, we review recent efforts in identifying genetic single nucleotide polymorphisms (SNPs) in DNA repair genes, which may have impact on AFB1-related HCC risk among Guangxiese population.

2. Epidemiology of AFB1-related HCC among Guangxi areas

In Guangxi, a known high AFB1 exposure area, HCC is the most common occurring cancer [5]. Epidemiologically, this type tumor is characterized as follows: (*a*) the incidence rate displaying a noticeable mountain shape, gradually increasing with age increasing before shape top and gradually decreasing with age increasing after shape top and (b) more than three times risk of HCC among males than among females, especially in the high AFB1-exposure areas (including Baise and Nanning) [5]. During 1990–1992, the incidence rates of this tumor in Guangxi area increased markedly compared between the late 1970s and the early 1980s (25.22 per 100,000 vs. 15.85 per 100,000), especially male Guangxiese population (**Figure 1A**) [9]. This might result from the increasing infective rate of hepatitis viruses and advance of diagnostic ability [10]. The following epidemiological investigations showed that the incidence rate of HCC among Guangxiese population significantly markedly decrease during 2004 and 2005 (mainly because of the control of hepatitis virus infection) (**Figure 1**) [9]. However, the incident rates of this tumor in high AFB1-exposure areas have little change. According to epidemiological investigation from AFB1-exposures areas, during May 2007–April 2008, incidence rates were 103.1/100,000 and 117.8/100,000 for Fusui in Nanning and Xiangzhou in Baise (two main high AFB1 exposure areas), respectively [11]. This is similar to the results before 10 years [11].

Because of the very poor prognosis, HCC is the first most common cause of death from cancer in Guangxi [9]. In the past 40 years, the total mortality rate of HCC gradually increased and followed by gradually decreased (**Figure 1B**), regardless of male or female population. Furthermore, this trend was not only associated with age but also more noticeable in male population than female population (**Figure 2**), possibly because male individuals featured more AFB1 exposure [4]. Supporting above-mentioned hypothesis, molecular epidemiological studies from high AFB1-exposure areas of Guangxi have exhibited that these individuals featuring more AFB1 exposure would face decreasing 5-year survival rate and increasing death risk [12–14].

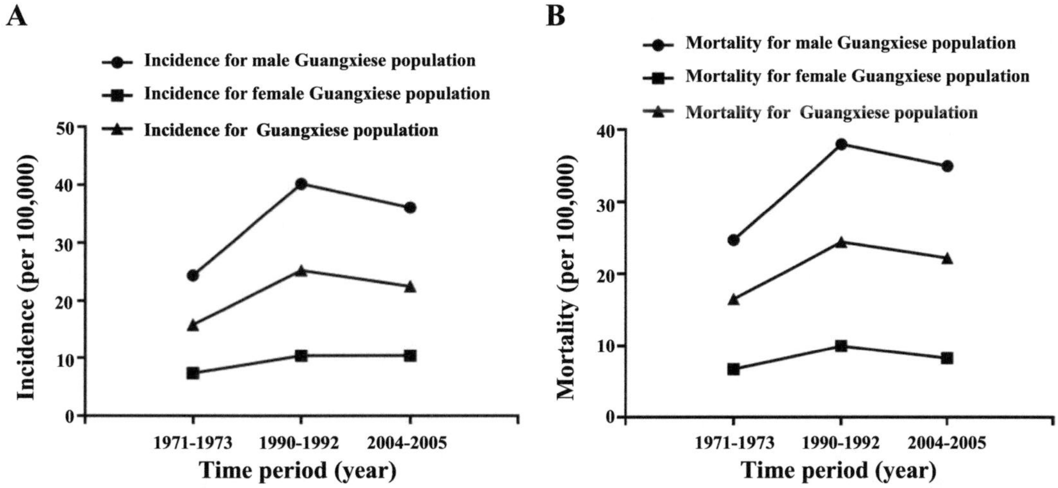

Figure 1. The incidence and mortality rates of hepatocellular carcinoma (HCC) in Guangxi during 1971 and 2005. Total incidence rate (A) and mortality rates (B), regardless of male or female population, were significantly increasing from during 1971 and 1973 to during 1990 and 1992. However, they would decrease during 2004 and 2005.

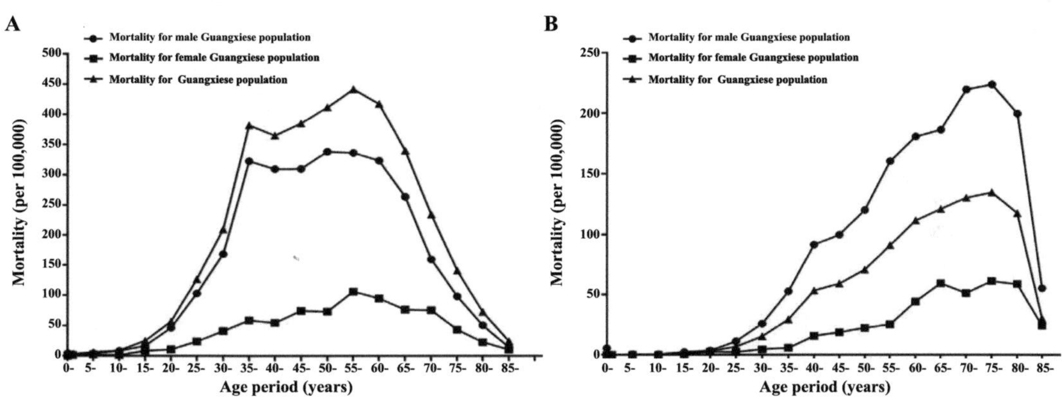

Figure 2. The gender and age distributions of hepatocellular carcinoma (HCC) mortality among Guangxiese population. (A) The gender and age distributions of HCC mortality between 1990 and 1992. (B) The gender and age distributions of HCC mortality between 2004 and 2005.

3. DNA damage induced byAFB1 and DNA repair

Several previous reviews have significantly summarized the toxicology of AFB1 [3–5, 15]. Generally, AFB1, an important mycotoxin and a category I known human carcinogen produced by *Aspergillus parasiticus* and *Aspergillus flavus* [4, 5], has been found as toxic contaminants of human food such as ground nuts and core in tropical areas as a result of fungal contamination during growth and after harvest which under hot and humid conditions [15]. Once this toxigenic agent is taken into body, it is metabolized by phase I detoxification enzymes to its reactive form, also called AFB1-8,9-epoxide (AFBO). This reactive product can also covalently bind to DNA and induce DNA damage, which might ultimately result to the development of HCC [16, 17].

AFB1-induced DNA damage types consist of DNA adducts, oxidative damage, and gene mutations. For AFB1-DNA adducts, AFB1-N^7-Gua adduct, the most common adduct type, is primarily identified and confirmed *in vivo* research studies [17–22], whereas the formamidopyridine AFB1 adduct (AFB1-FAPy) is a ring-opened DNA adduct [23, 24]. Because of the accumulations of AFB1-FAPy, it is characterized by a time-dependent and non-enzyme way and exhibits apparent persistence in DNA; it may be of biological basis of genes mutation. Furthermore, AFB1-N^7-Gua and AFB1-FAPy can induce error-prone DNA repair and result in the damage of DNA strands, including double-strand breaks (DSBs), single-strand breaks (SSBs), base pair substitution, frame shift mutations, and oxidation DNA damage such as 8-oxodeoxyguanosine (8-$_{oxyG}$) [25–28]. For genes mutations induced by AFB1 exposure, G:C > T:A mutation in codon 249 of TP53 gene has been frequently reported [29–36]. This mutation is tested in more than 40% of HCC from high-AFB1-exposure areas, but in either very rare or absent for those from low or null AFB1 exposure areas [36–39]. Therefore, G:C > T:A mutation in codon 249 of TP53 gene is regarded as the hotspot mutation caused by AFB1 and the molecular symbol of AFB1-related HCC [40–42].

DNA damage by AFB1 exposure, if not repaired, may cause genomic instability and ultimately result in cellular malignant transformation and tumor formation [20]. In human cells, several evolved surveillance mechanisms, including base excision repair (BER), nucleotide excision repair (NER), single-strand break repair (SSBR), and double-strand break repair (DSBR), can monitor the integrity of genome and repair and minimize the consequences of detrimental genome damage [3, 40]. DNA repair genes play an important role during aforementioned repair pathways of DNA damage; therefore, GSNPs in the DNA repair genes may be associated with risk of developing AFB1-related HCC [4].

4. Xeroderma pigmentosum C (XPC) GSNPs and AFB1-HCC among Guangxiese population

Xeroderma pigmentosum C (XPC) gene locates on chromosome 3p25 and spans 33kb. Its encoding protein consists of 940 amino acids and acts as a DNA damage recognition molecule during the global genome NER pathway [43, 44]. XPC can bind tightly with RAD23 homolog B (RAD23B, also called HR23B) to form a stable XPC/RAD23B complex. This complex can recognize DNA adducts formed by exogenous carcinogens such as AFB1 and binds to the DNA damage sites [44]. Thus, XPC may play a role in the pathogenesis of HCC-related AFB1. The pathological and cellular researches have shown that the abnormal expression of this gene is correlated with hepatocarcinogenesis [45]. Some studies have shown that GSNPs of XPC (rs2228001 (also called codon Lys939Gln polymorphism) can decrease DNA repair capacity related to AFB1-induced DNA damage [46–49]. In the past several decade years, a total of four studies from Guangxi area reported XPC rs2228001 polymorphism was involved in AFB1 detoxification (**Table 1**) [12, 49–51]. The first study

No.	Ref.	Year	AFB1 exposure[a]	Methods	Matching factor	Cases (*n*)	Controls (*n*)	Risk value[b] (OR)
1	Wu et al. [51]	2010	High	Case-control	Age, sex, HBV, HCV, race	98	157	1.46–2.08 ($P < 0.05$)
2	Long et al. [12]	2010	High	Case-control	Age, sex, HBV, HCV, race	1156	1402	1.25–1.81 ($P < 0.001$)
3	Li et al. [50]	2010	High	Case-control	No	500	507	1.20–1.81 ($P > 0.05$)
4	Yao et al. [49]	2014	High	Case-control	Age, sex, HBV, HCV, race	1486	1996	1.57–2.19 ($P < 0.001$)

[a]Defined by means of Henry et al. (Science, 1999).
[b]AFB1-related HCC risk will increase if OR > 1 and corresponding *P*-value < 0.05; will decrease if OR < 1 and corresponding *P*-value < 0.05; and will not change if OR is about 1 and/or corresponding *P*-value > 0.05.

Table 1. Characteristics of studies about GSNP at codon 939 of XPC and AFB1-related HCC risk.

conducted by Wu et al. [51] is from Baise area (a famous high AFB1 exposure area with high incidence rate of HCC). In this study, researchers investigated the association between XPC rs2228001 polymorphism and HCC risk via an hospital-based case-control study (including 98 HCC patients and 157 age-, sex-, race-, and hepatitis viruses-matching controls) method and found XPC rs2228001 polymorphism increased HCC risk of female individuals (odds ratios [ORs] were 5.44 with 95% CI 1.38–21.50), but not tumor risk of male population. Noticeably, they found a significant interaction of XPC variables and AFB1 exposure levels [51].

Results from the matching-design studies with large-size samples show that the mutant genotypes of XPC rs2228001 polymorphism increased about two times risk of HCC [12, 49]. The following quantitative analysis exhibited that AFB1 exposure interacted with risk genotypes of XPC rs2228001 polymorphism on HCC risk ($22.33 > 1.88 \times 8.69$ for the interaction of AFB1-exposure years and XPC risk genotypes and $18.38 > 1.11 \times 4.62$ for the interaction of AFB1-exposure levels and XPC risk genotypes) [12, 49]. Furthermore, mutant alleles were correlated with the decrease of XPC expression levels in cancerous tissues and with the overall survival of HCC patients [12]. However, another study also from Nanning area (another high AFB1 exposure area in Guangxi) exhibited that this polymorphism does not change HCC risk [50], possibly because it bases on nonmatching design and some confounders might affect their results. Interestingly, a significant risk value for HCC among female population was observed in the stratified analyses (OR = 2.17, 95% CI = 1.01–4.64), similar with findings from Wu et al. [51]. Given these different effects, we accomplished meta-analysis and found XPC rs2228001 polymorphism increased AFB1-related risk (combined OR = 1.89, $P < 0.01$). Therefore, these results demonstrate that GSNP at codon 939 of XPC gene is not only a genetic determinant in the development of HCC caused by AFB1 in Guangxiese population but also an independent prognostic factor influencing the survival of HCC, like AFB1 exposure.

5. Xeroderma pigmentosum D (XPD) GSNPs and AFB1-HCC among Guangxiese population

Xeroderma pigmentosum gene, contains 22 introns and 23 exons, locates on 19q13.3 and spans about 20 kb [3, 52]. Its encoded product is one of the TFIIH complexes (a DNA-dependent ATPase/helicase complex), it has classically been linked to the damage verification and the opening of the DNA helix step of NER pathway [53]. To date, molecular epidemiological studies on two GSNPs in this gene, namely, rs369191500 polymorphism (codon 312, Asp to Asn) and rs13181 polymorphism (codon 751, Lys to Gln), have been conducted by different laboratories [54]. Genotype-phenotype analyses have shown that these two GSNPs are associated with low DNA repair ability, which might modify DNA-adduct levels, p53 gene mutation, and risk of cancer [55, 56]. For genetic polymorphisms among Guangxiese population, a total of four epidemiological studies have been conducted via case-control design (**Table 2**). In 2009, Zeng et al. [57] investigated the association between XPD GSNPs and HCC and observed about 2.60-time risk of HCC for these with mutant genotypes of XPD codon 751. After that, results from Long et al. [58] and Yao et al. [49] have exhibited that the variants of XPD rs13181 polymorphism (including rs13181-LG and -GG) was significantly different between controls and HCC cases (26.3 vs. 35.9% for rs13181-LG and 8.6 vs. 20.1% for rs13181-GG, respectively, $P < 0.001$). Mutant alleles increased the

No.	Ref.	Year	AFB1 exposure[a]	Methods	Matching factor	Cases (*n*)	Controls (*n*)	Risk value[b] (OR)
1	Zeng et al. [57]	2009	High	Case-control	No	300	312	About 2.60 ($P < 0.001$)
2	Long et al. [58]	2009	High	Case-control	Age, sex, HBV, HCV, race	618	712	1.75–2.47 ($P < 0.001$)
3	Yao et al. [49]	2014	High	Case-control	Age, sex, HBV, HCV, race	1486	1996	2.19–4.27 ($P < 0.001$)
4	Hu et al. [59]	2016	High	Case-control	No	178	178	2.33–3.38 ($P < 0.05$)

[a] Defined by means of Henry et al. (Science, 1999).

[b] AFB1-related HCC risk will increase if OR > 1 and corresponding *P*-value < 0.05; will decrease if OR < 1 and corresponding *P*-value < 0.05; and will not change if OR is about 1 and/or corresponding *P*-value > 0.05.

Table 2. Characteristics of studies about genetic polymorphism at codon 751 of XPD and AFB1-related HCC risk.

risk of developing the cancer with a risk value of 1.75 (1.30–2.37) for Lys/Gln and 2.47 (1.62–3.76) for Gln/Gln, respectively [58]. Furthermore, the interactive effects of mutant genotypes of rs13181 polymorphism in XPD gene and AFB1 exposure on HCC risk were also found ($P_{interaction} < 0.05$) [49]. Recently, Hu et al. [59] have reported higher frequency of XPD codon 751 Gln alleles among HCC families than among non-HCC families. This suggests that genetic susceptibility resulting from XPD GSNPs might have a potential effect on AFB1-related HCC risk among Guangxiese population. Meta-analysis further improved the above-mentioned hypothesis [56]. However, the studies from molecular epidemiological studies exhibit that another GSNP of XPD is not significantly correlate with the risk of HCC related to AFB1 [49, 58].

6. The human 8-oxoguanine DNA glycosylase (hOGG1) GSNPs and AFB1-HCC among Guangxiese population

As described previously [60], DNA glycosylases play a central role in the BER pathway because they can recognize and catalyze the removal of damaged bases. Among having been reported GSNPs in DNA glycosylase-encoded genes, only hOGG1 correlates with DNA repair capacity [5, 61]. This gene consists of 7 exons and 6 introns and spans 17 kb on chromosome 3p26.2. It encodes a 546-amino acid protein, a specific DNA glycosylase that catalyzes the release of $8\text{-}_{oxy}G$ and the cleavage of DNA at the AP site (**Figure 3**) [61, 62]. The presence of several polymorphisms within hOGG1 locus is identified and only rs1052133 polymorphism (at codon 326, Ser → Cys) is suggested to modify DNA repair capacity [63–65]. Therefore, low capacity of $8\text{-}_{oxy}G$ repair resulting from hOGG1 326Cys polymorphism might contribute to the persistence of $8\text{-}_{oxy}G$ in genomic DNA *in vivo*, which, in turn, could be associated with increased cancer risk [66]. Several reports imply this polymorphism may be associated with HCC related to AFB1 exposure [67–70]. Through a hospital-based case-control study (including 500 cases with HCC and 507 healthy controls) conducted in Nanning area from Guangxi, Ji et al. [67] investigated the relationship between hOGG1 rs1052133 polymorphism and HCC risk and found significantly different distribution of three genotypes (Ser/Ser, Ser/Cys, and Cys/Cys) between cases and controls (71.40, 8.00, and 20.60% for patients with HCC, 84.22, 10.06, and 5.72% for controls). Regression logistic analysis shows that mutant alleles of this polymorphism increase AFB1-related HCC risk (OR = 2.14, 95% CI = 1.57–2.91). Molecular epidemiological studies from other researchers have also proved higher frequencies of Cys alleles in HCC cases than controls and this change increased HCC risk among Guangxiese population featuring AFB1-exposure history [69, 70]. Given that hOGG1 expression is significantly related to HCC carcinogenesis [71, 72], Peng et al. [68] explored the effects of hOGG1 rs1052133 polymorphism on $8\text{-}_{oxy}G$ levels and hOGG1 expression in Guangxiese population with AFB1 exposure. They observed that Cys alleles downregulated hOGG1 expression and increased $8\text{-}_{oxy}G$ levels. These findings suggested the pathogenic role of hOGG1 Cys326Ser polymorphism in the carcinogenesis of AFB1-related HCC.

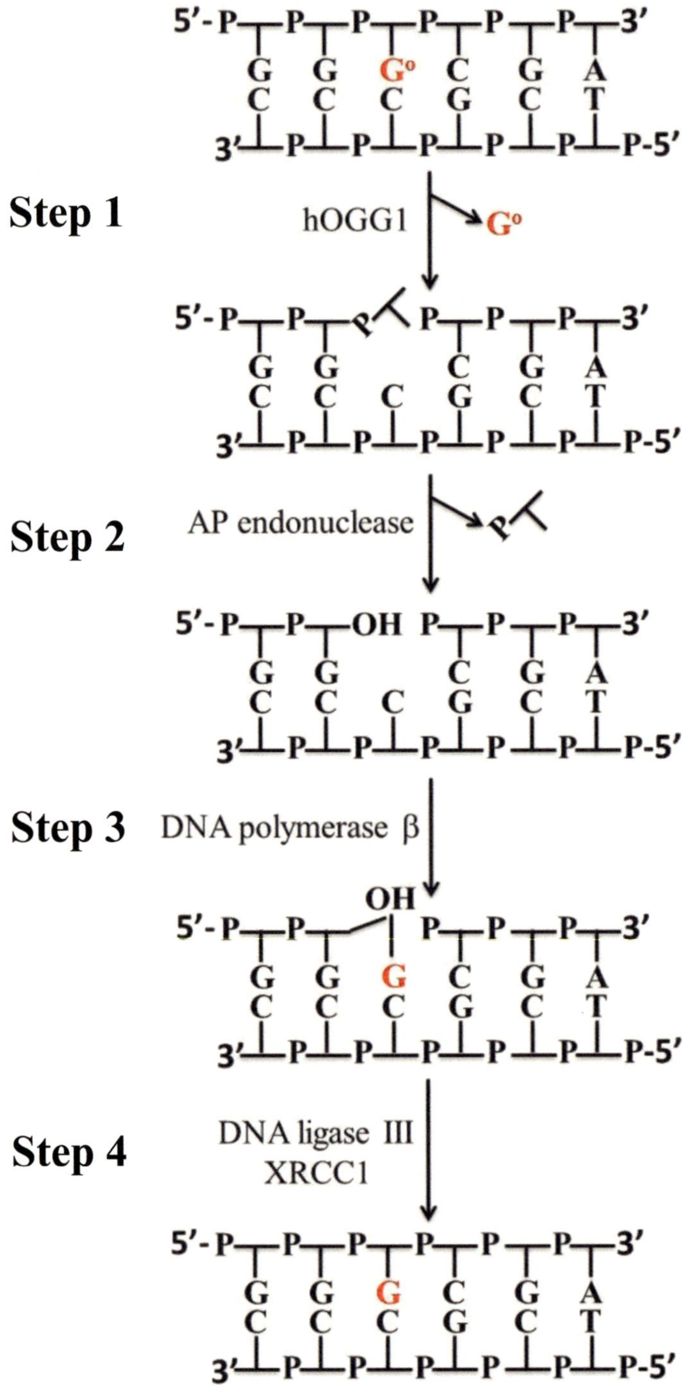

Figure 3. The base excision repair for oxidative DNA damage 8-oxyG in mammalian cells. In this repair pathway, human 8-oxoguanine DNA glycosylase (hOGG1) can catalyze the release of 8-oxyG (Red) and the cleavage of DNA at the AP site.

7. The XRCC1 GSNPs and AFB1-HCC among Guangxiese population

X-ray repair cross-complementing group 1 (XRCC1), also called RCC, spans about 32 kb on chromosome 19q13.2 and contains 17 exons and 16 introns. The encoding protein of XRCC1 acts as a scaffold protein in SSBR and BER pathways via the interaction with Pol β, DNA ligase III, and PARP [73]. According to data from SNP database, more than 50 GSNPs in the coding region of XRCC1 gene, which lead to amino acid substitution, have been identified. Of GSNPs, rs25487 polymorphism (at codon 399, Arg → Gln) is of special concern, because this GSNP resides in functionally significant regions and may decrease DNA repair activity and increase the risk of gene mutation cancers [3].

In Guangxi area, a total of five molecular epidemiological studies were found in PubMed Database, Web of Science Database, Wangfang Database, Google Database, and Weipu database (**Table 3**). In 2005, Long et al. [74] investigated the effects of XRCC1 rs25487 polymorphism on AFB1-related HCC risk. In their study, they included 140 patients with pathologically diagnosed HCC and 536 age-, sex-, race-, and hepatitis virus-matching controls and found significantly different distribution of three genotypes of XRCC1 rs25487 polymorphism (Arg/Arg, Arg/Gln, and Gln/Gln) between cases and controls (51.43, 45.00, and 3.57% for patients with HCC, 6.54, 29.66, and 2.88% for controls). Regression logistic analysis shows that mutant alleles of this polymorphism increase AFB1-related HCC risk (OR = 2.18, 95% CI = 1.27–3.74). They also observed more noticeable risk role for HCC under the conditions of individuals with both high AFB1 exposure and mutant genotypes of XRCC1 rs25487 polymorphism (risk value 1.84–10.87). The several following molecular epidemiological studies furthermore prove these results [49, 75, 77]. However, associations between

No.	Ref.	Year	AFB1 exposure[a]	Methods	Matching factor	Cases (n)	Controls (n)	Risk value[b] (OR)
1	Long et al. [74]	2005	High	Case-control	Age, sex, HBV, HCV, race	140	536	2.18 ($P = 0.0001$)
2	Long et al. [75]	2006	High	Case-control	Age, sex, HBV, HCV, race	257	649	2.47 ($P = 0.0001$)
3	Zeng et al. [76]	2010	High	Case-control	No	500	507	about 1 ($P > 0.05$)
4	He et al. [77]	2012	High	Case-control	Age, sex	119	119	2.50 ($P < 0.05$)
5	Yao et al. [49]	2014	High	Case-control	Age, sex, HBV, HCV, race	1486	1996	2.19–4.27 ($P < 0.001$)

Notes: [a] Defined by means of Henry et al. (Science, 1999, 286: 2453-2454).

[b] AFB1-related HCC risk will increase if OR > 1 and corresponding P-value < 0.05; will decrease if OR < 1 and corresponding P-value < 0.05; and will not change if OR is about 1 and/or corresponding P-value > 0.05.

Table 3. Characteristics of studies about genetic polymorphism at codon 399 of XRCC1 and AFB1-related HCC risk.

XRCC1 rs25487 polymorphism and individual susceptibility to HCC have been reported in a case-control study with the insignificant results [76]. This may be because of nonmatching design and the effects of confounders such as age, gender, race, and hepatitis viruses. Supporting aforementioned conclusions, meta-analysis from data in high AFB1 exposure areas also exhibited that these subjects with Gln alleles of XRCC1 rs25487 polymorphism had increasing HCC risk (OR > 1, $P < 0.01$) [78]. This suggests that XRCC1 rs25487 polymorphism should be a risk biomarker of Guangxiese HCC related to AFB1 exposure.

8. The XRCC3 GSNPs and AFB1-HCC among Guangxiese population

X-ray repair cross-complementing group 3 (XRCC3) is an important paralogs of the strand-exchange protein RAD51 and is primarily found and cloned by functional complementation in the Chinese hamster cell line irs1SF. This gene spans about 17.8 kb on chromosome 14q32.33 and contains 10 exons. Functionally, XRCC3 can bind directly with DNA breaks and facilitate the formation of the RAD51 nucleoprotein filament and protein-protein interaction of RAD51 family members in the SSBR pathway [79]. In XRCC3-defective irs1SF hamster cells, spontaneous chromosomal aberrations, high sensitivity to cross-linking agents, mild sensitivity to gamma rays, and significantly attenuated Rad51 focus formation after gamma ray exposure were observed, which suggests that XRCC3 is crucial for the SSBR pathway [80].

Recent molecular epidemiological studies have shown that the function of XRCC3 is modified by its GSNPs. Of the known GSNPs, only rs2228001 polymorphism (at codon 241, Thr → Met) is of special concern, because this GSNP results the change Thr to Met at codon 241 [81–83]. Up to now, three reports from high AFB1-exposure areas of Guangxi supported the above-mentioned conclusions [49, 84, 85]. In the first frequent case-control study in Guangxi population [85], higher mutant frequencies at codon 241 of XRCC3 are observed among cases with HCC than controls (33.01 vs. 61.48%, $P < 0.001$). The results from logistic regression analysis further prove that this mutate increases about 2- to 10-time risk of HCC. The following two relatively larger sample size molecular epidemiological studies (study 1 conducted by Long et al. [84] consisting of 491 patients with HCC and 862 healthy controls; study 2 from Yao et al. [49] including 1486 cases and 1996 controls) were accomplished in high AFB1 exposure. Similar to data from the first study, individuals having the mutant genotypes of XRCC3 rs2228001 polymorphism would feature higher risk of developing HCC. Interactive analysis of risk genotypes and AFB1 exposure further demonstrated that this allele multiplicatively interacted with AFB1 exposure in the process of hepatotumorigenesis [49]. Taken together, these results suggest that the GSNPs in XRCC3 gene, such as rs2228001 polymorphism, might a genetic determinant in the HCC carcinogenesis caused by AFB1 exposure among Guangxiese population.

9. The XRCC7 GSNPs and AFB1-HCC among Guangxiese population

X-ray repair cross-complementing 7 (XRCC7), also called protein kinase DNA-activated catalytic polypeptide (PRKDC), spans about 197 kb on 8q11.21 and contains 85 exons. Protein encoded by his gene is a member of the PI3/PI4-kinase family and acts as the catalytic subunit of the DNA-dependent protein kinase (DNA-PK). Functionally, it interacts with the Ku70/Ku80 heterodimer protein in the nonhomologous end joining (NHEJ) repair and recombination [86–88]. More than 200 of GSNPs have been reported in the XRCC7 gene, some of which are reported to affect tumorigenesis of malignant tumors [89–93]. In Guangxi area, several reports imply XRCC7 rs7003908 polymorphism (T to G) may be associated with HCC related to AFB1 exposure [49, 94]. Through a hospital-based case-control study (including 348 cases with HCC and 597 age-, gender-, race-, and hepatitis viruses-matched healthy controls) conducted in high AFB1 exposure area from Guangxi, Long et al. [94] investigated the association between XRCC7 rs7003908 polymorphism and HCC risk and found significantly different distribution of three genotypes (rs7003908-TT, -TG, and -GG) between cases and controls (25.9, 44.5, and 29.6% for patients with HCC, 58.1, 30.0, and 11.9% for controls). Regression logistic analysis shows that mutant alleles of this polymorphism increase AFB1-related HCC risk, with risk value of 3.45 (2.40–4.94) for rs7003908-TG and 5.04 (3.28–7.76) for rs7003908-GG, respectively. Furthermore, this GSNP was also related to higher the amounts of DNA adducts induced by AFB1 ($r = 0.142$) [94]. Interestingly, it also multiplicatively interacts with AFB1-exposure variable (interactive value: OR = 1.74; 95% CI = 1.66–1.82; $P = 2.21 \times 10^{-133}$) [49]. Taken together, these data exhibited that the XRCC7 rs7003908 polymorphism might modify AFB1-related HCC risk via decreasing NHEJ capacity. However, more studies are inquired to support this conclusion.

10. The XRCC4 GSNPs and AFB1-HCC among Guangxiese population

X-ray repair cross-complementing 4 (XRCC4, also known as SSMED) is an important NHEJ pathway gene locating on 5q14.2 and spanning about 293 kb. This gene is a generally expressed protein of 334 amino acids residues and functions together with DNA ligase IV and DNA-PK in the repair of DNA double-strand breaks. XRCC4 plays an important role in both nonhomologous end joining and the completion of V(D)J recombination [95, 96]. Increasing evidence has shown that mutations in XRCC4 can cause short stature, microcephaly, and endocrine dysfunction (SSMED) resulting from more-deficient NHEJ capacity [97, 98]. This suggests that the low repair capacity of this gene from genetic changes might be associated with cancer risk [99, 100]. Up to now, only two GSPs in the XRCC4 gene, namely, rs28383151 (at codon 56, Ala to Thr) and rs3734091 (at codon 247, Ala to Ser), have reported to be correlated with risk of AFB1-related HCC among Guangxiese population [13, 14, 49]. In these studies, Long et al. [13, 14] have examined the association between genetic polymorphisms (Ala56Thr and Ala247Ser) in XRCC4 and risk of HCC in a large case-control study in at-risk Guangxiese population. Genotypes were determined in 1499 patients with HCC and 2045 individually matched controls. We observed that individuals with Thr/Thr genotype at Arg194Trp site and Ser/Ser genotype at Ala247Ser site of XRCC4 had about twofold and threefold increased risk for the cancer compared with wild types, respectively. Furthermore, when risk genotypes of XRCC4 and AFB1-exposure were combined, this risk role was more noticeable, with the adjusted OR being11.26 (95% CI, 8.36–15.18) for rs28383151 polymorphism and 14.43 (95% CI, 7.98–26.09) for rs3734091 polymorphism, respectively. Interactive analysis further exhibited this multiplicative interaction (interactive OR = 1.64, 95% CI = 1.55–1.73, 6.41×10^{-73}) [49].

Functional exploration showed that these two polymorphisms increased AFB1-DNA adducts levels and TP53M risk, and AFB1-related HCC prognosis, suggesting they should be important modified factors of AFB1 toxicological effects [5, 13, 14]. Together, these results imply that XRCC4 rs28383151 and rs3734091 polymorphisms might play a role in the carcinogenesis of the liver under the conditions of AFB1 exposure.

11. Future directions

In the past decades, great progress has been made in understanding the molecular mechanisms of the GSNPs affecting risk of AFB1-related HCC. However, we are still far from a comprehensive view of this effect. The molecular mechanism about GSNPs in the DNA repair genes modifying the risk of HCC caused by AFB1 remains largely unknown. Although several reports have displayed that GSNPs may progress tumorigenesis of AFB1-related HCC via downregulating expression of DNA repair genes, breaking the structure of DNA repair proteins, or decreasing the function of DNA repair genes, more direct evidence is still missing. Disclosing the roles of different phenotypes of DNA repair genes will greatly benefit our understanding of pathological mechanisms of GSNPs affecting AFB1-related HCC risk, and will shed important light on the prevention values for individuals with risk types.

12. Conclusion

Like most other human cancers, HCC is a complex disease attributed to environment variation and genetic susceptive factors. In high incidence areas of HCC in Guangxi, AFB1 is an important environment variation. In the process of AFB1 hepatocarcinogenesis, DNA damage induced by AFB1 exposure plays a central role because of their genotoxicity and interactions with genetic susceptive factors. Numerous studies reviewed in this chapter have demonstrated that the hereditary variations in DNA repair genes (including XRCC1, XRCC3, XRCC4, XRCC7, hOGG1, XPC, and XPD) are related to the susceptibility to AFB1-related HCC among Chinese population. These molecular epidemiological studies have significantly contributed to our knowledge of the importance of genetic polymorphisms in DNA repair genes in the etiology of HCC related to AFB1 exposure. It would be expected that genetic susceptibility factors involved in DNA repair genes for HCC could serve as useful biomarkers for identifying at-risk individuals and, therefore, targeting prevention of this malignant tumor.

However, there are several issues to be noted. Because of conflicting data existing in the same ethnic population in view of between some genotypes of DNA repair genes and the risk of HCC related to AFB1, the conclusions should first be drawn carefully. For example, whether the XRCC1 Arg399Gln polymorphism is a risk factor or not remains controversial and further studies are needed. Second, because of the difference in population frequencies corresponding to genetic polymorphisms that depend on ethnicity, caution should be taken, particularly in extrapolating these data to other ethnic populations, especially from other high AFB1-exposure areas. Third, when risk of a specific polymorphism is considered, AFB1 exposure should be stressed because AFB1 exposure may differ from areas to areas and from individuals to individuals. Last, in view of that fact the development of AFB1-related HCC is "polygenic," a panel of susceptive biomarkers are warranted to define individuals at high risk for this cancer.

Acknowledgements

This study was supported in part by the National Natural Science Foundation of China (Nos. 81572353, 81372639, 81472243, 81660495, and 81460423), the Innovation Program of Guangxi Municipal Education Department (Nos. 201204LX674 and 201204LX324), the Natural Science Foundation of Guangxi (Nos. 2016GXNSFDA380003, 2015GXNSFAA139223, 2013GXNSFAA019251, 2014GXNSFDA118021, and 2014GXNSFAA118144), Innovation Program of Guangxi Health Department (No. Z2013781), Research Program of Guangxi Clinic Research Center of Hepatobiliary Diseases (No. 2016-11), and Open Research Program from Molecular Immunity Study Room Involving in Acute & Severe Diseases in Guangxi Colleges and Universities (Nos. kfkt20160062 and kfkt20160063).

Abbreviations

8-_{oxyG}	8-oxodeoxyguanosine
AFB1	aflatoxin B1
AFBO	AFB1-8,9-epoxide
AFB1-FAPy	8,9-dihydro-8-(2,6-diamino-4-oxo-3,4-dihydropyrimid-5-yl formamide)-9-hydroxy-AFB1
AFB1-N^7-Gua	(8,9-dihydro-8-N^7-guanyl-9-hydroxy-AFB1)
BER	base excision repair
DSBR	double-strand break repair
DSBs	double-strand breaks
GSNP	genetic single nucleotide polymorphism
HCC	hepatocellular carcinoma
HR	hazard ratio
hOGG1	human 8-oxoguanine DNA glycosylase
NER	nucleotide excision repair
NHEJ	nonhomologous end joining
OR	odds ratio
SSBs	single-strand breaks
SSBR	single-strand break repair
SSMED	short stature, microcephaly, and endocrine dysfunction

TP53M	the hotspot mutation at codon 249 of TP53 gene;
XPC	xeroderma pigmentosum C
XPD	xeroderma pigmentosum D
XRCC1	X-ray repair cross-complementing group 1
XRCC3	X-ray repair cross-complementing group 3
XRCC4	X-ray repair cross-complementing group 4
XRCC7	X-ray repair cross-complementing group 7

Author details

Xue-Ming Wu[1†], Zhi-Feng Xi[2†], Jun Lu[2†], Xing-Zhizi Wang[1†], Tian-Qi Zhang[1†], Xiao-Ying Huang[1†], Jin-Guang Yao[1†], Chao Wang[3†], Zhong-Heng Wei[4†], Chun-Ying Luo[1†], Bing-Chen Huang[1†], Qun-Qing Xu[5†], Wen-Pei Yang[6†], Qiang Xia[2*] and Xi-Dai Long[1,2*]

*Address all correspondence to: sjtulongxd@263.net or xiaqiang@sjtu.edu.cn

1 Department of Pathology, the Affiliated Hospital of Youjiang Medical College for Nationalities (AHYMCN), Baise, China

2 Department of Liver Surgery, Ren Ji Hospital, School of Medicine, Shanghai Jiao Tong University, Shanghai, China

3 Department of Medicine, AHYMCN, Baise, China

4 Department of Tumor, AHYMCN, Baise, China

5 Department of Central Test, Youjiang Medical College for Nationalities, Baise, China

6 Department of Basic Medicine, Youjiang Medical College for Nationalities, Baise, China

† These authors contributed equally to this work.

References

[1] Torre LA, Bray F, Siegel RL, Ferlay J, Lortet-Tieulent J, Jemal A. Global cancer statistics, 2012. CA A Cancer Journal for Clinicians. 2015;**65**:87-108. DOI: 10.3322/caac.21262

[2] Chen W, Zheng R, Baade PD, Zhang S, Zeng H, Bray F, Jemal A, Yu XQ, He J. Cancer statistics in China, 2015. CA A Cancer Journal for Clinicians. 2016;**66**:115-132. DOI: 10.3322/caac.21338

[3] Xia Q, Huang XY, Xue F, Zhang JJ, Zhai B, Kong DC, Wang C, Huang ZQ, Long XD. Genetic polymorphisms of DNA repair genes and DNA repair capacity related to aflatoxin b1 (AFB1)-induced DNA damages. In: Chen C, editor. New Research Directions in DNA Repair. 1st ed. Rijeka: InTech; 2013. pp. 377-412. DOI: 10.5772/53967

[4] Long XD, Yao JG, Zeng Z, Huang CH, Huang ZS, Huang YZ, Ban FZ, Huang XY, Yao LM, Fan LD, Fu GH. DNA repair capacity-related to genetic polymorphisms of DNA repair genes and aflatoxin B1-related hepatocellular carcinoma among Chinese population. In: Kruman I, editor. DNA Repair. Rijeka: InTech; 2011. pp. 505-524. DOI: 10.5772/20792

[5] Long XD, Yao JD, Yang Q, Huang CH, Liao P, Nong LG, Tang YJ, Huang XY, Wang C, Wu XM, Huang BC, Ban FZ, Zeng LX, Ma Y, Zhai B, Zhang JQ, Xue F, Lu CX, Xia Q. Polymorphisms of DNA repair genes and toxicological effects of aflatoxin B1 exposure In: Faulkner AG, editor. Aflatoxins: Food Sources, Occurrence and Toxicological Effects. 1st ed. New York: Nova Science Publishers; 2014. pp. 107-124. DOI: 978-1-63117-298-4

[6] Clifford RJ, Zhang J, Meerzaman DM, Lyu MS, Hu Y, Cultraro CM, Finney RP, Kelley JM, Efroni S, Greenblum SI, Nguyen CV, Rowe WL, Sharma S, Wu G, Yan C, Zhang H, Chung YH, Kim JA, Park NH, Song IH, Buetow KH. Genetic variations at loci involved in the immune response are risk factors for hepatocellular carcinoma. Hepatology. 2010;**52**:2034-2043. DOI: 10.1002/hep.23943

[7] Dominguez-Malagon H, Gaytan-Graham S. Hepatocellular carcinoma: An update. Ultrastructural Pathology. 2001;**25**:497-516. DOI: 10.1080/25.497516

[8] Long XD, Tang YH, Qu DY, Ma Y. The toxicity and role of aflatoxin B1 and DNA repair (corresponding DNA repair enzymes). Youjiang Medical College for Nationalities Xue Bao. 2006;**28**:278-280. DOI: 10.3969/j.issn.1001-5817.2006.02.092

[9] Zhang CY, Huang TR, Yu JH, Zhang ZQ, Li JL, Deng W, Ye SY, Zhou DN, He ZF. Epidemiological analysis of primary liver cancer in the early 21st century in Guangxi province of China. Chinese Journal of Cancer. 2010;**29**:545-550. DOI: 10.3969/j.issn.0253-4304.2000.04.003

[10] Huang ZB, Wu ZB, Xu GC. A study on serum epidemiology of several hepatitis viruses in Guangxi areas with high incident areas of liver cancer. Guangxi Medical Unveristy Xue Bao. 2000;**17**:79. DOI: 10.3969/j.issn.1005-930X.2000.01.037

[11] Ma AM, Luo YX, Wan JL, Long XD, Huang YZ. An investigative analysis of incidence, prevention, and treatment of hepatocellular carcinoma in Xiangzhou, Baise, Guangxi Autonomous Region, China. Youjiang Minzu Yixueyuan Bao. 2010;**32**:165-166. DOI: 10.3969/j.issn.1001-5817.2010.02.024

[12] Long XD, Ma Y, Zhou YF, Ma AM, Fu GH. Polymorphism in xeroderma pigmentosum complementation group C codon 939 and aflatoxin B1-related hepatocellular carcinoma in the Guangxi population. Hepatology. 2010;**52**:1301-1309. DOI: 10.1002/hep.23807

[13] Long XD, Zhao D, Wang C, Huang XY, Yao JG, Ma Y, Wei ZH, Liu M, Zeng LX, Mo XQ, Zhang JJ, Xue F, Zhai B, Xia Q. Genetic polymorphisms in DNA repair genes XRCC4 and XRCC5 and aflatoxin B1-related hepatocellular carcinoma. Epidemiology. 2013;**24**:671-681. DOI: 10.1097/EDE.0b013e31829d2744

[14] Long XD, Yao JG, Zeng Z, Ma Y, Huang XY, Wei ZH, Liu M, Zhang JJ, Xue F, Zhai B, Xia Q. Polymorphisms in the coding region of X-ray repair complementing group 4 and aflatoxin B1-related hepatocellular carcinoma. Hepatology. 2013;**58**:171-181. DOI: 10.1002/hep.26311

[15] Kensler TW, Roebuck BD, Wogan GN, Groopman JD. Aflatoxin: A 50-year odyssey of mechanistic and translational toxicology. Toxicological Sciences: An Official Journal of the Society of Toxicology. 2011;**120**(Suppl 1):S28–S48. DOI: 10.1093/toxsci/kfq283

[16] Guengerich FP, Johnson WW, Shimada T, Ueng YF, Yamazaki H, Langouet S. Activation and detoxication of aflatoxin B1. Mutation Research. 1998;**402**:121-128. DOI: S0027-5107(97)00289-3

[17] Ben Rejeb I, Arduini F, Arvinte A, Amine A, Gargouri M, Micheli L, Bala C, Moscone D, Palleschi G. Development of a bio-electrochemical assay for AFB1 detection in olive oil. Biosensors and Bioelectronics. 2009;**24**:1962-1968. DOI: 10.1016/j.bios.2008.10.002

[18] Giri I, Stone MP. Wobble DC. dA pairing 5' to the cationic guanine N7 8,9-dihydro-8-(N7-guanyl)-9-hydroxyaflatoxin B1 adduct: Implications for nontargeted AFB1 mutagenesis. Biochemistry. 2003;**42**:7023-7034. DOI: 10.1021/bi020688n

[19] Habib SL, Said B, Awad AT, Mostafa MH, Shank RC. Novel adenine adducts, N7-guanine-AFB1 adducts, and p53 mutations in patients with schistosomiasis and aflatoxin exposure. Cancer Detection and Prevention. 2006;**30**:491-498. DOI: 10.1016/j.cdp.2006.10.006

[20] Wang JS, Groopman JD. DNA damage by mycotoxins. Mutation Research. 1999;**424**:167-181. DOI: 01.2013/0027-5107.10064859

[21] Essigmann JM, Croy RG, Nadzan AM, Busby WF, Jr, Reinhold VN, Buchi G, Wogan GN. Structural identification of the major DNA adduct formed by aflatoxin B1 in vitro. Proceedings of the National Academy of Sciences of the United States of America. 1977;**74**:1870-1874. DOI: 10.2013/0027-8424.266709

[22] Croy RG, Essigmann JM, Reinhold VN, Wogan GN. Identification of the principal aflatoxin B1-DNA adduct formed in vivo in rat liver. Proceedings of the National Academy of Sciences of the United States of America. 1978;**75**:1745-1749. DOI: 10.2013/0027-8427.273905

[23] Croy RG, Wogan GN. Temporal patterns of covalent DNA adducts in rat liver after single and multiple doses of aflatoxin B1. Cancer Research. 1981;**41**:197-203. DOI: 10.2013/0008-5472.7448760

[24] Groopman JD, Croy RG, Wogan GN. In vitro reactions of aflatoxin B1-adducted DNA. Proceedings of the National Academy of Sciences of the United States of America. 1981;**78**:5445-5449. DOI: 10.2013/0027-8424.6795633

[25] Chen JD, Liu CJ, Lee PH, Chen PJ, Lai MY, Kao JH, Chen DS. Hepatitis B genotypes correlate with tumor recurrence after curative resection of hepatocellular carcinoma. Clinical Gastroenterology and Hepatology. 2004;**2**:64-71. DOI: S1542356503002933

[26] Gradelet S, Le Bon AM, Berges R, Suschetet M, Astorg P. Dietary carotenoids inhibit aflatoxin B1-induced liver preneoplastic foci and DNA damage in the rat: Role of the modulation of aflatoxin B1 metabolism. Carcinogenesis. 1998;**19**:403-411. DOI: 10.2013/0143-3334. 9525273

[27] Farombi EO, Adepoju BF, Ola-Davies OE, Emerole GO. Chemoprevention of aflatoxin B1-induced genotoxicity and hepatic oxidative damage in rats by kolaviron, a natural bioflavonoid of Garcinia kola seeds. European Journal of Cancer Prevention: The Official Journal of the European Cancer Prevention Organisation. 2005;**14**:207-214. DOI: 10.2013/0959-8278. 15901988

[28] Liu J, Yang CF, Lee BL, Shen HM, Ang SG, Ong CN. Effect of *Salvia miltiorrhiza* on aflatoxin B1-induced oxidative stress in cultured rat hepatocytes. Free Radical Research. 1999;**31**:559-568. DOI: 10.2013/1071-5762.10630680

[29] Wild CP, Montesano R. A model of interaction: Aflatoxins and hepatitis viruses in liver cancer aetiology and prevention. Cancer Letters. 2009;**286**:22-28. DOI: 10.1016/j.canlet.2009.02.053

[30] Shen HM, Ong CN. Mutations of the p53 tumor suppressor gene and ras oncogenes in aflatoxin hepatocarcinogenesis. Mutation Research. 1996;**366**:23-44. DOI: 10.2013/0027-5107.8921985

[31] Golli-Bennour EE, Kouidhi B, Bouslimi A, Abid-Essefi S, Hassen W, Bacha H. Cytotoxicity and genotoxicity induced by aflatoxin B1, ochratoxin A, and their combination in cultured Vero cells. Journal of Biochemical and Molecular Toxicology. 2010;**24**:42-50. DOI: 10.1002/jbt.20310

[32] Paget V, Sichel F, Garon D, Lechevrel M. Aflatoxin B1-induced TP53 mutational pattern in normal human cells using the FASAY (functional analysis of separated alleles in yeast). Mutation Research. 2008;**656**:55-61. DOI: 10.1016/j.mrgentox.2008.07.009

[33] Van Vleet TR, Watterson TL, Klein PJ, Coulombe Jr. RA. Aflatoxin B1 alters the expression of p53 in cytochrome P450-expressing human lung cells. Toxicological Sciences. 2006;**89**:399-407. DOI: 10.1093/toxsci/kfj039

[34] Vahakangas K. TP53 mutations in workers exposed to occupational carcinogens. Human Mutation. 2003;**21**:240-251. DOI: 10.1002/humu.10182

[35] Staib F, Hussain SP, Hofseth LJ, Wang XW, Harris CC. TP53 and liver carcinogenesis. Human Mutation. 2003;**21**:201-216. DOI: 10.1002/humu.10176

[36] Chan KT, Hsieh DP, Lung ML. In vitro aflatoxin B1-induced p53 mutations. Cancer Letters. 2003;**199**:1-7. DOI: S0304383503003379

[37] Long XD, Ma Y, Huang HD, Yao JG, Qu de Y, Lu YL. Polymorphism of XRCC1 and the frequency of mutation in codon 249 of the p53 gene in hepatocellular carcinoma among Guangxi population, China. Molecular Carcinogenesis. 2008;**47**:295-300. DOI: 10.1002/mc.20384

[38] Li D, Cao Y, He L, Wang NJ, Gu JR. Aberrations of p53 gene in human hepatocellular carcinoma from China. Carcinogenesis. 1993;**14**:169-173. DOI: 10.2013/0143-3334. 8382111

[39] Kirk GD, Camus-Randon AM, Mendy M, Goedert JJ, Merle P, Trepo C, Brechot C, Hainaut P, Montesano R. Ser-249 p53 mutations in plasma DNA of patients with

hepatocellular carcinoma from the Gambia. Journal of the National Cancer Institute. 2000;**92**:148-153. DOI: 10.2013/0027-8874.10639517

[40] Aguilar F, Hussain SP, Cerutti P. Aflatoxin B1 induces the transversion of G-->T in codon 249 of the p53 tumor suppressor gene in human hepatocytes. Proceedings of the National Academy of Sciences of the United States of America. 1993;**90**:8586-8590. DOI: 10.2013/0027-8424.8397412

[41] Denissenko MF, Koudriakova TB, Smith L, O'Connor TR, Riggs AD, Pfeifer GP. The p53 codon 249 mutational hotspot in hepatocellular carcinoma is not related to selective formation or persistence of aflatoxin B1 adducts. Oncogene. 1998;**17**:3007-3014. DOI: 10.1038/sj.onc.1202214

[42] Duflot A, Hollstein M, Mehrotra R, Trepo C, Montesano R, Cova L. Absence of p53 mutation at codon 249 in duck hepatocellular carcinomas from the high incidence area of Qidong (China). Carcinogenesis. 1994;**15**:1353-1357. DOI: 10.2017/0143-3334.8033311

[43] Sugasawa K. XPC: Its product and biological roles. Advances in Experimental Medicine and Biology. 2008;**637**:47-56. DOI: 10.2016/0065-2598.19181110

[44] Nemzow L, Lubin A, Zhang L, Gong F. XPC: Going where no DNA damage sensor has gone before. DNA Repair (Amst). 2015;**36**:19-27. DOI: 10.1016/j.dnarep.2015.09.004

[45] Fautrel A, Andrieux L, Musso O, Boudjema K, Guillouzo A, Langouet S. Overexpression of the two nucleotide excision repair genes ERCC1 and XPC in human hepatocellular carcinoma. Journal of Hepatology. 2005;**43**:288-293. DOI: 10.1016/j.jhep.2005.02.020

[46] Strom SS, Estey E, Outschoorn UM, Garcia-Manero G. Acute myeloid leukemia outcome: Role of nucleotide excision repair polymorphisms in intermediate risk patients. Leuk Lymphoma. 2010;**51**:598-605. DOI: 10.3109/10428190903582804

[47] Khan SG, Yamanegi K, Zheng ZM, Boyle J, Imoto K, Oh KS, Baker CC, Gozukara E, Metin A, Kraemer KH. XPC branch-point sequence mutations disrupt U2 snRNP binding, resulting in abnormal pre-mRNA splicing in xeroderma pigmentosum patients. Human Mutation. 2010;**31**:167-175. DOI: 10.1002/humu.21166

[48] Gangwar R, Mandhani A, Mittal RD. XPC gene variants: A risk factor for recurrence of urothelial bladder carcinoma in patients on BCG immunotherapy. Journal of Cancer Research and Clinical Oncology. 2010;**136**:779-786. DOI: 10.1007/s00432-009-0717-y

[49] Yao JG, Huang XY, Long XD. Interaction of DNA repair gene polymorphisms and aflatoxin B1 in the risk of hepatocellular carcinoma. International Journal of Clinical and Experimental Pathology. 2014;**7**:6231-6244. DOI: 10.2016/1936-2625.25337275

[50] Li LM, Zeng XY, Ji L, Fan XJ, Li YQ, Hu XH, Qiu XQ, Yu HP. Association of XPC and XPG polymorphisms with the risk of hepatocellular carcinoma. Zhonghua gan zang bing za zhi = Zhonghua ganzangbing zazhi = Chinese Journal of Hepatology. 2010;**18**:271-275. DOI: 10.3760/cma.j.issn.1007-3418.2010.04.009

[51] Wu XM, Ma Y, Deng ZL, Long XD. The polymorphism at codon 939 of xeroderma pigmentosum C gene and hepatocellular carcinoma among Guangxi population. Zhonghua Xiaohua Zazhi. 2010;**30**:846-848. DOI: 10.3760/cma.j.issn.0254-1432.2010.11.018

[52] Van Houten B, Kuper J, Kisker C. Role of XPD in cellular functions: To TFIIH and beyond. DNA Repair (Amst). 2016;**44**:136-142. DOI: 10.1016/j.dnarep.2016.05.019

[53] Manuguerra M, Saletta F, Karagas MR, Berwick M, Veglia F, Vineis P, Matullo G. XRCC3 and XPD/ERCC2 single nucleotide polymorphisms and the risk of cancer: A HuGE review. American Journal of Epidemiology. 2006;**164**:297-302. DOI: 10.1093/aje/kwj189

[54] Sandoval-Carrillo A, Mendez-Hernandez EM, Vazquez-Alaniz F, Aguilar-Duran M, Tellez-Valencia A, Barraza-Salas M, Castellanos-Juarez FX, Llave-Leon OL, Salas-Pacheco JM. Polymorphisms in DNA repair genes (APEX1, XPD, XRCC1 and XRCC3) and risk of preeclampsia in a Mexican mestizo population. International Journal of Molecular Sciences. 2014;**15**:4273-4283. DOI: 10.3390/ijms15034273

[55] Guo XF, Wang J, Lei XF, Zeng YP, Dong WG. XPD Lys751Gln polymorphisms and the risk of esophageal cancer: An updated meta-analysis. Internal Medicine Journal. 2015;**54**:251-259. DOI: 10.2169/internalmedicine.54.3256

[56] Peng Q, Li S, Lao X, Chen Z, Li R, Qin X. Association between XPD Lys751Gln and Asp312Asn polymorphisms and hepatocellular carcinoma risk: A systematic review and meta-analysis. Medicine (Baltimore). 2014;**93**:e330. DOI: 10.1097/MD.0000000000000330

[57] Zeng XY, Qiu XQ, Ji L, Yu HP. Study on the relationship between hepatoceilular carcinoma and the interaction between polymorphisms in DNA repair gene XPD and environmental factors. Zhong Hua Liu Xing Bing Xue Za Zhi. 2009;**30**:702-705. DOI: 10.3760/cma.j.issn.0254-6450.2009.07.014

[58] Long XD, Ma Y, Zhou YF, Yao JG, Ban FZ, Huang YZ, Huang BC. XPD Codon 312 and 751 polymorphisms, and AFB1 exposure, and hepatocellular carcinoma risk. BMC Cancer. 2009;**9**:400. DOI: 10.1186/1471-2407-9-400

[59] Hu HB, Tang CL, Li YB, Qin WB, Lu WX. Genic polymorphisms of XPD and risk of liver cancer among Guangxi Zhuang population. Shan Dong Yi Yao. 2016;**56**:33-35. DOI: 10.3969/j.issn.1002-266X.2016.13.012

[60] Wallace SS. Base excision repair: A critical player in many games. DNA Repair (Amst). 2014;**19**:14-26. DOI: 10.1016/j.dnarep.2014.03.030

[61] Kuznetsov NA, Koval VV, Fedorova OS. Mechanism of recognition and repair of damaged DNA by human 8-oxoguanine DNA glycosylase hOGG1. Biochemistry (Mosc). 2011;**76**:118-130. DOI: 10.2016/1608-3040.21568844

[62] Boiteux S, Radicella JP. The human OGG1 gene: Structure, functions, and its implication in the process of carcinogenesis. Archives of Biochemistry and Biophysics. 2000;**377**:1-8. DOI: 10.1006/abbi.2000.1773

[63] Weiss JM, Goode EL, Ladiges WC, Ulrich CM. Polymorphic variation in hOGG1 and risk of cancer: A review of the functional and epidemiologic literature. Molecular Carcinogenesis. 2005;**42**:127-141. DOI: 10.1002/mc.20067

[64] Kohno T, Shinmura K, Tosaka M, Tani M, Kim SR, Sugimura H, Nohmi T, Kasai H, Yokota J. Genetic polymorphisms and alternative splicing of the hOGG1 gene, that is involved in the repair of 8-hydroxyguanine in damaged DNA. Oncogene. 1998;**16**:3219-3225. DOI: 10.1038/sj.onc.1201872

[65] Kamali M, Kargar S, Heiranizadeh N, Zare M, Kargar S, Zare Shehneh M, Neamatzadeh H. Lack of any Association between the Hogg1 Ser326Cys polymorphism and breast cancer risk: A systematic review and meta-analysis of 18 studies. Asian Pacific Journal of Cancer Prevention. 2017;**18**:245-251. DOI: 10.22034/APJCP.2017.18.1.245

[66] Wang W, Dang S, Li Y, Sun M, Jia X, Wang R, Liu J. hOGG1 Ser326Cys polymorphism and risk of hepatocellular carcinoma among East Asians: A meta-analysis. PLoS One. 2013;**8**:e60178. DOI: 10.1371/journal.pone.0060178

[67] Ji L, Zeng XY, Li LM, Qiu XQ, Chen SX, Yu HP. Interaction between the single-nucleotide polymorphism of DNA repair gene hOGG1 and HBV infection and its susceptibility to hepatocellular carcinoma. Journal of Hygiene Research. 2011;**40**:705-708. DOI: 10.2017/1000-8020.2011.06.017

[68] Peng T, Shen HM, Liu ZM, Yan LN, Peng MH, Li LQ, Liang RX, Wei ZL, Halliwell B, Ong CN. Oxidative DNA damage in peripheral leukocytes and its association with expression and polymorphisms of hOGG1: A study of adolescents in a high risk region for hepatocellular carcinoma in China. World Journal of Gastroenterology. 2003;**9**:2186-2193. DOI: 10.2016/1007-9327.14562375

[69] Yuan T, Wei J, Luo J, Liu M, Deng S, Chen P. Polymorphisms of base-excision repair genes hOGG1 326cys and XRCC1 280His increase hepatocellular carcinoma risk. Digestive Diseases and Sciences. 2012;**57**:2451-2457. DOI: 10.1007/s10620-012-2192-6

[70] Zhang H, He BC, He FC. Impact of DNA repair gene hOGG1 Ser326Cys polymorphism on the risk of hepatocellular carcinoma. Shijie Huaren xiaohua zazhi. 2006;**14**:2311-2314. DOI: 10.3969/j.issn.1009-3079.2006.23.010

[71] Cheng B, Jungst C, Lin J, Caselmann WH. Potential role of human DNA-repair enzymes hMTH1, hOGG1 and hMYHalpha in the hepatocarcinogenesis. Journal of Huazhong University of Science and Technology. Medical sciences. 2002;**22**:206-211, 215. DOI: 10.2016/1672-0733.12658805

[72] Su ZX, Li LQ, Peng T, Ye XP, Xiao KY, Shang LM. The implications of hOGG1 expression in hepatocellular carcinoma and cirrhosis tissues. China Medical Abstracts: Oncology. 2009;**1**:3-6. DOI: 10.3969/j.issn.1674-5671.2009.01.003

[73] London RE. The structural basis of XRCC1-mediated DNA repair. DNA Repair (Amst). 2015;**30**:90-103. DOI: 10.1016/j.dnarep.2015.02.005

[74] Long XD, Ma Y, Wei YP, Deng ZL. X-ray repair cross-complementing group 1 (XRCC1) Arg 399 Gln polymorphism and aflatoxin B1 (AFB1)-related hepatocellular carcinoma (HCC) in Guangxi population. Chinese Journal of Cancer Research. 2005;**17**:17-21. DOI: 10.1007/s11670-005-0004-7

[75] Long XD, Ma Y, Wei YP, Deng ZL. The polymorphisms of GSTM1, GSTT1, HYL1*2, and XRCC1, and aflatoxin B1-related hepatocellular carcinoma in Guangxi population, China. Hepatology Research. 2006;**36**:48-55. DOI: 10.1016/j.hepres.2006.06.004

[76] Zeng XY, Yu HP, Qiu XQ, Ji L, Li LM. A case-control study of polymorphism of XRCC1 gene and the risk of hepatocellular carcinoma. Zhonghua Ji Bing Kong Zhi Za Zhi. 2010;**14**:760-763. DOI: 10.3760/cma.j.issn.0254-6448.2010.11.018

[77] He GZ, Huang TR, Deng JH, Zhang CY, Li JL. Research on association between XRCC1Arg399Gln polymorphism and liver cancer. Guangxi Zhongyi Xueyuan Xuebao. 2012;**15**:1-3. DOI: 10.3969/j.issn.1008-7486.2012.03.001

[78] Chen BP, Long XD, Fu GH. Meta-analysis of XRCC1 Codon 399 polymorphism and susceptibility of hepatocellular carcinoma. Journal of Shanghai Jiao Tong University (Medical Science). 2011;**31**:1588-1602. DOI: 10.3969/j.issn.1674-8115.2011.11.018

[79] Bishop DK, Ear U, Bhattacharyya A, Calderone C, Beckett M, Weichselbaum RR, Shinohara A. Xrcc3 is required for assembly of Rad51 complexes in vivo. Journal of Biological Chemistry. 1998;**273**:21482-21488. DOI: 10.2016/0021-9258. 9705276

[80] Kawabata M, Kawabata T, Nishibori M. Role of recA/RAD51 family proteins in mammals. Acta Medica Okayama. 2005;**59**:1-9. DOI: 10.2016/0386-300X.PMID.15902993

[81] Cheng S, Wang L, Wang L, Wang Z. Association of XRCC3 gene rs861539 polymorphism with gastric cancer risk: Evidence from a case-control study and a meta-analysis. International Journal of Clinical and Experimental Pathology. 2015;**8**:1911-1919. DOI: 10.2016/1936-2625.10086

[82] Bei L, Xiao-Dong T, Yu-Fang G, Jian-Ping S, Zhao-Yu Y. DNA repair gene XRCC3 Thr241Met polymorphisms and lung cancer risk: A meta-analysis. Bull Cancer. 2015;**102**:332-339. DOI: 10.1016/j.bulcan.2015.02.003

[83] Zhang X, Zhang L, Tian C, Yang L, Wang Z. Genetic variants and risk of cervical cancer: Epidemiological evidence, meta-analysis and research review. British Journal of Obstetrics and Gynaecology. 2014;**121**:664-674. DOI: 10.1111/1471-0528.12638

[84] Long XD, Ma Y, Qu de Y, Liu YG, Huang ZQ, Huang YZ, Lin ZH, Wei NB, Zhou SC. The polymorphism of XRCC3 codon 241 and AFB1-related hepatocellular carcinoma in Guangxi population, China. Annals of Epidemiology. 2008;**18**:572-578. DOI: 10.1016/j.annepidem.2008.03.003

[85] Long XD, Ma Y, Deng ZL, Huang YZ, Wei NB. Association of the Thr241Met polymorphism of DNA repair gene XRCC3 with genetic susceptibility to AFB1-related

hepatocellular carcinoma in Guangxi population. Zhonghua Yi Xue Yi Chuan Xue Za Zhi. 2008;**25**:268-271. DOI: 940625058

[86] Chen BP, Li M, Asaithamby A. New insights into the roles of ATM and DNA-PKcs in the cellular response to oxidative stress. Cancer Letters. 2012;**327**:103-110. DOI: 10.1016/j.canlet.2011.12.004

[87] Shrivastav M, De Haro LP, Nickoloff JA. Regulation of DNA double-strand break repair pathway choice. Cell Research. 2008;**18**:134-147. DOI: 10.1038/cr.2007.111

[88] Jolly CJ, Cook AJ, Manis JP. Fixing DNA breaks during class switch recombination. The Journal of Experimental Medicine. 2008;**205**:509-513. DOI: 10.1084/jem.20080356

[89] Zhou C, Tang H, Yu J, Zhuang D, Zhang H. Blood-based DNA methylation of DNA repair genes in the non-homologous end-joining (NEHJ) pathway in patient with glioma. International journal of Clinical and Experimental Pathology. 2015;**8**:9463-9467. DOI: 10.2016/1936-2625.PMID.26464705

[90] Xiao M, Shen Y, Chen L, Liao Z, Wen F. The rs7003908 (T>G) polymorphism in the XRCC7 gene and the risk of cancers. Molecular Biology Reports. 2014;**41**:3577-3582. DOI: 10.1007/s11033-014-3220-8

[91] Jahantigh D, Salimi S, Mousavi M, Moossavi M, Mohammadoo-Khorasani M, Narooei-nejad M, Sandoughi M. Association between functional polymorphisms of DNA Double-Strand breaks in repair genes XRCC5, XRCC6 and XRCC7 with the risk of systemic lupus erythematosus in South East Iran. DNA Cell Biology. 2015;**34**:360-366. DOI: 10.1089/dna.2014.2465

[92] Hsieh YH, Chang WS, Tsai CW, Tsai JP, Hsu CM, Jeng LB, Bau DT. DNA double-strand break repair gene XRCC7 genotypes were associated with hepatocellular carcinoma risk in Taiwanese males and alcohol drinkers. Tumour Biology. 2015;**36**:4101-4106. DOI: 10.1007/s13277-014-2934-5

[93] Hsia TC, Chang WS, Chen WC, Liang SJ, Tu CY, Chen HJ, Liang JA, Tsai CW, Hsu CM, Tsai CH, Bau DT. Genotype of DNA double-strand break repair gene XRCC7 is associated with lung cancer risk in Taiwan males and smokers. Anticancer Research. 2014;**34**:7001-7005. DOI: 10.2016/0250-7005.PMID.25503126

[94] Long XD, Yao JG, Huang YZ, Huang XY, Ban FZ, Yao LM, Fan LD. DNA repair gene XRCC7 polymorphisms (rs#7003908 and rs#10109984) and hepatocellular carcinoma related to AFB1 exposure among Guangxi population, China. Hepatology Research. 2011;**41**:1085-1093. DOI: 10.1111/j.1872-034X.2011.00866.x

[95] Koike M, Yutoku Y, Koike A. Cloning, localization and focus formation at DNA damage sites of canine XRCC4. The Journal of Veterinary Medical Science. 2017;**78**:1865-1871. DOI: 10.1292/jvms.16-0381

[96] Hammel M, Yu Y, Radhakrishnan SK, Chokshi C, Tsai MS, Matsumoto Y, Kuzdovich M, Remesh SG, Fang S, Tomkinson AE, Lees-Miller SP, Tainer JA. An intrinsically disordered APLF links Ku, DNA-PKcs, and XRCC4-DNA Ligase IV in an extended flexible Non-homologous end joining complex. Journal of Biological Chemistry. 2016;**291**:26987-27006. DOI: 10.1074/jbc.M116.751867

[97] Mizuta R, Cheng HL, Gao Y, Alt FW. Molecular genetic characterization of XRCC4 function. International Immunology. 1997;**9**:1607-1613. DOI: 10.2016/0953-8178.PMID. 9352367

[98] Li Z, Otevrel T, Gao Y, Cheng HL, Seed B, Stamato TD, Taccioli GE, Alt FW. The XRCC4 gene encodes a novel protein involved in DNA double-strand break repair and V(D)J recombination. Cell. 1995;**83**:1079-1089. DOI: 0092-8674(95)90135-3

[99] Yang CH, Lin YD, Yen CY, Chuang LY, Chang HW. A systematic Gene-Gene and Gene-Environment interaction analysis of DNA repair genes XRCC1, XRCC2, XRCC3, XRCC4, and oral cancer risk. OMICS. 2015;**19**:238-247. DOI: 10.1089/omi.2014.0121

[100] Jung SW, Park NH, Shin JW, Park BR, Kim CJ, Lee JE, Shin ES, Kim JA, Chung YH. Polymorphisms of DNA repair genes in Korean hepatocellular carcinoma patients with chronic hepatitis B: Possible implications on survival. Journal of Hepatology. 2012;**57**:621-627. DOI: 10.1016/j.jhep.2012.04.039

Chapter 6

Rho-kinase Gene Polymorphisms in Related Disease States

Seniz Demiryürek and Abdullah Tuncay Demiryürek

Additional information is available at the end of the chapter

http://dx.doi.org/10.5772/intechopen.69200

Abstract

The Rho-kinase (ROCK) family members, consisting of ROCK1 and ROCK2, are serine-threonine kinases that are activated by small GTPases. ROCKs play central roles in the actin cytoskeleton organization and regulate a wide range of fundamental cellular functions, such as apoptosis, inflammatory responses, cell contractility, adhesion, migration, motility, proliferation, phagocytosis, and apoptosis. Accumulating evidence from basic and clinical studies supports the concept that ROCK plays important roles in many diseases and could be a potential therapeutic target for diverse disorders, including cardiovascular, neurologic, metabolic, autoimmune disorders, and cancers. Although there are only limited numbers of published studies related to *ROCK* polymorphisms in humans, the contribution of the genetic studies related to *ROCK* variants to the disease states is emerging. Identifying mutated genes or associated polymorphisms and evaluating their potential risks are important steps for understanding the genetic components and pathogenesis of diseases. Identification of functional mutations or polymorphisms could potentially help in the development of novel ROCK-specific therapies in related disease states.

Keywords: disorder, polymorphism, Rho-kinase, ROCK, variant

1. Introduction

Rho-kinase (ROCK) is a serine/threonine kinase that is activated by small Rho GTPase proteins. Two ROCK isoforms have been identified: ROCK1 and ROCK2. These ROCK isoforms are encoded by separate genes on human chromosomes 18q11.1 (ROCK1) and 2p24 (ROCK2). ROCK1 and ROCK2 enzymes contain 1354 and 1388 amino acids, respectively [1, 2]. Two isoforms have ~65% overall amino acid homology and ~92% homology in the kinase domain. The carboxy terminus of ROCK folds back onto the kinase domain, thereby forming an autoinhibitory loop that maintains the enzyme in an inactive state. Binding of GTP-bound, biochemically active Rho (such as RhoA/RhoB/RhoC) to the Rho-binding domain (RBD) disrupts the negative regulatory interaction between the catalytic domain and the autoinhibitory C-terminal region, resulting in activation of the enzyme in response to extracellular signals [1, 2]. On the other hand, RhoE interacts with the N-terminal region of ROCK1 and prevents Rho binding to RBD [3]. ROCK1 is cleaved by caspase-3, but ROCK2 can be cleaved by granzyme B or caspase-2 (**Figure 1**) [1, 2]. ROCK enzymes are likely to exist as dimers by parallel association at the coiled-coil domain and the dimerized kinase domain of ROCK appears to be in an active conformation in the absence of phosphorylation [4, 5].

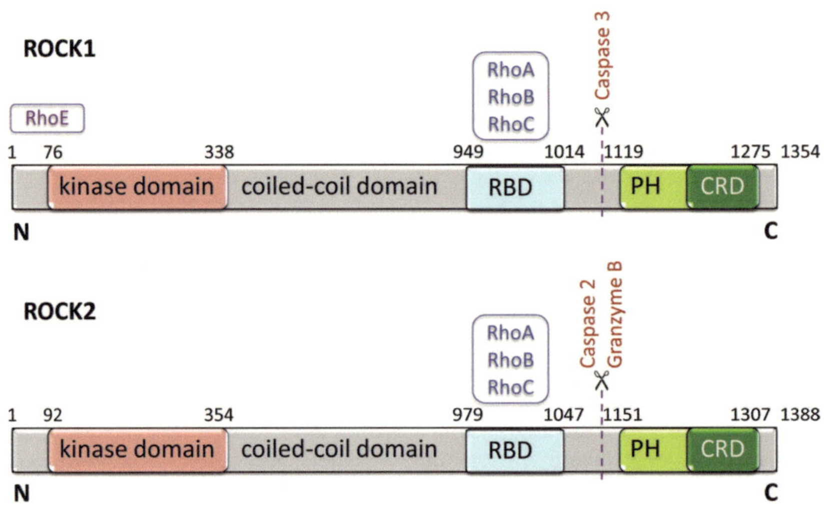

Figure 1. Schematic molecular structure and main regulators of ROCKs. ROCK sequences comprise a kinase domain located at the amino terminus of the protein, followed by a coiled-coil region containing the Rho-binding domain (RBD) and a pleckstrin homology (PH) domain with a cysteine-rich domain (CRD).

Although ROCK1 and ROCK2 are ubiquitously expressed, ROCK2 is highly expressed in the brain and the heart, whereas ROCK1 is preferentially expressed in the lung, liver, spleen, kidney, and testis [1, 6]. ROCK signaling has been implicated in a wide range of fundamental cellular functions including cell morphology, contraction, adhesion, motility, migration, proliferation, differentiation, invasion, metastasis, and apoptosis [1, 2]. ROCK can also regulate macrophage phagocytic activity and endothelial cell permeability, and it is known to play a role in inflammatory mechanisms and endothelial dysfunction [7, 8].

2. ROCK polymorphisms and disease susceptibility

There are only limited numbers of published studies related to *ROCK* polymorphisms in humans. However, the contribution of the genetic studies related to *ROCK* variants to the disease states is emerging.

2.1. Cancer

It has been demonstrated that *ROCK2* gene rs2230774 (Thr431Asn), but not rs1130757 (Arg83Lys), polymorphism is significantly associated with metastases of breast cancer [9]. Although homozygous carriers of the Thr431Thr genotype were more frequent, heterozygous carriers of the Thr431Asn genotype were less frequent among the metastatic patients than among controls. There was also an increase in Thr431 allele and decrease in Asn431 allele frequencies in patients with distant metastases. Furthermore, increased Thr431Thr genotype and Thr431 allele frequencies were found to be associated with negative estrogen and progesterone receptor status in the metastatic group [9]. This data suggest that Thr431Asn polymorphism of the *ROCK2* gene is a risk factor for the metastases of the breast cancer, and may help in predicting the prognosis. Indeed, activating *ROCK1* mutations (Y405*, S1126*, and P1193S) that increase cellular motility through actin cytoskeleton rearrangement have been identified in breast and lung carcinomas [10]. The Y405* and S1126* mutants, which lead to premature termination of translation at Tyr405 and Ser1126, were both identified in primary human breast cancers, whereas the third mutation, P1193S, which leads to a substitution of proline 1193 with serine, was identified from the established human non-small-cell lung carcinoma line NCI-H1770. rs11874761 rs8085504 rs2127958 rs17202375 rs288980 polymorphisms of the *ROCK1* gene were studied in patients with non-small cell lung cancer, but no association was observed [11]. Thus, no evidence was found to suggest that these polymorphisms play a significant role in lung cancer susceptibility [11]. Recently, a nonsense mutation (G285*) in *ROCK1* that introduces a premature stop codon at amino acid 285, and a *ROCK2* mutation (S457N) has been identified in gastric cancer patients with peritoneal carcinomatosis [12]. Collectively, these results may suggest the importance of the ROCK gene in breast, lung, and gastric carcinomas.

There are some controversial results about the association between the *ROCK* polymorphisms and colorectal carcinoma. Significant associations between *ROCK1* (rs73963110 and rs35996865) and *ROCK2* gene polymorphisms (rs2290156, rs10178332, rs35768389, rs10929732 and rs34945852) with colorectal cancer development have been detected [13]. However, no marked associations were found between *ROCK2* gene rs965665, rs2230774, rs6755196, and rs1515219 polymorphisms and the risk of developing colorectal cancer [13]. ROCK and p53 immunohistochemical stainings were found to be markedly elevated in the tumor tissue. There were also significant correlations between vascular and perineural invasions with ROCK2 or p53 protein expressions [13]. These data showed that the *ROCK1* and *ROCK2* genes might be a risk factor for colorectal cancer development, and that genetic polymorphism in these genes may modify individual susceptibility to colorectal cancer in the Turkish population [13]. However, none of the allelic or genotypic variants of the four *ROCK1* (rs35996865, rs73963110, rs2127958, and rs288980) and five *ROCK2* (rs12692437, rs7563468, rs35768389, rs17463896, and rs16857265) polymorphisms was found to be associated with the occurrence of colorectal cancer or with the development of regional lymph node metastasis in an Italian population [14]. It is noteworthy that no evidence of an association was found for *ROCK2* rs35768389 or for *ROCK1* rs73963110 variants, which have been previously described as relevant to colorectal cancer development in a Turkish cohort [13]. On the other hand, Zucchini et al. [14]. found that the *ROCK1* rs35996865 G variant allele was significantly more frequent in male patients than in the control group. This finding points to a possible gender-related modulation by the *ROCK1* gene in colorectal cancer susceptibility.

Although there were no significant associations between *ROCK2* gene polymorphisms [rs2290156, rs965665, rs10178332, rs2230774 (Thr431Asn), rs2230774 (Thr431Ser), rs6755196, and rs726843] and mantle cell lymphoma cases, ROCK1 protein and gene expressions were markedly increased in lymph node tissues of the patients [15]. Demonstration of no significant associations between *ROCK2* gene polymorphisms and mantle cell lymphoma cases may be due to the differences in pathogenesis between different types of cancer as well as the small number of cases in this study [15].

ROCK1 gene rs35996865 polymorphism was significantly associated with the increasing risk of clear cell renal cell carcinoma in a Chinese population [16]. However, no significant associations were found with *ROCK1* gene rs8089974 and rs11874761 polymorphisms. Results of this study indicate that the risk of clear cell renal cell carcinoma is increased in participants with G allele of rs35996865.

2.2. Cardiovascular diseases

Seasholtz et al. [17] reported that rs2230774 (Thr431Asn) polymorphism at *ROCK2* gene predicts increased blood pressure, systemic vascular resistance, and resistance in response to the endogenous renin-angiotensin system in twins. The Asn/Asn genotype was associated with a greater resting systolic, diastolic, and mean blood pressures. Systemic vascular resistance was found to be higher in Asn/Asn individuals, and aldosterone secretion was lowest in Asn/Asn homozygotes [17]. Rankinen et al. [18] showed that a major haplotype block at the *ROCK2* locus (containing the minor alleles of rs965665, rs10178332, rs6755196, and rs10929732) is recessively associated with a lower risk of hypertension. However, it has been shown that *ROCK2* Thr431Asn polymorphism does not exhibit any significant allele or genotype association with hypertension in a Chinese Han population [19]. Consistently, another Chinese population study did not detect the association between *ROCK2* gene polymorphisms and hypertension [20]. Liu et al. [20] tested the association between coronary artery disease and *ROCK2* gene rs978906, rs2230774 (Thr431Asn), rs56304104 polymorphisms, but no significant association was detected in a Chinese population. This study also does not support a major role for these three *ROCK2* polymorphisms in determining blood pressure levels. Thus, results of this analysis do not support common variants in the coding region of *ROCK2* to have a major effect to coronary artery disease susceptibility.

Significant associations were observed for GG genotype of rs978906, AA genotype of rs6753921, GG genotype of rs10495582, and AA genotype of rs2230774 (Thr431Asn) polymorphisms with high-altitude essential hypertension in Indian high-altitude native Ladakhi population [21]. Haplotype GAGA composed of variant alleles was found to be in higher proportion in cases [21]. Other six polymorphisms (rs2290156, rs10167277, rs10929727, rs6716817, rs4477886, and rs10929728) were also studied, but no marked changes were noted in this study [21]. Associations of *ROCK2* gene polymorphisms with elevated systolic blood pressure levels suggest the involvement of these four polymorphisms in high-altitude essential hypertension.

Peterson et al. [22] evaluated allelic variants [rs12622447, rs10929728, rs1868584, rs6716817, rs2230774 (Thr431Asn), rs5829297, rs4027164, and rs17366517] or haplotypic associations of *ROCK2* in women with preeclempsia in a Finnish population and did not detect any significant association, implying that *ROCK2* gene could not be a functional target for the regulation of preeclempsia. It is concluded that common genetic variations in *ROCK2* are unlikely to make a major contribution to the risk of preeclampsia in the Finnish population. However, *ROCK2* gene intronic rs1868584 variant is reported to be associated with cardiovascular disease and hypertension [23].

The major alleles of rs978906 (A allele) and rs2230774 (C allele) of *ROCK2* gene were found to be significantly associated with arterial stiffness in a Chinese population residing in Taiwan [24]. They found that the A allele of rs978906 has reduced repression of miR-1183 resulting in significantly higher ROCK2 expression levels than the G allele. It has been proposed that people carrying the A allele are prone to arterial stiffness because their ROCK2 levels tend to be high [24]. Thus, these two functional polymorphisms of *ROCK2* gene can increase the susceptibility of arterial stiffness by affecting ROCK2 levels and activity in the Chinese population.

Yoo et al. [25] demonstrated that the genotype frequencies of five polymorphisms (rs978906, rs2271621, rs2230774, rs1515219 and rs3771106) of *ROCK2*, in the vasospastic angina group, were not significantly different from that in the control group in the Korean population. The only marked difference was noted in haplotype analysis [25]. The haplotype GTCTG was significantly associated with a decreased risk of vasospastic angina, suggesting that the *ROCK2* gene might be involved in the pathogenesis of vasospastic angina in the Korean population.

No association of the *ROCK2* gene rs2230774 (Thr431Asn) polymorphism with the development of cardiac septal defects in pediatric patients has been reported [26], suggesting that this polymorphism is not a contributing factor to the susceptibility of atrial or ventricular septal defects.

Palomino Doza et al. [27] investigated the role of genetic variations in *ROCK1* on the risk of tetralogy of Fallot in British Caucasian patients, and found that *ROCK1* gene rs288979 and rs56085230 (Tyr269Tyr) variants were significantly associated with tetralogy of Fallot. In this study, *ROCK1* gene rs2292296 (Leu1097Phe), rs7237677, rs7227454, rs288989, rs45449301 (Ile432Val), rs288979, rs17202368, rs17202375, rs2271255 (Lys222Glu), rs1481280, rs8085504, rs398528, rs112165707 (Ser595Ser), and rs45562542 (Thr773Ser) polymorphisms were also studied, but no significant changes were determined [27].

2.3. Autoimmune diseases

Significant differences between systemic sclerosis patients and control group were observed with regard to rs35996865 polymorphism of the *ROCK1* gene and rs10178332 polymorphism of the *ROCK2* gene [28]. CC genotype frequency of the rs35996865 polymorphism was found to be extremely low in patients with Raynaud's phenomenon [28]. A significant difference between systemic sclerosis patients and control group was observed in G allele and GG genotype distributions of alteration in the *ROCK2* gene rs10178332 polymorphism. Additionally, GG allele frequency was significantly low in patients with Raynaud's phenomenon and lung involvement [28]. In this study, rs112108028 (Pro1164Leu) and rs1045144 for *ROCK1*; rs2230774 (Thr431Ser), rs2230774 (Thr431Asn), rs35768389 (Asp601Val), rs726843, rs2290156, rs965665, rs6755196, and rs10929732 for *ROCK2* gene polymorphisms were also examined, but no marked associations were noted. These results strongly suggest that rs35996865 and rs10178332 polymorphisms may be important risk factors for the development of systemic sclerosis.

It has been reported that *ROCK2* gene rs35768389 (Asp601Val) polymorphism is associated with Behçet's disease [29]. There are marked elevations in both TA genotype and A allele frequencies of this polymorphism in patients group. Although CC genotype of rs1515219 polymorphism was more frequent, CT genotype was less frequent among the patients with Behçet's disease. There was an increase in C allele frequency in patients [29]. Additionally, high AC and TT haplotype frequencies, and an increase in peripheral blood mRNA *ROCK2* gene expression were observed in cases with Behçet's disease. However, no associations were found with rs726843, rs2290156, rs965665, rs10178332, rs2230774, rs6755196, rs10929732, and rs34945852 polymorphisms [29]. These results strongly suggest that *ROCK2* gene polymorphisms may act as a contributing factor to the individual susceptibility of Behçet's disease.

ROCK1 gene polymorphisms may also have a significant impact on susceptibility to Behçet's disease. In the presence of CC genotype for rs73963110, CT genotype for rs111874856 (Val355Ile), and TC genotype for rs112130712 (Lys1054Arg) polymorphisms, the risk of Behçet's disease increased 12.13-, 15.05-, and 16.28-fold, respectively [30]. A lower frequency of the GA genotype of the rs112108028 (Pro1164Leu) polymorphism was associated with increased risk of Behçet's disease. Moreover, all these polymorphisms showed marked associations with the manifestations of Behçet's disease. Oguz et al. [30] showed that TC and CC genotypes and C allele of the rs73963110 polymorphism, TC genotype and C allele of the rs112130712 polymorphism, CT genotype and T allele of the rs111874856 polymorphism, and GG genotype and G allele of the rs112108028 polymorphism may increase the susceptibility to Behçet's disease. Although CTCG, CCTG, and TCTG haplotype frequencies were high in the patient group, TTCA haplotype frequency was low in Behçet's disease. Interestingly, CCTG and TCTG haplotypes were absent in the control group, while they had 9.5 and 6.8% frequencies in cases with Behçet's disease, respectively [30]. These two haplotypes can be advocated as a biomarker for early prediction of developing Behçet's disease in a Turkish population. However, no marked associations were detected between rs35996865, rs111312709 (Thr792Ala), and rs2271255 (Lys222Glu) polymorphisms and Behçet's disease [30]. Taken together, these data showed that *ROCK* gene appears to be a risk factor for Behçet's disease, and genetic polymorphisms in *ROCK* genes modify individual susceptibility to Behçet's disease. These findings may also provide important insight into the future development or use of potential therapeutic approaches, such as ROCK inhibitors, for patients with Behçet's disease.

There is also evidence that *ROCK2* gene intronic rs1868584 variant was shown to be associated with rheumatoid arthritis [23].

2.4. Ocular diseases

There are only two published association studies related to *ROCK* gene polymorphisms in ocular diseases. No evidence for an association of *ROCK2* gene rs2230774 (Thr431Asn) and rs1130757 (Arg83Lys) polymorphisms with diabetic retinopathy has been reported in a Turkish Population [31]. Additionally, the haplotypes are not significantly associated with diabetic retinopathy as shown in this study [31]. Moreover, another recent study demonstrated that the polymorphisms for the *ROCK1* (rs35996865) and *ROCK2* [rs2290156, rs965665, rs10178332, rs2230774 (Thr431Asn), rs2230774 (Thr431Ser), rs6755196, and rs726843] genes are not associated with the increased risk of development of primary open-angle glaucoma in a Turkish population [32]. There were also no marked associations between the haplotype frequencies and primary open-angle glaucoma. Collectively, these results suggest that studied *ROCK1* and *ROCK2* gene polymorphisms are not contributing factors to the susceptibility of diabetic retinopathy or primary open-angle glaucoma.

2.5. Ischemic stroke

In a large prospective study, associations of *ROCK1* gene variants with the risk of ischemic stroke have been observed in healthy Caucasian women [33]. Seven (rs7239317, rs2127958, rs1481280, rs1006881, rs11874761, rs10083915, and rs11873284) of the tagging single nucleotide polymorphisms evaluated in *ROCK1* gene were associated significantly with the risk of ischemic stroke [33]. rs288980 polymorphism was also studied, but no marked association was observed. Thus, *ROCK1* gene variation may influence the risk of ischemic stroke. In contrast, none of the polymorphisms (rs921322, rs8996, rs6753921, rs2230774, rs1515219, rs6716817, rs10203916, rs6755337, and rs12622447) in *ROCK2* were associated with the risk of ischemic stroke [33]. These findings may highlight the potential prognostic utility of *ROCK1*-associated gene variation in the prediction of the risk of ischemic stroke.

2.6. Metabolic syndrome

ROCK1 gene rs35996865 polymorphism and *ROCK2* gene rs2230774 (Thr431Asn) polymorphism are markedly associated with the obesity-related metabolic syndrome in a Turkish population [34]. However, no significant associations with the other 9 *ROCK* polymorphisms [*ROCK1*: rs73963110, rs112108028 (Pro1164Leu), and rs111312709 (Thr792Ala), *ROCK2*: rs2230774 (Thr431Ser), rs726843, rs2290156, rs965665, rs10178332, and rs6755196] have been observed [34]. These results suggest that CA and AA genotypes and A allele of the rs35996865 polymorphism, and CC genotype and C allele of the rs2230774 (Thr431Asn) polymorphism may increase the individual susceptibility to metabolic syndrome.

2.7. Respiratory distress syndrome

There is evidence that *ROCK1* gene rs2271255 (Lys222Glu) and rs35996865 polymorphisms, and *ROCK2* gene rs726843, rs2290156, rs10178332, rs35768389 (Asp601Val) polymorphisms are significantly associated with respiratory distress syndrome, and that these polymorphisms could be a risk factor for the development of neonatal respiratory distress syndrome [35]. High odds ratios were observed with these polymorphisms. However, no associations were found with rs73963110, rs1515219, rs965665, rs2230774 (Thr431Asn), rs6755196, and rs10929732 polymorphisms. Additionally, 12 haplotypes (6 in *ROCK1* and 6 in *ROCK2*) were found to be markedly associated with respiratory distress syndrome. Interestingly, TGCA and TGCT haplotypes were only observed among the cases. Although none of the controls had TGCT haplotype, it was seen in 26% of the infants with respiratory distress syndrome [35]. It should be emphasized that rs2271255 (Lys222Glu) and rs726843 polymorphisms have not been associated with any other disease yet. Collectively, these results strongly suggest that *ROCK* gene polymorphisms may modify individual susceptibility to respiratory distress syndrome in neonates.

2.8. Kidney disease

It has been demonstrated that rs2230774 (Thr431Asn) polymorphism of *ROCK2* gene is significantly associated with chronic kidney disease in individuals with a low serum concentration of triglycerides, with the A allele being protective against this condition [36]. Rao et al. [37] showed that rs1515219 and rs2290156 polymorphisms of the *ROCK2* gene are associated with urinary albumin excretion in twin pairs.

2.9. Overactive bladder

Gurocak et al. [38] found that genotype and allele frequencies were not significantly different between the children with overactive bladder and the control group for *ROCK2* gene rs2230774 (Thr431Asn) polymorphism. It was concluded that this polymorphism has no impact on the response to anticholinergic treatment.

2.10. Epilepsy

Association of the Thr431Asn polymorphism with idiopathic generalized epilepsy has been investigated in a study [39]. Genotype distributions and the allele frequencies for the Thr431Asn polymorphism showed no significant differences between the control and epilepsy groups. Moreover, this polymorphism did not influence age of epilepsy onset, family history, single or combined drug treatments, or status epilepticus [39]. Therefore, these results suggest that the Asn431 *ROCK2* variant allele is not an important risk factor for the development of idiopathic generalized epilepsy and does not influence the main clinical characteristics of idiopathic generalized epilepsy.

2.11. Migraine

Uslu Kuzudisli et al. [40] have investigated the association of the Thr431Asn polymorphism with migraine in a Turkish population. No statistically significant association between a migraine and genotype distributions or the allele frequencies for the *ROCK2* gene Thr431Asn polymorphism was demonstrated. In addition, there were no marked differences in genotype and allele frequencies for the migraine without aura and migraine with aura subgroups when compared with control group [40]. These findings suggest that the *ROCK2* gene Thr431Asn polymorphism is not a risk factor for the migraine, and it is not involved in the migraine pathogenesis.

2.12. Diabetes

It has been reported that *ROCK2* gene rs2230774 (Thr431Asn) and rs1130757 (Arg83Lys) polymorphisms were not associated with the risk of diabetes (mainly type-2) [31], suggesting that these polymorphisms are not a contributing factor to the susceptibility of diabetes in a Turkish population. However, Ross [23] presented evidence for the association of *ROCK2* rs1868584 variant with type-1 diabetes.

2.13. High altitude pulmonary edema

Pandey et al. [41] investigated a total of 13 *ROCK2* gene polymorphisms (rs978906, rs6753921, rs2290156, rs10495582, rs2230774, rs10167277, rs13393192, rs10929727, rs6716817, rs4477886, rs41264193, rs12622447, and rs10929728), but one polymorphism (rs10929728) emerged significant among the study groups. A significant association was observed for C allele of the rs10929728 with high altitude pulmonary edema [41]. Thus, an overrepresentation of *ROCK2* rs10929728C demonstrated the role of this allele in increasing the risk susceptibility to high altitude pulmonary edema. These data may suggest that stress-activated *ROCK2* gene has a role in predisposing an individual to high altitude pulmonary edema.

2.14. Psychiatric disorders

ROCK2 rs1868584 polymorphism was shown to be associated with bipolar disorder [23]. No associations between *ROCK1* gene rs8085654, rs288980, and rs1481280 polymorphism and schizophrenia have been reported in a Japanese population [42]. No correlations were also detected between these *ROCK1* genotypes and Brief Psychiatric Rating Scale scores, amounts of antipsychotics, or age at onset in that study.

Tables 1 and **2** show the significant and insignificant associations of *ROCK* polymorphisms with disease states.

Disease	Significant association	Ref.	Insignificant association	Ref.
Breast cancer	Y405*, S1126*	[10]		
Lung cancer	P1193S	[10]	rs11874761, rs8085504, rs2127958, rs17202375, rs288980	[11]
Gastric cancer	G285*	[12]		
Colorectal cancer	rs73963110, rs35996865	[13]	rs35768389, rs73963110, rs2127958, rs288980	[14]
	rs35996865 (in male patients)	[14]		
	V1309*	[43]		
Clear cell renal cell carcinoma	rs35996865	[16]	rs8089974, rs11874761	[16]
Tetralogy of Fallot	rs288979, rs56085230 (Tyr269Tyr)	[27]	rs2292296 (Leu1097Phe), rs7237677, rs7227454, rs288989, rs45449301 (Ile432Val), rs288979, rs17202368, rs17202375, rs2271255 (Lys222Glu), rs1481280, rs8085504, rs398528, rs112165707 (Ser595Ser), rs45562542 (Thr773Ser)	[27]

Disease	Significant association	Ref.	Insignificant association	Ref.
Systemic sclerosis	rs35996865	[28]	rs112108028 (Pro1164Leu), rs1045144	[28]
Behçet's disease	rs73963110, rs111874856 (Val355Ile), rs112130712 (Lys1054Arg), rs112108028 (Pro1164Leu)	[30]	rs35996865, rs111312709 (Thr792Ala), rs2271255 (Lys222Glu)	[30]
Primary open-angle glaucoma			rs35996865	[32]
Ischemic stroke	rs7239317, rs2127958, rs1481280, rs1006881, rs11874761, rs10083915, rs11873284	[33]	rs288980	[33]
Obesity-related metabolic syndrome	rs35996865	[34]	rs73963110, rs112108028 (Pro1164Leu), rs111312709 (Thr792Ala),	[34]
Respiratory distress syndrome	rs2271255 (Lys222Glu), rs35996865	[35]	rs73963110	[35]
Schizophrenia			rs8085654, rs288980, rs1481280	[42]

Table 1. Significant and insignificant associations between *ROCK1* variants and disease susceptibility.

Disease	Significant association	Ref.	Insignificant association	Ref.
Breast cancer	rs2230774 (Thr431Asn)	[9]	rs1130757 (Arg83Lys)	[9]
Gastric cancer	S457N	[12]		
Colorectal cancer	rs2290156, rs10178332, rs35768389, rs10929732, rs34945852	[13]	rs965665, rs2230774, rs6755196, rs1515219	[13]
			rs12692437, rs7563468, rs35768389, rs17463896, rs16857265	[14]
Mantle cell lymphoma			rs2290156, rs965665, rs10178332, rs2230774 (Thr431Asn), rs2230774 (Thr431Ser), rs6755196, rs726843	[15]
Hypertension	rs2230774 (Thr431Asn)	[17]	rs2230774 (Thr431Asn)	[19]
	rs965665, rs10178332, rs6755196, rs10929732	[18]	rs978906, rs2230774 (Thr431Asn), rs56304104	[20]
	rs1868584	[23]		
High-altitude essential hypertension	rs978906, rs6753921, rs10495582, rs2230774 (Thr431Asn)	[21]	rs2290156, rs10167277, rs10929727, rs6716817, rs4477886, rs10929728	[21]
Preeclampsia			rs12622447, rs10929728, rs1868584, rs6716817, rs2230774 (Thr431Asn), rs5829297, rs4027164, rs17366517	[22]
Arterial stiffness	rs978906, rs2230774 (Thr431Asn)	[24]		
Vasospastic angina	GTCTG haplotype	[25]	rs978906, rs2271621, rs2230774, rs1515219, rs3771106	[25]

Disease	Significant association	Ref.	Insignificant association	Ref.
Cardiac septal defects			rs2230774 (Thr431Asn)	[26]
Systemic sclerosis	rs10178332	[28]	rs2230774 (Thr431Ser), rs2230774 (Thr431Asn), rs35768389 (Asp601Val), rs726843, rs2290156, rs965665, rs6755196, rs10929732	[28]
Behçet's disease	rs35768389 (Asp601Val), rs1515219	[29]	rs726843, rs2290156, rs965665, rs10178332, rs2230774, rs6755196, rs10929732, rs34945852	[29]
Rheumatoid arthritis	rs1868584	[23]		
Diabetic retinopathy			rs2230774 (Thr431Asn), rs1130757 (Arg83Lys)	[31]
Primary open-angle glaucoma			rs2290156, rs965665, rs10178332, rs2230774 (Thr431Asn), rs2230774 (Thr431Ser), rs6755196, rs726843	[32]
Ischemic stroke			rs921322, rs8996, rs6753921, rs2230774, rs1515219, rs6716817, rs10203916, rs6755337, rs12622447	[33]
Obesity-related metabolic syndrome	rs2230774 (Thr431Asn)	[34]	rs2230774 (Thr431Ser), rs726843, rs2290156, rs965665, rs10178332, rs6755196	[34]
Respiratory distress syndrome	rs726843, rs2290156, rs10178332, rs35768389 (Asp601Val)	[35]	rs1515219, rs965665, rs2230774 (Thr431Asn), rs6755196, rs10929732	[35]
Chronic kidney disease	rs2230774 (Thr431Asn)	[36]		
Urinary albumin excretion	rs1515219, rs2290156	[37]		
Overactive bladder			rs2230774 (Thr431Asn)	[38]
Idiopathic generalized epilepsy			rs2230774 (Thr431Asn)	[39]
Migraine			rs2230774 (Thr431Asn)	[40]
Diabetes	rs1868584 (with type-1 diabetes)	[23]	rs2230774 (Thr431Asn), rs1130757 (Arg83Lys)	[31]
High altitude pulmonary edema	rs10929728	[41]	rs978906, rs6753921, rs2290156, rs10495582, rs2230774, rs10167277, rs13393192, rs10929727, rs6716817, rs4477886, rs41264193, rs12622447, rs10929728	[41]
Bipolar disorder	rs1868584	[23]		

Table 2. Significant and insignificant associations between *ROCK2* variants and disease susceptibility.

3. Structure or function of the ROCK enzymes affected by polymorphisms

The Thr431Asn polymorphism lies immediately carboxyl-terminal to the start of the putative coiled-coil region and encodes an amino acid substitution in the predicted coiled-coil domain of the protein, which is associated with ROCK2/ROCK2 parallel homodimerization and Rho binding. Asp601Val polymorphism is also located on the coiled-coil region. Because the dimeric structure of ROCK is essential for normal *in vivo* function [4, 5], changes in the coiled-coil region could be hypothesized to effect dimerization, Rho binding, and thereby ROCK activation and phosphorylation of its substrates. Indeed, it has been demonstrated for rs2230774 (Thr431Asn) polymorphism that cells transfected with C allele constructs have significantly higher ROCK activities than those with A allele constructs [24]. Moreover, the average leukocyte ROCK activity was found to be highest in CC genotype, followed by AC and then lowest in AA [24]. Taken together, non-synonymous polymorphism rs2230774 (Thr431Asn) influences ROCK2 activity.

Three *ROCK1* mutations (Y405*, S1126*, and P1193S) attenuate the autoinhibitory domain at the carboxy-terminal end of the protein and enhance kinase activity [10]. In a colorectal cancer study, the *ROCK1* mutation (typically c.3921delA leading to V1309*) is also predicted to partially delete the autoinhibitory domain [43]. *ROCK1* nonsense mutation (G285*) introduces a premature stop codon at the 285th amino acid of ROCK1, leading to the truncation of ~79% of ROCK1 [12]. The lack of a Rho-binding domain by the *ROCK1* mutation could impair the Rho/ROCK pathway [12]. Therefore, this mutation may cause the loss-of-function of ROCK1, because most of the functional domains, including the Rho-binding domain, are truncated by the mutation. The rs56085230 (Tyr269Tyr) variant is synonymous and located within the kinase motif of the protein which might influence splicing [27]. *ROCK2* gene rs978906 polymorphism located at 3′-UTR is predicted to influence microRNA(miR)-1183 binding to ROCK2 [24]. Thus, 3′-UTR rs978906 polymorphism affects the ROCK2 protein synthesis by interfering miR-1183 binding. miR-1183 may modulate the disease states by fine tuning the ROCK2 protein expression.

It has been reported that polymorphism can change the binding of the transcription factors to the gene. Pandey et al. [41] found that the variant allele rs10929728C of the *ROCK2* gene binds to a transcription factor Nkx-2, but the wild-type allele rs10929728T binds to CdxA. Bioinformatic analysis also revealed that serum response factor, a transcription factor, binding site was found for the variant allele G of the *ROCK2* gene rs10495582 polymorphism [21]. Serum response factor is known to promote the transcriptional expression of ROCK2 [44]. In general, the structural or functional changes of the ROCK enzymes affected by polymorphisms are mostly unknown and require further studies.

4. Conclusions

There are some inconsistent results with the association studies, which can be explained in part by population stratification, ethnic differences, selection bias, genotyping errors, or other factors. The incomplete polymorphism coverage likely does not represent the entire gene and therefore may not fully describe the contribution of *ROCK* genes. In the future, systematic and large prospective studies or meta-analysis are warranted to evaluate thoroughly the role of *ROCK1* and *ROCK2* genes in the genetic predisposition to disease. The structure or function of the ROCK enzymes affected by polymorphisms is mostly unknown, and functional studies would be very helpful in elucidating the involvement of ROCK in disease pathogenesis. Further validations from larger, independent cohorts as well as perspective studies are also required to verify presently known associations in different ethnic groups. Furthermore, identification of functional mutations could potentially help in the development of ROCK-specific therapies for ROCK-related disease states.

Author details

Seniz Demiryürek[1] and Abdullah Tuncay Demiryürek[2]*

*Address all correspondence to: demiryurek@gantep.edu.tr

1 Faculty of Medicine, Department of Physiology, University of Gaziantep, Gaziantep, Turkey

2 Faculty of Medicine, Department of Medical Pharmacology, University of Gaziantep, Gaziantep, Turkey

References

[1] Amano M, Nakayama M, Kaibuchi K. Rho-kinase/ROCK: A key regulator of the cytoskeleton and cell polarity. Cytoskeleton (Hoboken). 2010;**67**(9):545-554. DOI: 10.1002/cm.20472

[2] Julian L, Olson MF. Rho-associated coiled-coil containing kinases (ROCK): structure, regulation, and functions. Small GTPases. 2014;**5**:e29846. DOI: 10.4161/sgtp.29846

[3] Komander D, Garg R, Wan PT, Ridley AJ, Barford D. Mechanism of multi-site phosphorylation from a ROCK-I:RhoE complex structure. The EMBO Journal. 2008;**27**(23):3175-3185. DOI: 10.1038/emboj.2008.226

[4] Doran JD, Liu X, Taslimi P, Saadat A, Fox T. New insights into the structure-function relationships of Rho-associated kinase: A thermodynamic and hydrodynamic study of the dimer-to-monomer transition and its kinetic implications. Biochemical Journal. 2004;**384**(Pt 2):255-262. DOI: 10.1042/BJ20040344

[5] Yamaguchi H, Kasa M, Amano M, Kaibuchi K, Hakoshima T. Molecular mechanism for the regulation of rho-kinase by dimerization and its inhibition by fasudil. Structure. 2006;**14**(3):589-600. DOI: 10.1016/j.str.2005.11.024

[6] Nakagawa O, Fujisawa K, Ishizaki T, Saito Y, Nakao K, Narumiya S. ROCK-I and ROCK-II, two isoforms of Rho-associated coiled-coil forming protein serine/threonine kinase in mice. FEBS Letters. 1996;**392**(2):189-193. DOI: 10.1016/0014-5793(96)00811-3

[7] Yao L, Romero MJ, Toque HA, Yang G, Caldwell RB, Caldwell RW. The role of RhoA/Rho kinase pathway in endothelial dysfunction. Journal of Cardiovascular Disease Research. 2010;**1**(4):165-170. DOI: 10.4103/0975-3583.74258

[8] Zhou Q, Gensch C, Liao JK. Rho-associated coiled-coil-forming kinases (ROCKs): Potential targets for the treatment of atherosclerosis and vascular disease. Trends in Pharmacological Sciences. 2011;**32**(3):167-173. DOI: 10.1016/j.tips.2010.12.006

[9] Kalender ME, Demiryürek S, Oztuzcu S, Kizilyer A, Demiryürek AT, Sevinc A, Dikilitas M, Yildiz R, Camci C. Association between the Thr431Asn polymorphism of the ROCK2 gene and risk of developing metastases of breast cancer. Oncology Research. 2010;**18**(11-12):583-591. DOI: 10.3727/096504010X12767359113767

[10] Lochhead PA, Wickman G, Mezna M, Olson MF. Activating ROCK1 somatic mutations in human cancer. Oncogene. 2010;**29**(17):2591-2598. DOI: 10.1038/onc.2010.3

[11] Cebrián A, Taron M, Sala N, Ardanaz E, Chirlaque MD, Larrañaga N, Redondo ML, Sánchez MJ, Gómez del Pulgar T, Camps C, Rosell R, González CA, Lacal JC. Variants in phospholipid metabolism and upstream regulators and non-small cell lung cancer susceptibility. Clinical and Translational Oncology. 2014;**16**(1):107-112. DOI: 10.1007/s12094-013-1080-7

[12] Lim B, Kim C, Kim JH, Kwon WS, Lee WS, Kim JM, Park JY, Kim HS, Park KH, Kim TS, Park JL, Chung HC, Rha SY, Kim SY. Genetic alterations and their clinical implications in gastric cancer peritoneal carcinomatosis revealed by whole-exome sequencing of malignant ascites. Oncotarget. 2016;**7**(7):8055-8066. DOI: 10.18632/oncotarget.6977

[13] Sari I, Berberoglu B, Ozkara E, Oztuzcu S, Camci C, Demiryurek AT. Role of rho-kinase gene polymorphisms and protein expressions in colorectal cancer development. Pathobiology. 2013;**80**(3):138-145. DOI: 10.1159/000341395

[14] Zucchini C, Martinelli M, De Sanctis P, Rodia MT, Mattei G, Ugolini G, Montroni I, Ghignone F, Solmi R. Possible gender-related modulation by the ROCK1 gene in colorectal cancer susceptibility. Pathobiology. 2015;**82**(6):252-258. DOI: 10.1159/000439405

[15] Yanardag Acik D, Yılmaz M, Sarı I, Oztuzcu S, Sayıner ZA, Subari S, Demiryürek AT. Investigation of Rho-kinase expressions and polymorphisms in mantle cell lymphoma patients. Turkish Journal of Hematology. 2016;**33**(2):141-147. DOI: 10.4274/tjh.2015.0193

[16] Zhao R, Liu K, Huang Z, Wang J, Pan Y, Huang Y, Deng X, Liu J, Qin C, Cheng G, Hua L, Li J, Yin C. Genetic variants in caveolin-1 and RhoA/ROCK1 are associated with clear cell renal cell carcinoma risk in a Chinese population. PLoS One. 2015;**10**(6):e0128771. DOI: 10.1371/journal.pone.0128771

[17] Seasholtz TM, Wessel J, Rao F, Rana BK, Khandrika S, Kennedy BP, Lillie EO, Ziegler MG, Smith DW, Schork NJ, Brown JH, O'Connor DT. Rho kinase polymorphism influences blood pressure and systemic vascular resistance in human twins: Role of heredity. Hypertension. 2006;**47**(5):937-947. DOI: 10.1161/01.HYP.0000217364.45622.f0

[18] Rankinen T, Church T, Rice T, Markward N, Blair SN, Bouchard C. A major haplotype block at the rho-associated kinase 2 locus is associated with a lower risk of hypertension in a recessive manner: The HYPGENE study. Hypertension Research. 2008;**31**(8):1651-1657. DOI: 10.1291/hypres.31.1651

[19] Zhao Q, Wang L, Yang W, Chen S, Huang J, Fan Z, Li H, Lu X, Gu D. Interactions among genetic variants from contractile pathway of vascular smooth muscle cell in essential hypertension susceptibility of Chinese Han population. Pharmacogenetics and Genomics. 2008;**18**(6):459-466. DOI: 10.1097/FPC.0b013e3282f97fb2

[20] Liu L, Cao Y, Cui G, Li Z, Sun J, Zhang L, Chen C, Wang Y, Wang P, Ding H, Wang DW. Association analysis of polymorphisms in ROCK2 with cardiovascular disease in a Chinese population. PLoS One. 2013;**8**(1):e53905. DOI: 10.1371/journal.pone.0053905

[21] Pandey P, Mohammad G, Singh Y, Pasha MA. Polymorphisms and haplotype of ROCK2 associate with high altitude essential hypertension in native high altitude Ladakhi Indian population: A preliminary study. Clinical and Experimental Hypertension. 2016;**38**(2):238-244. DOI: 10.3109/10641963.2015.1081231

[22] Peterson H, Laivuori H, Kerkelä E, Jiao H, Hiltunen L, Heino S, Tiala I, Knuutila S, Rasi V, Kere J, Kivinen K. ROCK2 allelic variants are not associated with pre-eclampsia susceptibility in the Finnish population. Molecular Human Reproduction. 2009;**15**(7):443-449. DOI: 10.1093/molehr/gap032

[23] Ross KA. Evidence for somatic gene conversion and deletion in bipolar disorder, Crohn's disease, coronary artery disease, hypertension, rheumatoid arthritis, type-1 diabetes, and type-2 diabetes. BMC Medicine. 2011;**9**:12. DOI: 10.1186/1741-7015-9-12

[24] Liao YC, Liu PY, Lin HF, Lin WY, Liao JK, Juo SH. Two functional polymorphisms of ROCK2 enhance arterial stiffening through inhibiting its activity and expression. Journal of Molecular and Cellular Cardiology. 2015;**79**:180-186. DOI: 10.1016/j.yjmcc.2014.11.023

[25] Yoo SY, Kim J, Cheong S, Shin DH, Jang J, Lee C, Tahk SJ, Shin JH, Choi SY, Yoon MH. Rho-associated kinase 2 polymorphism in patients with vasospastic angina. Korean Circulation Journal. 2012;**42**(6):406-413. DOI: 10.4070/kcj.2012.42.6.406

[26] Aksoy M, Uygun H, Baspinar O, Demiryurek S, Oztuzcu S, Cengiz B, Irdem A, Araz NC. Is there any association between childhood cardiac septal defects and ROCK2 gene polymorphism?. Genetics and Molecular Research. 2014;**13**(1):1949-1954. DOI: 10.4238/2014.March.17.22

[27] Palomino Doza J, Topf A, Bentham J, Bhattacharya S, Cosgrove C, Brook JD, Granados-Riveron J, Bu'Lock FA, O'Sullivan J, Stuart AG, Parsons J, Relton C, Goodship J, Henderson DJ, Keavney B. Low-frequency intermediate penetrance variants in the ROCK1 gene predispose to Tetralogy of Fallot. BMC Genetics. 2013;**14**:57. DOI: 10.1186/1471-2156-14-57

[28] Pehlivan Y, Yolbas S, Cetin GY, Alibaz-Oner F, Cagatay Y, Yilmaz N, Oztuzcu S, Donmez S, Ozgen M, Koca SS, Pamuk ON, Sayarlıoglu M, Kisacik B, Direskeneli H, Demiryurek AT, Onat AM. Investigation of the association between Rho/Rho-kinase gene polymorphisms and systemic sclerosis. Rheumatology International. 2016;**36**(3):421-427. DOI: 10.1007/s00296-015-3400-4

[29] Oguz E, Alasehirli B, Pehlivan Y, Onat AM, Oztuzcu S, Ozkara E, Kisacik B, Camci C, Demiryürek AT. Association between Rho-kinase (ROCK2) gene polymorphisms

and Behçet's disease. Translational Research. 2012;**160**(6):428-434. DOI: 10.1016/j.trsl.2012.08.002

[30] Oguz E, Demiryürek AT, Pehlivan Y, Kisacik B, Ozkara E, Oztuzcu S, Alasehirli B, Onat AM. Association of Rho-kinase 1 (ROCK1) gene polymorphisms with Behçet's disease. Molecular Diagnosis & Therapy. 2014;**18**(4):419-426. DOI: 10.1007/s40291-014-0092-5

[31] Demiryurek AT, Erbagci I, Oztuzcu S, Alasehirli B, Ozkara E, Seker M, Sönmez A, Ozsan M, Camci C. Lack of association between the Thr431Asn and Arg83Lys polymorphisms of the ROCK2 gene and diabetic retinopathy. Current Eye Research. 2010;**35**(12):1128-1134. DOI: 10.3109/02713683.2010.507903

[32] Demiryürek S, Okumus S, Bozgeyik İ, Oztuzcu S, Coskun E, Mat E, Durucu E, Tatar MG, Erbagci İ, Gürler B, Demiryürek AT. Investigation of the Rho-kinase gene polymorphism in primary open-angle glaucoma. Ophthalmic Genetics. 2016;**37**(1):9-13. DOI: 10.3109/13816810.2014.895016

[33] Zee RY, Wang QM, Chasman DI, Ridker PM, Liao JK. Gene variations of ROCKs and risk of ischaemic stroke: The Women's Genome Health Study. Clinical Science (Lond). 2014;**126**(12):829-835. DOI: 10.1042/CS20130652

[34] Tabur S, Oztuzcu S, Oguz E, Korkmaz H, Eroglu S, Ozkaya M, Demiryürek AT. Association of Rho/Rho-kinase gene polymorphisms and expressions with obesity-related metabolic syndrome. European Review for Medical and Pharmacological Sciences. 2015; **19**(9):1680-1688

[35] Kaya G, Sivasli E, Oztuzcu S, Melekoglu NA, Ozkara E, Sarikabadayi U, Demiryürek AT. Association of Rho-kinase gene polymorphisms with respiratory distress syndrome in preterm neonates. Pediatrics & Neonatology. 2017;**58**(1):36-42. DOI: 10.1016/j.pedneo.2015.12.006

[36] Yoshida T, Kato K, Yokoi K, Oguri M, Watanabe S, Metoki N, Yoshida H, Satoh K, Aoyagi Y, Nishigaki Y, Nozawa Y, Yamada Y. Association of genetic variants with chronic kidney disease in individuals with different lipid profiles. International Journal of Molecular Medicine. 2009;**24**(2):233-246. DOI: 10.3892/ijmm_00000226

[37] Rao F, Wessel J, Wen G, Zhang L, Rana BK, Kennedy BP, Greenwood TA, Salem RM, Chen Y, Khandrika S, Hamilton BA, Smith DW, Holstein-Rathlou NH, Ziegler MG, Schork NJ, O'Connor DT. Renal albumin excretion: Twin studies identify influences of heredity, environment, and adrenergic pathway polymorphism. Hypertension. 2007;**49**:1015-1031. DOI: 10.1161/HYPERTENSIONAHA.106.081679

[38] Gurocak S, Konac E, Ure I, Senol C, Onen IH, Sozen S, Menevse A. The impact of gene polymorphisms on the success of anticholinergic treatment in children with overactive bladder. Disease Markers. 2015;**2015**:732686. DOI: 10.1155/2015/732686

[39] Yigiter R, Bozkurt H, Oztuzcu S, Demiryürek S, Demir T, Uslu Kuzudisli S, Yilmaz M, Demiryürek AT. No evidence for an association between ROCK2 gene Thr431Asn

polymorphism and idiopathic generalized epilepsy: Preliminary findings. Journal of Neurological Sciences [Turkish]. 2013;**30**(3):494-501

[40] Uslu Kuzudisli S, Yilmaz M, Gül Z, Demiryürek S, Yigiter R, Bozkurt H, Akcali A, Neyal M, Bagci C, Cengiz B, Oztuzcu S, Demiryürek AT. Investigation of the Rho-kinase 2 gene Thr431Asn polymorphism in migraine. Neurology India. 2014;**62**(1):9-14. DOI: 10.4103/0028-3886.128241

[41] Pandey P, Mohammad G, Singh Y, Qadar Pasha MA. ROCK2 and MYLK variants under hypobaric hypoxic environment of high altitude associate with high altitude pulmonary edema and adaptation. The Application of Clinical Genetics. 2015;**8**:257-267. DOI: 10.2147/TACG.S90215

[42] Nakataki M, Numata S, Iga J, Tayoshi S, Tayoshi-Shibuya S, Song H, Tanahashi T, Itakura M, Ueno S, Ohmori T. No association between Rho-associated coiled-coil forming protein serine/threonine kinase1 gene and schizophrenia in the Japanese population. Psychiatric Genetics. 2009;**19**(3):162. DOI: 10.1097/YPG.0b013e32832a5030

[43] Alhopuro P, Sammalkorpi H, Niittymäki I, Biström M, Raitila A, Saharinen J, Nousiainen K, Lehtonen HJ, Heliövaara E, Puhakka J, Tuupanen S, Sousa S, Seruca R, Ferreira AM, Hofstra RM, Mecklin JP, Järvinen H, Ristimäki A, Orntoft TF, Hautaniemi S, Arango D, Karhu A, Aaltonen LA. Candidate driver genes in microsatellite-unstable colorectal cancer. International Journal of Cancer. 2012;**130**(7):1558-1566. DOI: 10.1002/ijc.26167

[44] Liu HW, Halayko AJ, Fernandes DJ, Harmon GS, McCauley JA, Kocieniewski P, McConville J, Fu Y, Forsythe SM, Kogut P, Bellam S, Dowell M, Churchill J, Lesso H, Kassiri K, Mitchell RW, Hershenson MB, Camoretti-Mercado B, Solway J. The RhoA/Rho kinase pathway regulates nuclear localization of serum response factor. American Journal of Respiratory Cell and Molecular Biology. 2003;**29**(1):39-47. DOI: 10.1165/rcmb.2002-0206OC

Chapter 7

Mitochondrial DNA Damage in Atherosclerosis

Igor A. Sobenin

Additional information is available at the end of the chapter

http://dx.doi.org/10.5772/intechopen.69622

Abstract

The defects in the mitochondrial genome are associated with different pathologies, including atherosclerosis. It is generally believed that atherosclerosis leads to premature cell senescence, but there is increasing evidence that cell senescence, the biomarker of which is the mutational load of mitochondrial genome, is itself a mechanistic factor of atherogenesis. The basic scientific problem addressed is an examination of functional consequences of mitochondrial DNA (mtDNA) damage based on the analysis of variability of mitochondrial genome. The paper is devoted to identification of genetic markers of mtDNA mutation burden, molecular and cellular markers of disorders in functional properties of cells arising from mutations in the mitochondrial genome, and identification of combinations of genetic markers that lead to violation of functional properties of human monocyte-macrophages. New data are presented, which resulted from whole genome sequencing of mtDNA from atherosclerotic lesions of arterial intima, the analysis of the relationship of mtDNA damage with the changes in cellular composition of arterial intima and expression of apoptosis- and inflammation-related genes, retrieving the data on mitochondrial genome variability in patients with atherosclerosis, and the study of functional activity of human blood monocytes differing substantially by the degree of mtDNA mutation burden.

Keywords: atherosclerosis, mitochondrial DNA, mitochondrial dysfunction, mutations, predisposition

1. Introduction

The defects in the mitochondrial genome are often associated with various human pathologies. There is the evidence that such a relationship can be in the case of atherosclerosis. The nature and the mechanisms of this association remain unclear. The basic scientific problem, to which the given chapter is aimed, is the study of functional consequences of mtDNA damage based on the analysis of variability of the mitochondrial genome. The disclosure of those associations will provide new knowledge on atherogenesis as an age-related degenerative pathological process and will create a basis for development of new approaches to the diagnosis, prevention, and treatment of atherosclerosis.

Chronic age-related degenerative diseases account for the major share of mortality in society. The most frequent pathology is atherosclerosis, which is classified as a typical disease of aging, and its prevalence in the elderly reaches 100%. It is generally believed that atherosclerosis leads to premature biological aging of cells, but there exists also the increasing evidence that cell aging, one of the indicators of which is the mutational load of mitochondrial genome, is a mechanistic factor of atherogenesis. In such a case, the association of mitochondrial DNA (mtDNA) variability with the disturbances in the functional properties of the artery wall cells participating in atherogenesis remains poorly understood. The results of the study of the association of mtDNA damage and functional properties of cells based on the analysis of the mitochondrial genome variability will make it possible to establish the features and patterns of the pathology of vascular aging and to justify the assumption that the prevention of accelerated cell aging is a therapeutic target in atherosclerosis.

Mammalian cells contain dozens, hundreds, and even thousands of mtDNA copies. It was previously assumed that all mtDNA molecules are identical at birth [1, 2]. However, later studies have shown that about 25% of healthy people inherit a mixture of wild-type and variant mtDNA (the phenomenon of heteroplasmy) and the latter may imply potentially pathogenic variants in the coding region of mtDNA [3, 4]. The mitochondrial genome is characterized by exaggerated instability, with an estimated mutation rate of at least 5–15 times higher than that of the nuclear genome. This is partly a result of proximity to the electron transport chain, which is the main intracellular source of free oxygen radicals, and partly due to relatively limited protection and reparation of mtDNA mechanisms [5]. The high frequency of mutations determines the high level of mtDNA variability, as well as the appearance of somatic mutations of mtDNA with the aging of human organism [6]. The proportion of mutant copies of mtDNA carrying both inherited and somatic mutations may be changed during lifetime due to unequal separation of mitochondrial genotypes during cytokinesis in dividing cells (vegetative segregation) or in nondividing cells during mtDNA replication. An increase in the degree of heteroplasmy represents a kind of "clonal expansion" of low-level inherited variants, which occurs due to preferential replication of mtDNA carrying certain types of mutations [7]. Exceeding the critical threshold level of the degree of heteroplasmy of pathogenic mutations in the cell is manifested by biochemical defects in the mitochondrial respiratory chain [8]. The high level of mtDNA mutations manifests itself in the form of multi-system mitochondrial diseases [9] and degenerative age-related diseases and undoubtedly contributes to biological aging processes [10].

The basic scientific problem addressed by this chapter is an examination of functional consequences of mitochondrial DNA (mtDNA) damage based on the analysis of variability of mitochondrial genome. The described results are devoted to identification of genetic markers of mutational load of mitochondrial genome, molecular and cellular mechanisms of disorders in functional properties of cells arising from mutations in the mitochondrial genome, and identification of combinations of genetic markers that lead to violation of functional properties of human monocyte-macrophages.

2. The markers of mitochondrial DNA mutation load in atherosclerotic lesions

It has been shown earlier that several mutations of mitochondrial genome have significantly higher prevalence and mean value in lipofibrous plaques as compared to non-atherosclerotic intima and therefore are associated with atherosclerosis [11–13].

In continuation of the above studies, the samples of human thoracic aorta (32 samples, 19 men, 13 women aged 53–78 years old) were taken at autopsy performed within 6–16 h after sudden death. After macroscopic identification of unaffected and atherosclerotic areas of the aorta (initial lesions, fatty streaks, lipofibrous and fibrous plaques), autopsy aortic samples (2 × 2 cm, 4–9 sites per autopsy sample) were excised for further studies. In addition, five aortas were subjected to complete morphological mapping, that is, from whole samples approximately 8 × 12 cm in size, 25–56 sites differing by the degree of atherosclerotic lesion were obtained. The total of 297 samples was obtained. Histological and immunocytochemical analysis of the samples was carried out; DNA and RNA were isolated from aortic intima. For the analysis of mtDNA mutations, the pyrosequencing technology was used.

The analysis of heteroplasmy of mitochondrial genome of cells from unaffected and atherosclerotic regions of aortic intima was performed for 42 mutations previously known from the MITOMAP database (m.652delG, m.652insG, m. 716T>G, m. 750A>G, m.961insC, m. 961delC, M.1555A>G, m.3256C>T, m.3258T>C, m.3271T>C, m.3280A>G, m.3285C>T, m. 3316G>A, m.3336T>C, m. 5132insAA, m.5178C>A, m.5540G>A, m.5692T>C, m.5814T>C, m.6489C>A, m.8362T>G, m.8363G>A, m.8993T>G, M.8993T>C, m.9379G>A, m.9480del15, m. 9537insC, m.12315G>A, m.13513G>A, m.14459G>A, m.14482C>G, m.14482C>A, M.14484T>C, m.14487T>C, m.14709T>C, m.14846G>A, m.15059G>A, m.15084G>A, m.15452C>A, m.15498del24, m.15723G>A, and m.15762G>A). Thus, most of the mitochondrial DNA genes encoding enzymes (9 of 13) were covered, except for the *MT-CO2* (subunit II of cytochrome oxidase C), *MT-ND3* (subunit 3 of dihydronicotinamide adenine dinucleotide (NADH) dehydrogenase), and *MT-ND4L* and *MT-ND4* (subunits 4L and 4 of NADH dehydrogenases). Seven of the 22 genes encoding transport RNA and *MT-RNR1* gene encoding 12S ribosomal RNA were also covered. Forty examined mutations were heteroplasmic, and two (m.8362T>G and m.8363G>A) were homoplasmic by the absence of a mutant allele in atherosclerotic lesions.

The analysis showed that mtDNA variants m.652delG, m.3256C>T, m.12315G>A, m.14459G>A, and m.15059G>A were significantly associated with the lipofibrous plaque ($p < 0.05$), and for m.13513G>A and m.14846G>A, the association was significant at the level of $p < 0.1$. Variants m.1555A>G and m.5178C>A were antiatherosclerotic with respect to lipofibrous plaque at $p < 0.05$. In addition to formal statistical analysis, the approach was used where the prevalence was used to determine the difference between the indices of heteroplasmy in normal and atherosclerotic lesions in samples obtained from the same donor of autopsy material. As a result, 11 mtDNA mutations belonging to 8 mitochondrial genes were detected, those encoding 12S rRNA; tRNA-Leu (UUR recognition codon); tRNA-Leu (CUN recognition codon); subunits 1, 2, 5, and 6 of NADH dehydrogenase; and cytochrome B, which were associated with lipofibrous plaques [12–14]. To evaluate the relationship of these mtDNA variants identified as potential markers of atherosclerosis, the study was performed on the autopsy material with complete morphological and mutational mapping.

It was found that the same mtDNA variants associated with the advanced atherosclerotic lesions are also associated with the initial atherosclerotic lesions (fatty dots and fatty streaks). The mutation m.13513G>A was antiatherosclerotic, as it correlated negatively with the degree of atherosclerotic lesion. Mutation m.1555A>G negatively correlated with initial atherosclerotic lesions and lipofibrous plaques ($p < 0.05$), and mutation m.14846G>A—with lipofibrous plaques. Lipofibrous and fibrous plaques tended to positive correlation with m.652delG mutation at $p < 0.1$, which being absent in unaffected intima and in the initial atherosclerotic lesions. The presence of fibrous plaques positively correlated with mtDNA mutations m.3256C>T and m.5178C>A and negatively correlated with m.12315G>A [14].

To determine the relationship between the mutational load and the degree of atherosclerotic lesion, a linear regression analysis was performed. For each mutation in each aorta, the distribution of the heteroplasmy level was assessed, and interquartile boundaries were determined. When estimating the integral mutation burden for 11 mutations, the linear regression model reached statistical significance at $p < 0.001$. Given the sufficient number of degrees of freedom, it can be assumed that the degree of atherosclerotic lesion is associated with integral mutation burden caused by these mutations at 99.9% probability of error-free prediction. The sensitivity and specificity for each of the mutations associated with atherosclerosis were studied. The analysis was carried out by constructing receiver operating characteristic (ROC) curves with subsequent measurement of the area under the curve, which allowed to describe the explanatory properties of genetic markers. For this analysis, the rank values (quartile numbers) of the heteroplasmy were summed according to the sign of the beta coefficient obtained in the regression analysis. The obtained parameter was assumed as mutation burden. Using this model, sensitivity was 88.2% ($p < 0.05$, 95% confidence interval from 74.6 to 95.3). The specificity was 77.1% ($p < 0.05$, 95% confidence interval from 70.8 to 87.3). Thus, the integral mutation burden assessed by 11 mtDNA variants was associated with 88.2% of the cases of atherosclerotic lesions in the morphologically mapped aortas [14].

Further, whole genome sequencing of mtDNA from unaffected and atherosclerotic intima of the thoracic aorta, obtained in autopsy (11 cases) within 6–16 h after sudden death, was carried out using next-generation sequencing (NGS) technology on the Roche 454 GS Junior Titanium platform (Roche Applied Science, USA). The following samples were analyzed: unaffected areas of intima ($n = 12$), initial lesions ($n = 14$), fatty streaks ($n = 15$), lipofibrous plaques ($n = 13$), and fibrous plaques ($n = 12$). The following parameters were achieved: the mean reading length, 458 bp; the mean number of readings, 18,734; and the mean number of nucleotides read in one sample, 8.65 million bp. The mean percent of mapped readings reached 93%. To detect heteroplasmic mutations of mtDNA, sequences with more than 300-fold coverage of the mitochondrial genome were taken, thus allowing reliable detection of mutations with a level of heteroplasmy of at least 1% in the presence of direct and reverse readings of the mutant allele.

It has been established that the mitochondrial genome has a significant individual variability and has a much larger number of heteroplasmic mutations than was previously assumed in the literature. Most mitochondrial DNA mutations found by whole genome sequencing had a low degree of heteroplasmy, but the results of the analysis suggest that there are both general and individual variants associated with atherosclerotic lesions [15].

Thus, heteroplasmic mtDNA mutations associated with atherosclerotic lesions were identified by NGS, and the integral mutation burden of the mitochondrial genome was assessed. Ten heteroplasmic mutations of mtDNA were detected that occurred simultaneously in different parts of the intima of the aorta (m.368A>G, m.751delA, m.8404T>C, m.8485G>C, m.9720delT, m.10663delT, m.14160G>A, m.14207delG, m.16086T>C, and m.16389G>A). The level of heteroplasmy of these mutations ranged from 2 to 26%, with more than half of the values not exceeding 6%. Among the heteroplasmic mutations found, the majority occurred in the coding region, namely, in the mitochondrial 12S-RNA genes, the ATP synthase subunit 8, the cytochrome oxidase subunits 3 and 4L, and the NADH dehydrogenase subunit 6. One mutation was synonymous, and the rest were either deletions or missense mutations. For mutations occurring in genes encoding mitochondrial respiratory chain proteins, the levels of heteroplasmy did not exceed 15%, while mutations in the hypervariable segment 1 (HVS1) and in adjacent noncoding region were characterized by heteroplasmy values of 20–26% [15].

The distribution of mtDNA mutations in various parts of the aortic intima was of a mosaic nature, and in some cases, even neighboring parts of the intima were characterized by different compositions of heteroplasmic mutations. Unaffected areas of the intima and areas with initial lesions (fatty dots) were characterized by an almost complete absence of heteroplasmic mutations of mtDNA. In areas with fatty streaks and fibrous and lipofibrous plaques, heteroplasmic variants were more common, and the levels of heteroplasmy increased. The highest frequency of heteroplasmic mutations was found in lipofibrous plaques, while in areas with fatty streaks in close proximity to lipofibrous plaques, an increased frequency of mutations was also observed. The fact of the presence of heteroplasmic deletions, previously not described in the literature (m.9720delT, m.10663delT, and m.14207delG in the coding region of mtDNA with a level of heteroplasmy up to 15%), was revealed. Because of the reading frame shift, the presence of deletions in mtDNA should lead to completely defective synthesis of the mtDNA-encoded proteins, and the level of heteroplasmy at a 15% for deletion means that the synthesis of respiratory chain proteins should be reduced by 15%. It should be noted that heteroplasmic deletions in the coding region of mtDNA were detected only in fatty streaks and lipofibrous plaques. As an example, the distribution of m.9720delT mutation, the deletion in the gene encoding cytochrome oxidase subunit 3, may be described: it was found with a similar level of heteroplasmy (12–15%) only in areas with fatty streaks and lipofibrous plaques, located relatively close to each other [15].

Taking into account the results of pyrosequencing and whole genome sequencing of mtDNA, the genes were identified, the damage of which due to point mutations is observed in atherosclerotic lesions, and heteroplasmic mtDNA mutations were revealed being associated with atherosclerotic lesions: m.368A>G (*MT-HV2* gene, hypervariable segment 2), M.652delG, m.751delA, m.1555A>G (*MT-RNR1* gene, 12S ribosomal RNA), m.3256C>T

(*MT-TL1* gene, leucine tRNA-recognition codon L-UUA/G), m.5178C>A (*MT-ND2* gene, subunit 2 of NADH dehydrogenase), m.8404T>C, m.8485G>C (*MT-ATP8* gene, subunit 8 ATP synthase F0), m.9720delT (*MT-CO3* gene, subunit III of cytochrome C oxidase), m.10663delT (*MT-ND4L* gene, subunit 4L NADH dehydrogenase), m.12315G>A (*MT-TL2* gene, leucine tRNA-L-CUN recognition codon), m.13513G>A (*MT-ND5* gene, subunit 5 NADH dehydrogenase), m.14160G>A, m.14207delG, m.14459G>A (*MT-ND6* gene, subunit 6 NADH dehydrogenase), m.14846G>A (*MT-CYB* gene, cytochrome b), m.16086T>C (*MT-HV1* gene, hypervariable segment 1), and m.16389G>A (*MT-7SDNA* gene, 7S DNA). It has been established that the best indicator of the association between mtDNA mutant variants and the type of atherosclerotic lesion is integral (total) mutation burden, which belongs to the below-described pattern of the first type (bell-shaped relationship with the type of atherosclerotic lesion with the maximum at fatty types of lesions—fatty streaks and lipofibrous plaques).

3. Cellular composition of atherosclerotic lesions

The use of a set of antibodies covering most of the cells found in the intima made it possible to characterize the qualitative and quantitative changes that occur with resident intimal cells and cells of hematogenous origin in the same site of the vessel. By the results of immunocytochemical typing, the proportion of smooth muscle cells containing α-actin was determined, which was about half of the total cell population in both normal and atherosclerotic intima. In the row "unaffected intima—initial lesions—fatty streak—lipofibrous plaque—fibrous plaque," the proportion of cells expressing smooth muscle α-actin was 46.7% (SD = 9.8), 47.2% (SD = 7.9), 42.2% (SD = 9.2), 47.0% (SD = 9.9), and 42.4% (SD = 9.0), respectively. Accordingly, the rest of the cells (about 50% of the total population) could not be identified with this smooth muscle cell marker. About two-thirds of the cells of the muscular-elastic intimal sublayer were positively stained with anti-smooth muscle α-actin antibodies, whereas in the proteoglycan (subendothelial) intimal sublayer, the percentage of cells containing α-actin was significantly lower. Cells of hematogenous origin (lymphocytes and macrophages) were localized only in the subendothelial part of the intima in the proteoglycan sublayer. Their proportion increased in atherosclerotic lesions and accounted for about 20% of all cells. The percentage of cells expressing CD68, the antigen of macrophages, increased with the progression of atherosclerotic lesion: 3.9% (SD = 1.7), 6.1% (SD = 6.3), 13.2% (SD = 3.2), 13.1% (SD = 6.3), and 18.2% (SD = 8.8), respectively [16].

Resident intimal cells also expressed antigens uncommon for the typical smooth muscle cells of intima media. In areas with advanced atherosclerotic lesions (fatty streaks and lipofibrous and fibrous plaques), the cells expressing 2A7 antigen characteristic for pericytes from active regions of angiogenesis were present. In unaffected intima, such cells could not be identified. The proportion of cells expressing the antigen of activated pericytes (2A7) increased with the progression of atherosclerotic lesion in the row "unaffected intima—initial lesions—fatty streak—lipofibrous plaque—fibrous plaque": 0.0% (SD = 0.2), 1.2% (SD = 1.3), 3.0% (SD = 2.8), 27.0% (SD = 9.9), and 24.0% (SD = 8.6). The maximum proportion of 2A7-positive cells was reached in the lipofibrous plaques. In addition to antibodies against 2A7 antigen, antipericytic antibodies 3G5 characteristic for resting pericytes were used. In atherosclerotic lesions, the number of cells expressing 3G5 antigen was significantly less than in intact intima. The proportion of cells expressing 3G5 antigen decreased with progression of atherosclerotic lesion in the row "unaffected intima—initial lesions—fatty streak—lipofibrous plaque—fibrous plaque": 31.3% (SD = 7.0), 16.3% (SD = 4.5), 11.7% (SD = 8.0), 5.0% (SD = 2.8), and 3.9% (SD = 3.6). The total number of cells expressing antigens 2A7 and 3G5 remained relatively constant, but their ratio varied. The total number of 3G5-positive cells and 2A7-positive cells was about 30% of the entire cell population in the areas of unaffected intima and atherosclerotic plaques. In the initial lesions and fatty streaks, the number of resting and activated pericytes was a smaller part. This pattern of expression of two pericyte antigens allows us to assume that when atherosclerotic lesions are formed, the functional state of the pericyte-like cells of the proteoglycan intima sublayer changes, accompanied by a change in the antigens that they express. With double immunocytochemical staining, the CD68 antigen of macrophages was expressed not only in cells of hematogenic origin but also in some resident subendothelial cells. This suggests that the presence of CD68 antigen is not only a sign of monocytic origin of cells but also a marker of their phagocytic activity, which increases when atherosclerotic lesions are formed [16].

Thus, smooth muscle cells, macrophages, and lymphocytes are present both in unaffected arterial intima and in the areas of atherosclerotic lesions. In contrast to popular beliefs, no predominance of monocyte-macrophages among cells inhabiting atherosclerotic lesion has been detected. There is a special type of cells expressing pericytic antigens, the number of which constitutes a significant proportion of intimal cells. Pericyte-like cells, together with smooth muscle cells, represent the majority of cellular population of subendothelial intima. In the areas of atherosclerotic lesion, the behavior of pericyte-like cells changes—they capture lipids and begin to proliferate. This is accompanied by a change in expression of antigens specific for pericytes.

4. Expression of apoptosis-related genes in atherosclerotic lesions

In the aortic intima samples differing by the degree of atherosclerotic lesion, the mRNA expression level of several genes associated with apoptosis (*CASP3, CASP9, ENO1, NTN1, NTN4,* and *UNC5A)* was analyzed. The level of gene expression was evaluated by qPCR.

A monotonous decrease in the expression level of the mRNA of the *CASP3* gene depending on the degree of atherosclerotic lesion was observed. Maximum *CASP3* expression was in unaffected intima, the minimum—in fibrous plaques ($p = 0.0018$). The significant difference was found in the expression of the *CASP3* gene in fibrous plaque from that in unaffected areas ($p = 0.041$) and initial lesions ($p = 0.019$), but when compared with fatty streaks and lipofibrous plaques, statistically significant differences were not observed ($p = 0.098$ and $p = 0.061$, respectively). In a pairwise comparison of all other types of atherosclerotic lesions, there was no statistically significant difference in the expression of the mRNA of the *CASP3* gene. Significant correlation of *CASP3* gene expression in unaffected intima and initial lesions was shown (r = 0.643, p = 0.018), as well as in fatty streaks and lipofibrous plaques (r = 0.593, p = 0.033). The expression of the *CASP9* gene did not practically change in all types of atherosclerotic lesions when compared to unaffected areas, except for fatty streaks, where the expression level was almost doubled (p = 0.084, p = 0.030, p = 0.002, and p = 0.046 when compared to the unaffected intima, initial lesions, lipofibrous plaque, and fibrous plaque, respectively). In the samples of fatty streaks and lipofibrous plaques, a significant correlation of the expression of the *CASP9* gene was noted (r = 0.933, p = 0.031) [16].

It was found that the level of expression of the *ENO1* gene increased in areas with severe atherosclerotic lesions (lipofibrous and fibrous plaques) at p = 0.021. In the initial types of atherosclerotic lesions, the expression of the mRNA of the *ENO1* gene did not differ significantly from that in the intact intima (p = 0.916 and p = 0.209 for the initial lesions and fatty streaks, respectively). When comparing the level of expression in lipofibrous plaques and atherosclerotic lesions, no statistically significant differences were found (p = 0.114). However, when compared with unaffected areas and initial atherosclerotic lesions, the expression of the mRNA of the *ENO1* gene significantly increased (p = 0.046 and p = 0.028 for the initial lesions and fatty streaks, respectively). The change in the level of expression of the *ENO1* gene in lipofibrous and fibrous plaques did not reach statistical significance (p = 0.080). The significant correlation was found for mRNA expression of *ENO1* gene in unaffected areas and initial lesions (r = 0.618, p = 0.024), unaffected areas and fatty streaks (r = 0.818, p = 0.001), initial lesions and fatty streaks (r = 0.655, p = 0.011), initial lesions and lipofibrous plaques (r = 0.554, p = 0.040), as well as for fatty streaks and lipofibrous plaques (r = 0.629, p = 0.021). It was found that the expression level of the mRNA of the *NTN1* gene is practically the same in unaffected intima and initial lesions (p = 0.929), and in the fatty streaks it increases insignificantly (p = 0.239, p = 0.817 when compared with the unaffected tissue and initial lesions, respectively). A sharp decrease in the expression of the *NTN1* gene was observed in lipofibrous plaques (p = 0.014, p = 0.004, and p = 0.016 when compared with intact unaffected intima, initial lesions, and fatty streaks, respectively), as well as in fibrous plaques (p = 0.016, p = 0.006, and p = 0.050 when compared with unaffected intima, initial lesions, and fatty streaks, respectively). When comparing the expression of the mRNA of the *NTN1* gene in lipofibrous and fibrous plaques, no statistically significant differences were revealed (p = 0.490). A significant correlation of the level of expression of the NTN1 gene in unaffected areas and initial lesions (r = 0.888, $p < 0.001$), as well as in unchanged intima and fatty streaks (r = 0.674, p = 0.016), was found.

There were no significant changes in the level of expression of the mRNA of the *NTN4* gene in all the types of atherosclerotic lesions examined in comparison with unaffected intima. The significant correlation of *NTN4* gene expression in unaffected intima and initial lesions (r = 0.775, p = 0.002) and initial lesions and fatty streaks (r = 0.592, p = 0.033) was revealed. The expression profile of the *UNC5A* gene resembled the changes in the expression level of the mRNA of the *CAPS9* and *NTN1* genes. The highest level of expression was observed in the areas of fatty streaks, while in the areas of unaffected intima, initial lesions, and lipofibrous plaques, the level of mRNA expression did not practically change. The lowest level of expression was observed in fibrous plaques. Statistically significant changes in the expression of *UNC5A* gene mRNA were observed in fibrous and lipofibrous plaques (p = 0.046), in fibrous plaques and fatty streaks (p = 0.025), as well as in fibrous plaques and initial lesions

($p = 0.016$). A significant correlation of the expression level of the *UNC5A* gene in the initial lesions and fatty streaks ($r = 0.827$, $p < 0.001$), initial lesions and lipofibrous plaques ($r = 0.833$, $p < 0.001$), fatty streaks and lipofibrous plaques ($r = 0.744$, $p < 0.001$), and lipofibrous and fibrous plaques ($r = 0.961$, $p = 0.009$) was observed.

The presented data of immunocytochemical analysis of changes in cellular composition in atherosclerotic lesions can partly explain the patterns of changes in the expression of apoptosis-related genes. It can be assumed that if the most significant changes in the cellular composition, namely, an increase in the proportion of cells of hematogenic origin, are observed in atherosclerotic plaques, the activation of pericyte-like cells is accompanied by corresponding changes in the expression of *CASP3, CASP9, ENO1, NTN1* and *UNC5A* genes. Reduction in the expression of *CASP3, NTN1,* and *UNC5A* genes may be due to the predominance of necrotic processes and cell death in atherosclerotic plaques. Although cell death in atherosclerosis occurs in several ways (necrosis, autophagy, and apoptosis), the latter mechanism is best described for the processes of cellular aging. Apoptosis is believed to be increased not only in senescent vascular cells but also in smooth muscle cells and other types of cells that inhabit atherosclerotic plaques. Thus, it is believed that the majority of cell deaths occurring in necrotic zones of plaques are associated with apoptosis. However, there are discrepancies such as a decrease in the expression of apoptotic biomarkers in advanced atherosclerotic lesions, which is explained by the hypothesis that many apoptotic cells lose their key markers of origin, which complicates their precise identification. Nevertheless, we consider the possibility that the changes in the expression of apoptosis-related genes in atherosclerosis are much more dependent on changes in the composition of cells than on loss of markers by aged cells.

5. Expression of inflammation-related genes in atherosclerosis

The expression of genes associated with inflammation (*TNF-α, CCL18, CD14, IL-1β, CASP1,* and *APAF-1*) was measured and analyzed. The results of qPCR analysis showed that both in the intact intima of the human aorta and in atherosclerotic lesions, expression of the pro-inflammatory cytokine TNF-α and anti-inflammatory cytokine/chemokine CCL18 is observed. Quantitative differences are observed between the values obtained for unaffected and atherosclerotic regions. In the unaffected intima, the values obtained for both cytokines did not differ. However, even in the initial lesion, the expression level of CCL18 was 2.6% relatively to the reference housekeeping genes, whereas for TNF-α, it did not reach 2%. In advanced fatty lesions, the gap between the values for both cytokines increased. Thus, in the fatty streaks, the expression level of CCL18 was approximately 10%, and of TNF-α, it was 1.8%; in the lipofibrous plaque, the expression levels were 11.4% and 1.8%, respectively. In the fibrous plaque, the level of expression of the studied genes was reduced, but the differences for pro-inflammatory and anti-inflammatory cytokines remained, accounting for 7.4% for CCL18 and 1.1% for TNF-α, respectively. Similar changes in fibrotic plaques can be explained by a decrease in cellularity in this type of lesion. The bell-shaped dependence of mRNA expression of *TNF-α* gene on the type of atherosclerotic lesion was found with a maximum attributable to early fatty lesions (in the initial lesions, 2.1-fold increase in expression, and in fatty streaks and lipofibrous plaques, 1.9-fold increase). The mRNA expression of the pro-inflammatory cytokine *TNF-α* gene in fibrous plaques was not significantly different from that in unaffected regions. The bell-shaped dependence was observed for the expression of the mRNA of the anti-inflammatory chemokine *CCL18* gene (2.2-fold increase in expression in the initial lesions, 7.6-fold increase in fatty streaks, 9.4-fold in lipofibrous plaques, and 5-fold increase in fibrous plaques). In all types of atherosclerotic lesions, the expression of the mRNA of the *CCL18* gene was significantly higher than in the intact intimal.

Rather poorly expressed bell-shaped dependence was observed for the expression of the mRNA of the *CD14* gene (the marker of monocytes migrated into intima from the blood). In the initial lesions, the *CD14* gene expression did not increase: in fatty streaks it increased by 2.3-fold; in lipofibrous plaques, by 1.8-fold; and in fibrous plaques, by 1.6-fold. The expression of *IL-1β* gene mRNA, in whole, increased steadily as the degree of atherosclerotic lesion increased: in the initial lesions, expression was increased by 9.6-fold; in fatty streaks, by 5.6-fold; in lipofibrous plaques, by 10.3-fold; and in fibrous plaques, by 26.0-fold. The expression of the mRNA of the *CASP1* gene was relatively stable in the initial lesions and fatty streaks and did not change significantly in comparison with the unaffected areas, but decreased in advanced atherosclerotic lesions: in lypofibrous plaques by 1.9-fold and in fibrous plaques by 2.2-fold as compared to the norm. The mRNA expression of the *APAF-1* gene was relatively stable in the initial lesions, fatty streaks, and lipofibrous plaques but was significantly decreased in fibrous plaques—by 1.6 times—as compared to the norm. There was no significant relationship between the levels of mRNA expression of *IL-1β*, *CASP1*, and *APAF-1* genes and the degree of atherosclerotic lesion.

6. Interaction of mitochondrial DNA mutation burden, cellular composition, and expression of apoptosis- and inflammation-related genes in atherosclerotic lesions

An analysis was made to examine the relationship between the mtDNA variability, the qualitative and quantitative changes in intimal cell composition that occur in atherosclerosis, and the expression of apoptosis- and inflammation-related genes. The analysis used an adaptive neural network model based on artificial neural networks and the theory of neuro-fuzzy interactions [17]. It was found that there are rather similar but interdependent patterns of association of variables with the type of atherosclerotic lesion. The pattern of the first type (the bell-shaped relationship with the maximum for fatty lesions) combines and similarly characterizes the mRNA expression of *CAPS9*, *NTN1*, and *UNC5A* apoptosis-related genes; the mRNA expression of the *TNF-α*, *CCL18*, and *CD14* inflammation-related genes; the CDLC+/CD14+ cells of the hematogenic origin; the degree of heteroplasmy by mtDNA variants m.1555A>G, m.14846G>A, m.14459G>A, m.751delA, m.8485G>C, m.9720delT, m.10663delT, m.8404T>C, and m.14207delG; as well as the total mutation burden of the mitochondrial genome. The pattern of the second type (the increase with the maximum attributable to fibrotic lesions) combines and similarly characterizes the mRNA expression of the apoptosis-related gene

ENO1, the mRNA expression of the *IL-1β* inflammation-related gene, the content of CD68+ cells of hematogenic origin and 2A7+ pericyte-like cells, and the degree of heteroplasmy for mtDNA variants m.652delG, m.3256C>T, m.5178C>A, m.14160G>A, m.16086T>C, m.368A>G, and m.16389G>A. The pattern of the third type (reduction with a minimum occurring in the fibrotic type of lesion) combines and similarly characterizes the mRNA expression of the *CAPS9* apoptosis-related gene and partly the *NTN1* and *UNC5A* genes (the two indicators belong to two patterns), the mRNA expression of the inflammation-related genes *CASP1* and *APAF-1*, the content of 3G5+ pericyte-like cells, and the degree of heteroplasmy for mtDNA variants m.13513G>A and m.12315G>A. The pattern of the fourth type (lack of interrelation or disordered neuro-fuzzy association of parameters with the type of lesion) combines and similarly characterizes the mRNA expression of the apoptosis-related gene *NTN4*, in part the mRNA expression of the *CASP1* inflammation-related gene (belonging to the two patterns), smooth muscle actin α-positive resident cells, and the degree of heteroplasmy for mtDNA variants m.716T>G, m.3316G>A, m.3336C>T, m.5132delAA, m.6489C>A, m.9379G>A, m.9480del15, m.14482C>G, and m.14487T>C.

Thus, at least three groups of nonequilibrium interactions were identified: between the mtDNA mutation burden and mRNA expression of *TNF-α*, *CCL18*, and *CASP9* genes; between cell composition and mRNA expression of *TNF-α*, *CCL18*, *ENO1*, and *UNC5A* genes; and between the mtDNA mutation burden and the cellular composition, in particular, the ratio of 2A7- and 3G5-positive cells.

7. Mitochondrial genome variability and subclinical atherosclerosis

The study of the degree of mtDNA heteroplasmy by detected atherosclerosis-related mutations was performed in nonrelative women. At the first stage of the study, 183 apparently healthy women were screened. Study participants had no clinical manifestations of cardiovascular diseases, and an ultrasonographic examination of carotid arteries was performed, followed by a quantitative measurement of carotid intima-media thickness (cIMT). The participants of the study were genotyped for 37 heteroplasmic mtDNA variants. In this study, five mutations of the mitochondrial genome m.3256C>T, m.14709G>A, m.12315G>A, m.13513G>A, and m.14846G>A were in focus, and the level of heteroplasmy was associated with the degree of preclinical atherosclerosis. The total mutation burden of the mitochondrial genome assessed by these mutations accounted for 68% of the cIMT variability, while the combination of conventional risk factors for cardiovascular disease accounted for only 8% of the variability of cIMT. Data were obtained on the correlation of the degree of heteroplasmy in these mutations with each other, which indicated the predominantly hereditary nature of these mutations, as well as the existence of proatherosclerotic haplotypes of the mitochondrial genome [18].

Further, those women with a high mtDNA mutation burden, who were asked to participate in genetic screening of the maternal relatives, were selected. In total, 37 families (1 family of 4 generations, 27 families of 3 generations, 7 families of 2 generations) were examined. Monocytes were isolated from the mononuclear fraction by affinity separation using magnetic

CD14 affinity microparticles on LS Separation Columns (Miltenyi Biotec, Germany). Genotyping was carried out on heteroplasmic variants m.1555A>G, m.5178C>A, m.3256C>T, m.13513G>A, m.12315G>A, m.14846G>A, and m.15059G>A. The choice of mtDNA variants was due to their high occurrence and the level of heteroplasmy sufficient for evaluation in the mathematical model of inheritance of mutations. Heteroplasmy of mtDNA by selected variants was determined by qPCR. The probability of the hereditary nature of these variants was calculated, as well as the probability that the above variants are mutations that arise in any generation and may be transmitted by the maternal line with accumulation from generation to generation.

When analyzing the results of genotyping mtDNA samples from maternal relatives, it was established that the probability of hereditary nature of variant m.1555A>G approximates to 100%; m.5178C>A, 100%; m.3256C>T, 92%; m.13513G>A, 99%; m.12315G>A, 99%; m.14846G>A, 100%; and m.15059G>A, 96%. The probability that the above variants may be somatic arising in any generation, for variant m.1555A>G accounted for 8%; m.5178C>A, for 5%; m.3256C>T, for 19%; m.13513G>A, for 10%; m.12315G>A, for 12%; m.14846G>A, for 4%; and m.15059G>A, for 11%. Thus, the prevalent variants of the mitochondrial genome are thought to be heritable with a high degree of probability.

The differences in the degree of mtDNA heteroplasmy in various types of blood cells (monocytes, neutrophils, lymphocytes, platelets, and the total fraction of leukocytes) obtained from non-related individuals were studied. Seventy-one study participants (32 men, 39 women) were examined. The leukocyte fraction of cells was obtained from the whole citrated blood by gradient centrifugation using Ficoll-Paque (GE Healthcare Life Sciences, UK). Blood cells of various types were isolated from the leukocyte fraction by affinity separation using magnetic affinity microparticles on LS Separation Columns (Miltenyi Biotec, Germany). Heteroplasmy of mitochondrial genome was determined by pyrosequencing of short-chain mtDNA fragments by mtDNA variants m.13513G>A, m.3256C>T, m.3336T>C, m.12315G>A, and m.1555A>G. There were no significant differences in the level of heteroplasmy of these mutations studied between different types of blood cells from the same participant within the study. The only statistically significant difference was observed between neutrophils and lymphocytes by mutation m.1555A>G. The obtained data indicate that these mutations are not accumulated during differentiation of blood cells, but more probably are inherent in the progenitor cells in the bone marrow. Thus, for the studies of single nucleotide substitutions of mtDNA in various pathologies, it is possible to use whole fraction of white blood cells rather than certain types of them [19].

Further, the variability of mtDNA from blood leukocytes was evaluated by NGS (Roche 454 GS Junior Titanium platform) in a sample of 80 non-related study participants (37 healthy individuals and 43 patients with subclinical carotid atherosclerosis, the diagnosis being established by ultrasound scanning of the common carotid arteries and measurement of cIMT). Arterial hypertension, diabetes mellitus, and myocardial infarction were criteria of exclusion in sample formation. Despite of the relatively low percentage of mapped readings during sequencing, the mean 70-fold mitochondrial genome coverage was provided sufficiently to detect single nucleotide substitutions. The possibility of sequencing using Roche 454 technology made it possible to determine as accurately as possible the haplogroup of the mitochondrial genome, considering all single nucleotide substitutions throughout the mtDNA. As a result, mitochondrial haplogroups H, U, T, and J were the most common (85.7% of cases), which corresponds to general data from the Russian population. Haplogroups I, W, R, and D were represented only among persons with preclinical atherosclerosis. In turn, haplogroups N, V, and M were found only among apparently healthy individuals. When calculating the odds ratio for preclinical atherosclerosis, it was established that belonging to haplogroup H is associated with an increased risk of atherosclerosis ($\chi^2 = 3.97$, $p = 0.046$, OR = 2.76, 95% confidence interval 1.01–7.58). Belonging to haplogroups T and U was associated with reduced risk of subclinical carotid atherosclerosis (OR = 0.31 and OR = 0.57, respectively). The increased risk of atherosclerosis and its clinical manifestations (e.g., myocardial infarction) in representatives of haplogroup H may be associated with the differences in the functional activity of mitochondria [20, 21].

According to the data of whole mtDNA sequencing, the list of variants of the mitochondrial genome presumably determining the individual genetic predisposition to atherosclerosis was compiled. The methodology used to assess the variability of the mitochondrial genome as a marker of predisposition to atherosclerosis involved the use of data on the presence of 12 mtDNA variants and considered the calculation of the cumulative mutation burden for those mtDNA variants.

The ROC analysis was performed to assess the diagnostic effectiveness of this method for estimating the total mutation burden of mtDNA to determine the predisposition to atherosclerosis. The following results were obtained: the area under the curve was 0.791, sensitivity of the test was 73.3%, and specificity of the test was 75.0%. The accuracy of the method was 74.0%, the proportion of true positive results was 42.9%, and the proportion of true negative results was 31.1%. The odds ratio for the risk of atherosclerosis was 8.25 (95% confidence interval 2.9–23.29), and the relative risk was 2.41. The relationship between mtDNA variants and their combinations with atherosclerosis, conventional risk factors for cardiovascular diseases, and age-gender variation was characterized. There were no significant differences between the mean values of blood lipids, both between persons belonging to different haplogroups and between groups with the presence and absence of preclinical atherosclerosis. Nevertheless, the mean value of low-density lipoprotein (LDL) to high-density lipoprotein (HDL) ratio in the group of patients with preclinical atherosclerosis was slightly increased in comparison with healthy subjects (3.0 ± 1.7 versus 2.7 ± 1.1, $p < 0.05$). There was no correlation between mtDNA variants and their combinations with conventional cardiovascular risk factors and age-gender variation (Sobenin et al., not published).

8. Mitochondrial DNA mutation burden and functional activity of cells

Based on the results of whole genome sequencing and pyrosequencing of mtDNA from normal and atherosclerotic sites of intima of the aorta, as well as of genotyping of mtDNA from the blood cells of the above study participants, valuable information was obtained on proatherosclerotic mtDNA variants (m.652delG, m.3256C>T, m12315G>A, m.14459G>A, m.15059G>A, m.368A>G, m.751delA, m.8404T>C, m.8485G>C, m.9720delT, m.14160G>A, m.14207delG, M.16086T>C, and m.16389G>A) and antiatherosclerotic mtDNA variants (m.1555A>G, m.5178C>A, m.13513G>A, and m.14846G>A). These data were used to determine whether the study participants belonged to persons with a low, neutral, or high mtDNA mutation burden, as judged by combinations of the proatherosclerotic or antiatherosclerotic alleles of mtDNA variants, or the highest possible matching to Cambridge reference sequence of the mitochondrial human genome, version NC_012920.1. Of the examined and genotyped persons (a total of 525 subjects), 139 (26.5%) met the above criteria. Of these, 97 subjects signed informed consent and donated venous blood for the study of functional activity of blood monocytes. Among them, 32 were included in the group with a low mtDNA mutation burden; 29, in the group with a neutral mtDNA genotype; and 36, in the group with a high mtDNA mutation burden (Sobenin, personal communication).

It is known that atherosclerotic phenotype at the cellular level for cells actively involved in the formation of atherosclerotic lesions is characterized by increased proliferative activity, increased protein and connective tissue matrix synthesis, and accumulation of esterified cholesterol. Recently, the markers of cell activation by pro-inflammatory (M1) and anti-inflammatory (M2) types, reflecting the processes of chronic inflammation in atherogenesis, have been added to phenotype description.

Mononuclear cells were isolated from the leukocyte fraction by affinity separation using magnetic CD14 affinity microparticles on LS Separation Columns (Miltenyi Biotec, Germany) and cultured in serum-free X-Vivo 10 medium (Lonza). To stimulate cell activation into pro-inflammatory phenotype, interferon-gamma was added to the medium at a final concentration of 100 ng/ml (1-day incubation). To stimulate cell activation into anti-inflammatory phenotype, interleukin-4 was added to the medium at a final concentration of 10 ng/ml (6-days incubation). After incubation, concentrations of TNF-α (the marker of activation into pro-inflammatory phenotype) and chemokine CCL18 (the marker of activation into anti-inflammatory phenotype) were measured in culture medium by enzyme-linked immunosorbent assay (ELISA) technique. To measure the expression of *TNF-α* and *CCL18* genes, mRNA was extracted from cells. To determine the ability of cells to accumulate cholesterol, the cells were incubated in the presence of modified low-density lipoprotein (LDL) (100 μg/ml culture medium) obtained from the blood of patients with coronary heart disease by gradient ultracentrifugation followed by isolation of the fraction of modified lipoproteins by affinity chromatography on ricin-agglutinin Sepharose (Sigma, USA). To determine proliferative activity, the cultured cells were incubated for 24 h in the presence of 10 μCi/ml of [^{3}H]-thymidine. To determine the synthetic activity, the cells were incubated for 24 h in the presence of 10 μCi/ml [^{14}C]-leucine. To determine the synthesis of the connective tissue matrix components (collagen), the cells were incubated for 24 h in the presence of 5 μCi/ml [^{3}H]-proline. The measurement of the respiration rate of mitochondria was carried out by oximetry; the coefficient of respiratory control and the phosphorylation coefficient characterizing the rate of ATP synthesis were determined. The determination of the rate of oxygen uptake by cells was carried out with Clarke oxygen electrode on Oxygraph Plus System instrument (Hansatech Instruments, UK); 2,4-dinitrophenol (0.2 mM) blocking the synthesis of adenosine triphosphate (ADP) was used as an uncoupler of oxidative phosphorylation. The measurement of endogenous respiration of cells was carried out on intact non-permeabilized cells and provided an overall assessment of cell respiration using endogenous substrates.

Significant differences were found between the cells for such parameters as proliferative activity, synthetic activity, synthesis of matrix components (collagen), the ability of cells to accumulate cholesterol from modified low-density lipoproteins, stimulated secretion of anti-inflammatory chemokine CCL18, *TNF-α* gene expression, *CCL18* gene expression, and mitochondrial dysfunction markers (respiratory control and phosphorylation coefficients, oxygen consumption rate). At the same time, the cells did not differ significantly in the basal secretion of TNF-α and CCL18, as well as in the stimulated secretion of TNF-α (Sobenin, personal communication). The data were analyzed using an adaptive neural network model to identify the relationship between mtDNA damage and functional impairment of cells. It was necessary to consider the ambiguity of the results obtained, which was due to the complexity of combinations of phenotypic traits, to high individual variability of cellular properties from different donors, and to far-reaching individual combinations of mtDNA variants, which were employed to classify the cells by the degree of the mtDNA mutation burden. The considered mtDNA variants were in the loci belonging to the hypervariable segments 1 and 2; loci responsible for the coding of the 12S and 16S subunits of ribosomal RNA; leucine tRNA; subunits 2, 4, 5, and 6 of NADH dehydrogenase; subunits I and III of cytochrome C oxidase; subunit 8 ATP synthetase F0; cytochrome b; as well as a membrane-bound site. Thus, the analysis belonged to a class of fuzzy, poorly formalized problems and was carried out using the theory of fuzzy sets and neuro-fuzzy approaches that potentially can analyze the nonequilibrium interaction of many genotypic and phenotypic characteristics.

The cells with a low and neutral mtDNA mutation burden did not differ significantly by proliferative and synthetic activity. The cells with a high mtDNA mutation burden were characterized by 1.8-fold increased proliferative activity ($p < 0.001$) and 1.4-fold increased synthetic activity ($p < 0.001$). However, in analyzing the synthesis of collagen (the main protein component of the connective tissue matrix), it turned out that in cells with a high mtDNA mutation burden, matrix synthesis was significantly decreased both in comparison with the cells with a neutral mtDNA mutation burden (by 1.3-fold) and cells with a low mtDNA mutation burden (by 1.1-fold) ($p = 0.022$) (Sobenin, not published).

The ability of cells to accumulate cholesterol from modified low-density lipoprotein was the highest in cells with a high mtDNA mutation burden; the intracellular cholesterol content increased by 1.7-fold in comparison with control cells, $p < 0.001$. At the same time, the cells with a low or neutral mtDNA mutation burden poorly accumulated cholesterol; in some cases, there was no significant increase of cholesterol level in cells, and if the accumulation of cholesterol occurred, it was rather moderate (by 1.15- to 1.35-fold). The accumulation of cholesterol correlated with the mtDNA mutation burden ($r = 0.721$, $p < 0.001$) and proliferative activity of cells ($r = 0.483$, $p < 0.001$), but not with synthetic activity. Proliferative activity did not correlate with synthetic activity.

Thus, by traditional cellular markers of atherosclerosis (fibrosis, proliferation, lipidosis), the cells with a high mtDNA mutation burden typically demonstrated proatherosclerotic phenotype, except for the dissonance with respect to collagen synthesis (Sobenin, not published). On the one hand, monocytes-macrophages are not professional producers of matrix in tissues, but on the other hand, this dissonance may reflect the dysregulation of cell adaptation, possibly related specifically to the presence of a high mtDNA mutation burden. Indirect confirmation of the latter assumption may be the characteristics of cell activation by an anti-inflammatory or pro-inflammatory phenotype.

The cells did not differ significantly by basal secretion of TNF-α (the marker of pro-inflammatory type of activation); there was a tendency to decrease of basal TNF-α secretion in the row "low-neutral-high mtDNA mutation burden," which did not reach statistical significance ($p = 0.19$). Stimulated by interferon-gamma secretion of TNF-α also did not differ significantly; there was a tendency to decrease of stimulated TNF-α secretion in the row "low-neutral-high mtDNA mutation burden," which also did not reach statistical significance ($p = 0.18$). The degree of stimulation of the secretion of TNF-α (the ratio of stimulated secretion to basal) was the same in all types of cells. Stimulated secretion of TNF-α negatively correlated with proliferative activity ($r = -0.235$; $p = 0.021$).

Basal secretion of CCL18 (the marker of anti-inflammatory type of activation) was practically absent, which is normal, as the cells usually do not secrete CCL18 in the absence of stimulation. The cells with a neutral mtDNA mutation burden were the best responders to stimulation with interleukin-4 ($p = 0.038$), while the cells with a low or high mtDNA mutation burden poorly responded to stimulation and did not differ in the extent of response. The stimulated secretion of CCL18 did not correlate with any of other cellular markers of atherosclerosis.

Ambiguous dissonance was observed not only at the level of expression of the product but also at the level of expression of the coding genes. The expression of the *TNF-α* gene was the highest in cells with a high mtDNA mutation burden, and the lowest in cells with a neutral mtDNA mutation burden, and did not correlate with either the degree of mtDNA mutation burden or the basal or stimulated TNF-α secretion. In contrast, the expression of *CCL18* gene significantly increased in the row "low-neutral-high mtDNA mutation burden" and correlated with the degree of mtDNA mutation burden ($r = 0.782$, $p < 0.001$), but not with stimulated CCL18 secretion.

Among the remaining characteristics, the expression of the *TNF-α* gene correlated only with the accumulation of cholesterol in the cells ($r = 0.347$, $p < 0.001$). *CCL18* gene expression negatively correlated with stimulated secretion of TNF-α ($r = -0.211$, $p = 0.038$), and synthesis of matrix components ($r = -0.201$; $p = 0.048$) positively correlated with proliferative activity of cells ($r = 0.486$; $p < 0.001$) and the accumulation of cholesterol caused by modified low-density lipoproteins ($r = 0.487$; $p < 0.001$).

Obviously, such combinations of phenotypic cellular markers of atherosclerosis and mtDNA mutation burden should be associated with mitochondrial dysfunction. Indeed, such a dysfunction was detected, and it was increasing in the row "low-neutral-high mtDNA mutation burden," by manifesting the decrease of the coefficient of respiratory control, the phosphorylation coefficient, and the rate of oxygen consumption. Correlation coefficients between these indices were $r = -0.692$ ($p < 0.001$), $r = -0.934$ ($p < 0.001$), and $r = -0.697$ ($p < 0.001$), respectively. The rate of oxygen uptake in cultured cells with a low mtDNA mutation burden when inhibited by an uncoupler of oxidative phosphorylation decreased significantly slower than in cells with neutral or high mtDNA mutation burden. Such results of mitochondrial dysfunction assessment were quite predictable, since the studied mutations of the mitochondrial genome should influence the efficiency of oxidative phosphorylation in the mitochondria by the nature of mutations. It should be noted that the parameters of mitochondrial dysfunction were associated with several phenotypic cellular markers of atherosclerosis. Thus, the coefficient of respiratory control negatively correlated with the proliferative activity of cells ($r = -0.461$, $p < 0.001$), the synthetic activity of cells ($r = -0.222$; $p = 0.029$), the accumulation of intracellular cholesterol ($r = -0.489$; $p < 0.001$), and the expression of the *CCL18* gene ($r = -0.453$, $p < 0.001$) and positively correlated with stimulated secretion of TNF-α ($r = 0.253$, $p = 0.012$). There was a positive correlation with both the phosphorylation coefficient ($r = 0.607$, $p < 0.001$) and the rate of oxygen consumption ($r = 0.513$, $p < 0.001$). The phosphorylation coefficient negatively correlated with proliferative activity of cells ($r = -0.645$, $p < 0.001$), the synthetic activity of cells ($r = -0.352$, $p < 0.001$), the accumulation of intracellular cholesterol ($r = -0.678$, $p < 0.001$), and the *CCL18* gene expression ($r = -0.615$, $p < 0.001$) and positively correlated with the rate of oxygen consumption ($r = 0.668$; $p < 0.001$). Finally, the oxygen absorption rate negatively correlated with the proliferative activity of cells ($r = -0.450$, $p < 0.001$), the synthetic activity of cells ($r = -0.396$, $p < 0.001$), the accumulation of intracellular cholesterol ($r = -0.535$; $p < 0.001$), and the expression of *CCL18* gene ($r = -0.457$, $p < 0.001$) (Sobenin et al., not published).

In the analysis of the relationship between mtDNA damage and functional impairment of cells with the use of an adaptive neural network model, the similar and interdependent patterns of relationships were identified (Sobenin et al., not published). The pattern of type 1 is compliant to the typical atherosclerotic phenotype (increased proliferation, increased synthetic activity, the ability of cells to accumulate cholesterol, the unchanged expression of *TNF-α* and *CCL18* genes, high cell activation both into pro-inflammatory and anti-inflammatory phenotypes, and evident mitochondrial dysfunction). This pattern is characterized by the presence of combinations of homoplasmic mtDNA variants m.930G, m.7028C, and m.11251A and heteroplasmic mtDNA variants m.652delG, m.751delA, m.3256C>T, m.12315G>A, and m.14459G>A. The pattern of type 2 represents an atypical atherosclerotic phenotype (increased proliferation without increased synthetic activity, the ability of cells to accumulate cholesterol, increased expression of *TNF-α* and *CCL18* genes, low cell activation into pro-inflammatory phenotype, high cell activation into anti-inflammatory phenotype, and evident mitochondrial dysfunction). This pattern is characterized by the presence of combinations of homoplasmic mtDNA variants m.73A, m.930G, and m.16296C and heteroplasmic mtDNA variants m.368A>G, m.652delG, m.3256C>T, m.8404T>C, m.8485G>C, m.12315G>A, m.14160G>A, and m.15059G>A. Finally, the pattern of type 3 represents normal (non-atherosclerotic) phenotype (low proliferative activity, low synthetic activity, low ability of cells to accumulate cholesterol, unchanged expression of *TNF-α* and *CCL18* genes, moderate equilibrium cell activation both into pro-inflammatory and anti-inflammatory phenotypes, and the absence of manifestations of mitochondrial dysfunction). This pattern is characterized by the presence of combinations of homoplasmic mtDNA variants m.5460A, m.11719G, m.14233A, and m.14766C and heteroplasmic mtDNA variants m.1555A>G, m.5178C>A, and m.14846G>A; however, in this pattern proatherosclerotic heteroplasmic mtDNA variants m.652delG and m.3256C>T nonrandomly occur.

9. Conclusions

The data obtained from the described studies allow to analyze the relationship of mtDNA damage and its variability; qualitative and quantitative changes in the cellular composition of arterial intima, occurring in atherosclerosis; as well as expression of apoptosis- and inflammation-related genes. In maternal relatives in 2–4 generations, the differences in the degree of mtDNA heteroplasmy in different types of blood cells obtained from the same individuals helped to identify heritable mutations accumulated in the cells, and somatic mutations arising during the life of the individual. The relationship of mtDNA variants with atherosclerosis, traditional risk factors for cardiovascular disease, and age-gender variation was identified and characterized. In cell culture studies, the relationship of individual mtDNA mutation burden with functional activity of cells was studied. Taken together, the results of these studies strongly support the hypothesis on proatherosclerotic role of mtDNA mutations in atherogenesis.

Acknowledgements

This study was supported by the Russian Science Foundation, Grant #14-14-01038.

The author also acknowledges the efforts of the research group members (Margarita A. Sazonova, PhD; Andrey V. Zhelankin, PhD; Tatiana V. Kirichenko, MD, PhD; Zukhra B. Khasanova, BS; Konstantin Y. Mitrofanov, BS; Vasily V. Sinyov, BS; Nikita G. Nikiforov, BS; and Valeria A. Barinova, BS) in described in studies.

Author details

Igor A. Sobenin

Address all correspondence to: igor.sobenin@gmail.com

Russian Cardiology Research and Production Complex, Moscow, Russia

References

[1] Taylor RW, Turnbull DM. Mitochondrial DNA mutations in human disease. Nature Reviews Genetics. 2005;**6**:389-402. DOI: 10.1038/nrg1606

[2] Parsons TJ, Muniec DS, Sullivan K, Woodyatt N, Alliston-Greiner R, Wilson MR, Berry DL, Holland KA, Weedn VW, Gill P, Holland MM. A high observed substitution rate in the human mitochondrial DNA control region. Nature Genetics. 1997;**15**:363-368. DOI: 10.1038/ng0497-363

[3] Li M, Schonberg A, Schaefer M, Schroeder R, Nasidze I, Stoneking M. Detecting heteroplasmy from high-throughput sequencing of complete human mitochondrial DNA genomes. American Journal of Human Genetics. 2010;**87**:237-249. DOI: 10.1016/j.ajhg.2010.07.014

[4] Elliott HR, Samuels DC, Eden JA, Relton CL, Chinnery PF. Pathogenic mitochondrial DNA mutations are common in the general population. American Journal of Human Genetics. 2008;**83**:254-260. 10.1016/j.ajhg.2008.07.004

[5] Wallace DC. Colloquium paper: Bioenergetics, the origins of complexity, and the ascent of man. Proceedings of the National Academy of Sciences of the United States of America. 2011;**107**(Suppl.2):8947-8953. DOI: 10.1073/pnas.0914635107

[6] Wallace DC. Mitochondrial DNA mutations in disease and aging. Environmental and Molecular Mutagenesis. 2010;**51**:440-450. DOI: 10.1002/em.20586

[7] Birky CW. Uniparental inheritance of organelle genes. Current Biology. 2008;**18**:R692–R695. DOI: 10.1016/j.cub.2008.06.049

[8] Schon EA, Bonilla E, DiMauro S. Mitochondrial DNA mutations and pathogenesis. Journal of Bioenergetics and Biomembranes. 1997;**29**:131-149. DOI: 10.1023/A:1022685929755

[9] Schaefer AM, McFarland R, Blakely EL, He L, Whittaker RG, Taylor RW, Chinnery PF, Turnbull DM. Prevalence of mitochondrial DNA disease in adults. Annals of Neurology. 2008;**63**:35-39. DOI: 10.1002/ana.21217

[10] Park CB, Larsson NG. Mitochondrial DNA mutations in disease and aging. Journal of Cell Biology. 2011;**193**:809-818. DOI: 10.1083/jcb.201010024

[11] Sazonova M, Budnikov E, Khasanova Z, Sobenin I, Postnov A, Orekhov A. Studies of the human aortic intima by a direct quantitative assay of mutant alleles in the mitochondrial genome. Atherosclerosis. 2009;**204**:184-190. DOI: 10.1016/j.atherosclerosis.2008.09.001

[12] Sobenin IA, Sazonova MA, Postnov AY, Bobryshev YV, Orekhov AN. Mitochondrial mutations are associated with atherosclerotic lesions in the human aorta. Clinical and Developmental Immunology. 2012;**2012**:832464. DOI: 10.1155/2012/832464

[13] Sobenin IA, Sazonova MA, Postnov AY, Bobryshev YV, Orekhov AN. Changes of mitochondria in atherosclerosis: possible determinant in the pathogenesis of the disease. Atherosclerosis. 2013;**227**:283-288. DOI: 10.1016/j.atherosclerosis.2013.01.006

[14] Sazonova MA, Sinyov VV, Barinova VA, Ryzhkova AI, Zhelankin AV, Postnov AY, Sobenin IA, Bobryshev YV, Orekhov AN. Mosaicism of mitochondrial genetic variation in atherosclerotic lesions of the human aorta. BioMed Research International. 2015;**2015**:825468. DOI: 10.1155/2015/825468

[15] Sazonova MA, Zhelankin AV, Barinova VA, Sinyov VV, Khasanova ZB, Postnov AY, Sobenin IA, Bobryshev YV, Orekhov AN. Dataset of mitochondrial genome variants associated with asymptomatic atherosclerosis. Data in Brief. 2016;**7**:1570-1575. DOI: 10.1016/j.dib.2016.04.055

[16] Sobenin IA, Bobryshev YV, Korobov GA, Borodachev EN, Postnov AY, Orekhov AN. Quantitative analysis of the expression of caspase 3 and caspase 9 in different types of atherosclerotic lesions in the human aorta. Experimental and Molecular Pathology. 2015;**99**:1-6. DOI: 10.1016/j.yexmp.2015.05.004

[17] Karpenko AP, Moor DA, Mukhlisulina DT. Multicriteria optimization based on neural network, fuzzy and neuro-fuzzy approximation of decision maker's utility function. Optical Memory and Neural Networks. 2012;**21**:1-10. DOI: 10.3103/S1060992X12010031

[18] Sazonova MA, Chicheva MM, Zhelankin AV, Sobenin IA, Bobryshev YV, Orekhov AN. Association of mutations in the mitochondrial genome with the subclinical carotid atherosclerosis in women. Experimental and Molecular Pathology. 2015;**99**:25-32. DOI: 10.1016/j.yexmp.2015.04.003

[19] Sinyov VV, Malyar NL, Kosogorova SA, Postnov AY, Orekhov AN, Sobenin IA, Sazonova MA. Mitochondrial genome variability in different types of human blood cells. International Research Journal. 2013;**19**:58-61. DOI: 10.18454/IRJ.2227-6017

[20] Zhelankin A, Khasanova Z, Barinova L, Sazonova M, Postnov A, Sobenin I. Mitochondrial DNA haplogroup H is associated with subclinical carotid atherosclerosis in Russian population. Journal of Hypertension. 2015;**33**(Suppl 1):e2. DOI: 10.1097/01.hjh.0000467356.04711.50

[21] Zhelankin AV, Sazonova MA, Khasanova ZB, Sinyov VV, Mitrofanov KY, Sobenin IA, Orekhov AN, Postnov AY. Analysis of mitochondrial haplogroups in persons with subclinical atherosclerosis based on high-throughput mtDNA sequencing. Patologicheskaia Fiziologiia i Eksperimentalnaia Terapiia. 2015;**59**:12-16

Chapter 8

Genetic Polymorphism of UDP-Glucuronosyltransferase

Huma Mehboob, Imtiaz Mahmood Tahir,
Tahira Iqbal, Naheed Akhter, Naveed Munir and
Muhammad Riaz

Additional information is available at the end of the chapter

http://dx.doi.org/10.5772/intechopen.69206

Abstract

Genetic polymorphism is referred to the discontinuous interspecies genetic variability among individuals having distinct alleles on a particular locus. Genetic polymorphism of genes encoding drug-metabolizing enzymes constitutes individual's susceptibility to drugs, affirmed by having discrete allelic frequencies by the individual, strengthening the concept of precision medicine. To combat with toxic consequences of drugs, the polymorphic genes associated with xenobiotic metabolism must be studied. Up to 70% xenobiotic elimination is believed to be dependent on UDP-glucuronosyltransferase (UGT), an enzyme encoded by polymorphic UGT1A and UGT2B genes. Both bimodal and trimodal distribution patterns of UGT have been reported in various human populations studied. Genetic polymorphisms of UGT may even lead to truncated and shorter gene with grossly diminished enzymatic activity. The extent of phenotypic alteration inflicted by genetic polymorphisms depends on its nature and position on gene locus. The different isoforms of UGT superfamily differ from each other regarding substrate specificity and selectivity. The incidence of genetic polymorphisms and associated altered gene functions results in inter-individual variability in metabolic clearance and elimination of drugs. Hence, the critical interaction between genetics and biotransformation of drugs has recently been the focus of pharmacology research.

Keywords: bilirubin, biotransformation, drug-metabolizing enzymes, SNP, UGT, xenobiotics

1. Introduction

Pharmacogenetics enables the personalized therapeutics based on genetic profiling and describes Patient's variation in response to therapy due to genetic factors. Pharmacogenetics is the study of inter-individual differences in the sequence of particular genes affecting drug metabolism [1]. Genetic polymorphism is the variation in the sequence of DNA among populations and individuals. Inter-ethnic variations in drug response are connected to polymorphisms with racial populations showing discrete allele frequencies and inconsistency from each other [2–4]. Genetic polymorphisms may occur by chance and they may be caused by some agents such as chemicals, radiations or viruses. In the human genome, the most common source and simple form of genetic polymorphism are the single-nucleotide polymorphism (SNP) and it contributes to 90% of human DNA polymorphisms. Genetic polymorphisms of drug-metabolizing enzymes (DMEs) can influence the biodisposition of drugs and thus alter the concentration of drugs in plasma and in target tissues [5].

In the human population, person-to-person variations in gene expression and functional activity of drug-metabolizing enzymes have been found to be associated with the change in their responses to toxicants, carcinogens and drugs [6]. Progress in pharmacogenetics has displayed that a series of drug-metabolizing enzymes have become essential to consider the biotransformation of drugs. Allelic variants with different catalytic functions have been recognized from common and wild-type allele as the number of drug-metabolizing enzymes is increased. In individualizing drug therapy, these specific genetic variants are valuable to phenotype/genotype an individual [7, 8]. Hence, the interplay of pharmacogenetics and biotransformation of drugs has recently been a focus of research.

2. Molecular bases

Genetic polymorphism within a population arises as a result of alteration in genes encoding metabolizing enzymes with a variant allele frequency of more than 1% [9]. For such genes, an allelic site has a number of single-nucleotide polymorphisms (SNPs) which may result in increased, reduced or even no enzyme function and their disrupted biological regulations through incorporating several mechanisms. A genotype is referred to a comprehensive study of an organism's particular genetic make-up while the associated observable traits of an individual describe its phenotype. However, keeping in view that a phenotype is influenced by the combination of genetic and environmental determinants, it may not always express a complete concordance with associated genotype [10].

3. SNPs and drug-metabolizing enzymes

Single-nucleotide polymorphism in genes of drug-metabolizing enzymes affects the response of drug to body and absorption, distribution, biotransformation, and excretion of drugs. These SNPs are a source of inter-individual and inter-ethnic differences. Some mutations in the coding region cause amino acid change, which results in alterations of enzyme activity, substrate selectivity and sometimes, protein stability. Ensuring functional differences causes different metabolizer phenotypes [11]. Pharmacogenetics analysis provides insight into mechanisms included in drug response, with the ultimate goal to achieve optimal drug efficacy and safety.

Drug-metabolizing enzymes (DMEs) have a significant role in biotransformation and final excretion of xenobiotics and drugs by increasing their hydrophilicity. Biotransformation of drugs is usually comprised of phase I (oxidation, reduction and hydrolysis) reactions carried out by cytochrome P450 enzyme, and phase II conjugation reactions involve glucuronidation by uridine diphosphate glucuronosyltransferases (UGTs), acetylation by N-acetyltransferase (NAT) and glutathione-S-transferase in the liver, with numerous proteins accountable for transportation. These phase I and phase II enzymes are highly polymorphic leading to variation in the level of enzyme expression *in vivo* [12].

The first polymorphism in drug-metabolizing enzyme was reported in patients more than 40 years ago with the incidence of side effects after administration of a recommended therapeutic dose of the drug [13]. An array of possible physiological and environmental factors has been assigned to human variability in drug response. The physiological features consist of hepatic and renal function, age, gender and bodyweight, whereas the environmental features include concomitant drug administration, contact to definite chemicals and dietary intake as well. Genetic factors have traced that individual's body respond to drug therapy in a different way as some people are well tolerated while others have harmful effects [12].

4. SNP-mediated metabolic modulation

The uridine diphosphate glucuronosyltransferases (UGTs) exist in almost all living beings counting microorganisms (viruses, bacteria), animals, plants and humans. UDP-glucuronosyltransferase is a microsomal enzyme carrying the glucuronidation of several exogenous (different carcinogens as well as drugs) and endogenous compounds (bilirubin; breakdown product of heme, hormones). Glucuronidation is a primary reaction for the removal of countless substrates and drug compounds. The genetic variations in UGT enzyme lead to its changed regulation and expression. The activities of UDP-glucuronosyltransferase contribute to pharmacological and physiologic consequences [14].

In humans, a main drug-metabolizing reaction called glucuronidation is catalysed by uridine diphospho glucuronosyltransferase enzyme (EC 2.4.1.17). Glucuronidation is the conjugation of small lipophilic molecules with uridine diphosphate (UDP) as a sugar donor, altering them into more water-soluble metabolites and accounts for 40–70% of xenobiotic elimination approximately [15]. UDP-glucuronosyltransferases are primarily expressed in the liver but are also distributed in various organs of the body, including the heart, kidney, thymus, spleen, olfactory epithelium, brain, intestine, adrenal glands and lungs. The expression of UGT is known to be affected by genetic polymorphism, physiological and environmental factors like age, diet, disease state, induction and inhibition by chemicals [16].

5. Classification of UGT

The superfamily UGT is divided into four subfamilies called UDP-glucuronosyltransferase 1, UDP-glucuronosyltransferase 2, UDP-glucuronosyltransferase 3 and UDP-glucuronosyltransferase 8. This classification is kept on sequence similarity at the level of amino acid. The isozymes of family UGT1A have the first exon that is spliced into two to five common exons and thus producing a C-terminal and N-terminal domain. The gene-specific promoter region is possessed by each member of UGT1A family [17]. The 13 isoenzymes of UGT1A gene (9 functional and 4 pseudogenes) are all originated due to alteration in exon 1 region of this gene located on chromosome 2q37 and 6 isoforms of UGT2B subfamily emerge to be encoded by a rigid cluster of separate genes located on chromosome 4 in humans [18].

6. UDP-glucuronosyltransferases (UGTs)

The covalent conjugation of sugar with the small organic molecule is brought about by a super family UDP-glucuronosyltransferase (UGT). This superfamily of UDP-glucuronosyltransferase enzyme has been explored in microorganisms (bacteria), plants and animals evolutionarily conserved and adapted to combat with the dynamic interaction with lipid-soluble compounds. The UDP-glucuronosyltransferases are protein in nature that is bound to the membrane and is confined to the smooth endoplasmic reticulum (SER) and nuclear compartment of the cell. They have a significant role in glucuronidation of many antibiotics and xenobiotics [14]. UGTs are synthesized as approximately 530 residues precursor containing an N-terminal signal peptide [19].

The mammalian UGT superfamily comprises of four families, and members of each of four families can also be recognized in various lower vertebrates. The UGT superfamily comprises of all glucosyltransferases that contain the UGT signature sequence (FVA)-(LIVMF)-(TS)-(HQ)-(SGAC)-G- X(2) -(STG)-X(2)- (DE)-X(6)-P-(LIVMFA)-(LIVMFA)-X(2)-P-(LMVFIQ)- X(2)- (DE)-Q, (X is any amino acid) [20], and add sugar to small lipophilic compounds. Glucuronidation of compounds forms a range of glucuronides containing functional groups (O-, N-, S- and C-), which significantly enhance the solubility of the parent drugs and terminates its biological effect [21].

7. Distribution of UDP-glucuronosyltransferases

Approximately, the drugs from all therapeutic classes containing an extensive range of acceptor groups pass through glucuronidation process. However, non-steroidal anti-inflammatory drugs and analgesic agents are usually metabolized by this mechanism. It is well recognized that the liver has the maximum abundance and array of UDP-glucuronosyltransferases [22, 23]. The members of UGT1A and UGT2B subfamilies are also found in many other tissues and organs incorporating the epithelium, brain, nasal cavity, stomach, small intestine, colon, kidneys, lungs, ovaries, mammary glands, testis and prostate gland, in addition to hepatic abundance [16, 23]. The kidneys and GIT (gastrointestinal tract; stomach, small intestine and colon) are the most important extra-hepatic sites in case of drug metabolism [24]. All members of the UGT1A and UGT2B families are expressed differentially in human liver with the exception of some members of both families including UGT1A5, 1A7, 1A8, 1A10 and 2A1 [25]. In contrast to the UGT1A and UGT2B, members of UGT3 family are principally expressed in thymus, testis and kidney with nearly untraceable expression in liver and GI tract [26].

8. Types of glucuronides

The UDP-glucuronosyltransferase enzyme catalyses the transfer of sugar glucuronic acid (GA) from uridine-diphospho-glucuronic acid (UDP-GA) to various exogenous as well as endogenous compounds containing hydroxyl, thiol, amine, carbonyl, carboxylic and hydroxylamine due to structural diversity of the substrates. Binding with glucuronic acid is a quantitatively most important phase II reaction and is a primary pathway in nature for detoxification of a wide range of drugs, dietary compounds, cancer causing agents and their oxidized metabolites, and a variety of environmental chemicals and thus excreting lipid-soluble waste compounds from the body in urine and bile [27, 28]. Glucuronidation of compounds

Polymorphic enzymes	Endogenous cofactor	Biochemical reactions involved	Specific substrate	Intermediate metabolites	References
Sulfotransferase (SULT)	Sulfate	Sulfation	Salbutamol	Salbutamol sulfate	[30]
UDP-glucuronosyltransferase (UGT)	UDP glucuronic acid	Glucuronidation	Morphine	Morphine-3-glucuronide	[31]
Glutathione-S-transferase (GST)	Glutathione	Glutathione conjugation	Doxorubicin	Glutathione metabolite	[32]
N-acetyltransferase (NAT)	Acetyl-CoA	Acetylation	SMX, caffeine	N-Ac SMX AFMU	[33, 34]
Methyltransferase (MT)	Methyl	Methylation	Mercaptopurine, captopril	Methyl metabolite	[35]

Table 1. Important polymorphic human DMEs, cofactors, biochemical reactions, substrates and their intermediate metabolites.

forms a range of glucuronides containing functional groups (O-, N-, S- and C-) which significantly enhance the solubility of the parent drugs and terminates its biological effect [21].

Substrates containing different functional groups chemically form different glucuronides like aliphatic alcohols and phenols form ether glucuronide, while those containing a $COOH^-$ group form ester glucuronides (acyl glucuronides). The compounds, which possess both phenolic and $COOH^-$ groups, can be transformed into both ether and ester glucuronides such as mycophenolic acid (MPA). Glucuronidation of amines (primary, secondary and tertiary) and sulfhydryl compounds result in the formation of N-glucuronides and S-glucuronides, respectively, whereas C-glucuronides are obtained from compounds containing carbonyl group. The most common and rare drug glucuronides in humans are O-glucuronides and C-glucuronides, respectively [29].

There are many enzymes in humans that are polymorphic in nature and metabolize a variety of drugs through biotransformation reactions presented in **Table 1**.

9. UGT isozymes

The large substrate specificity of each UGT isoform makes possible the glucuronidation of structurally isolated molecules. In humans, roughly (40–70%) drugs administered clinically undergo glucuronidation [36]. In humans, 19 UGT isoforms have been recognized, expressed and differentiated: 9 UGT1A members encoded by the UGT1A gene locus are positioned on chromosome number 2 and nine members of UGT2B family (7 members of UGT2B and 2 members of the UGT2A subfamily) are located on chromosome 4. The isoforms of the UGT1A and UGT2B families have a key role in dispensing lipophilic compounds because of their ability to glucuronidate an extensive array of structurally different substrates. Different UGT isoforms are involved in the formation of drug glucuronides but they reveal overlapping and unusual substrate selectivity and specificity. Individual UGTs differ from each other in sense of regulation and expression. UGT activity is known to be affected by physiological and environmental factors like age, diet, disease state, induction and inhibition of UDP-glucuronosyltransferase by chemicals, ethnicity, genetic polymorphism and hormonal level [37]. Some general conjugation reactions of glucuronidation carried by UGT are expressed through chemical equations A–F, given below [38].

A. R -OH + UDP -GA → UDP + R -O-GA

B. R – SH + UDP -GA → UDP + R - S-GA

C. R -NH_2 + UDP-GA → UDP + R NH–GA

D. R –CHO + UDP-GA → UDP + R -CO-GA

E. R -COOH + UDP-GA → UDP + R –CO–(OGA)

F. R -NHOH + UDP-GA → UDP + R -N–(OH)GA

10. Structural organization of UDP-glucuronosyltransferase 1

The UGT1A isoforms are encoded by a single intricate and complex locus that is organized similarly in all mammals. The nine functional proteins are encoded by UGT1A gene locus

(1A1, 1A3, 1A4, 1A5, 1A6, 1A7, 1A8, 1A9 and 1A10). In humans, the UGT1A gene size is about 200 kb located on chromosome 2q37 and encodes 13 isozymes. Each isoform has a distinctive promoter region, unique exon-1, and shares (2–5) four common exons [39]. Transcription is commenced at unique promoter. Consequently, each of the 13 transcripts has a unique 5′ end and a similar 3′ end, which is engaged in identification of the UDP-sugar molecule. The human UGT1A isoforms can be divided into four groups on the basis of sequence resemblance, amplification and divergence of gene: UGT1A1, UGT1A6 and UGT1A2P to 1A5 cluster and UGT1A7 to 1A13P cluster. Exons of UGT1A1 and UGT1A6 made proteins that are nearly 50% alike; conversely, within exons of 1A2P–1A5 and 1A7–1A13P clusters, the resulting proteins are more than 90% identical [17]. Four members (1A2P, 1A11P, 1A12P and 1A13P) of UGT2A subfamily have been recognized as pseudogenes since they have mutations that would avert their translation into functional proteins. It has been observed that complexity to the UGT1A locus produces another form of the common exon 5 so-called as 5b exon that can be merged into the human UGT1 proteins. The alternative forms produce mRNAs that encode smaller polypeptides of each UGT1 protein. These smaller proteins do not have a transmembrane part but keep their ability to confine themselves to smooth endoplasmic reticulum. These small UGT1 forms are non-functional and can heterodimerize with whole UGT1 form and lack their activity [40]. In human tissues, short-form UGT1 transcripts are largely distributed and expressed at considerable levels [41].

11. Function/effect of UGT1A isoforms

UGT1A1 is the most important isoform of UGT1A gene that brings about the glucuronidation of bilirubin (a breakdown product of haemoglobin) which required to be eliminated from the body. Genetic alterations in the UGT1A gene are presumed to have an intense effect on the health of affected individuals, particularly those that modify UGT1A1 activities and correspond to rare mutations. Sixty rare mutations have been well known as point mutations, deletions and insertions in UGT1A1 gene. Only a small number of these mutations are reported in common population with high frequency (up to 41%). These mutations called polymorphisms in TATA box region of UGT1A1 promoter produce variant alleles that lead to decrease in activity and rate of glucuronidation by UDP-glucuronosyltransferase [42–44]. These mutations in the UGT1 gene are correlated with two forms of the unconjugated hyperbilirubinemia syndromes. The wild type and common variant allele include six and seven repeats, respectively [45]. The UGT1A isoforms appeared to be expressed at a lower level in different populations of the world: approximately 0–3% in the Asian population, 2–13% in Caucasian population and up to 16–19% in Africans [44].

Paracetamol is being used as a probe drug to study slow and fast acetylation capacity of human [46], which is mainly cleared by hepatic glucuronidation from the body. Inter-individual variability in capacity to glucuronidate paracetamol and possible risk for liver damage could be explained by polymorphisms in genes encoding the paracetamol glucuronidation [47].

Court et al. used human liver samples for accessing paracetamol glucuronidation activity by UGT isoforms (1A1, 1A6, 1A9 and 2B15) that chiefly glucuronidate paracetamol.

Three single-nucleotide polymorphisms (rs10929303, rs1042640 and rs8330) positioned in 3' untranslated region of UGT1A1 were found to be associated with paracetamol glucuronidation activity. Consistently the highest glucuronidation activity is observed with SNP rs8330. This single-nucleotide polymorphism did not modify stability of mRNA and translation capacity [48].

In the pharmacokinetic studies, acetaminophen and SN-38 were used as phenotyping probes *in vivo* to check glucuronidation activity. Study subjects were given irinotecan and acetaminophen separately after a specific wash out period, and no association was observed between irinotecan and acetaminophen glucuronidation activity, proposing affinity for many different UGT1 isoforms [49, 50].

12. UDP-glucuronosyltransferase 2

The UGT2 gene family is further divided into two subfamilies on the basis of sequence resemblance: UGT2A and UGT2B. The genes in each subfamily usually have more than 70% sequence resemblance. The great level of resemblance makes it complex to establish orthologous associations between species in each subfamily. Therefore, a sequential numbering system based on their chronological order of discovery has been used for UGT2 genes [20]. In the human genome, the UGT2 family comprises of three UGT2A and six UGT2B members. The members of UGT2A subfamily are called pseudogenes as they do not form functional proteins. The members of UGT2B subfamily are encoded by separate and independent genes, including UGT2B4, UGT2B7, UGT2B10, UGT2B11, UGT2B15 and UGT2B17. The UGT2B genes emerge to be encoded by a firm group of genes located on chromosome number four [18].

The members of UGT2 family are supposed to be developed by replication of whole UGT2 gene. UGT2A3 gene has six distinct exons. However, UGT2A1 and UGT2A2 genes have a variable and shared exon structure similar to that of the UGT1A family. The UGT2 members also have first unique exon and a set of five shared (2–6) exons. The first 2 exons of each UGT2 gene encode a region of 241 amino acids similar to that of UGT1A gene locus [51].

13. Function and effect of UGT2B genes

UGT2B4 gene of UGT2 family plays an important role in biotransformation and glucuronidation of bile acids allowing their glucuronide efflux from hepatocytes *via* transporters such as multi-drug resistance-associated protein (MRP) 2 or MRP3 [52] and detoxification of many phenols [18, 53].

UGT2B4 gene is expressed in the chief metabolizing organ: liver and in several extrahepatic tissues [18, 54]. Polymorphism in the co-substrate binding region of UGT2B4 gene resulted in mutant allele, which causes change in position of amino acid from aspartate to glutamate at 458 codons [54]. The single change in position of amino acid alters the rate of glucuronidation. This variant allele is present in the Caucasian, African and Hispanic populations at a frequency varying between 0.17 and 0.38, whereas it is absent from the Asian population [54–56]. Lampe et al. used human liver samples to study polymorphisms in UGT2B4 gene. These polymorphisms cause a change in position of amino acids: from phenylalanine to leucine at codons 109 and 396. It was found that these polymorphisms are rare because they were absent in a big group of 272 individuals [56].

UGT2B15 gene showed glucuronidation activity towards steroid hormones, a number of classes of drugs and their metabolites [57–60]. A guanine to thymine replacement at codon 85 causes an amino acid change from aspartate to tyrosine in substrate binding site of UGT2B15 gene. The homozygous wild-type allele is not common in Caucasians as compared to the Asian, Hispanic and African populations. On the whole, 19–32% of the studied population have been found to bear homozygous variant allele. Levesque et al. studied the effect of UGT2B15 gene polymorphisms on function and enzyme activity *in vitro* using liver microsomes. The homozygous variant allele presented same reaction constant (K_m) values but the rate of reaction (V_{max}) is two times different for steroid hormones [58]. Court et al. determined the functional impact of UGT2B15 variants towards catalytic activities in HEK 293 cellular fractions by using S-oxazepam as probe drug. The glucuronidation activity of homozygous wild-type allele for S-oxazepam was five times more than homozygous variant allele UGT2B15*2 [59].

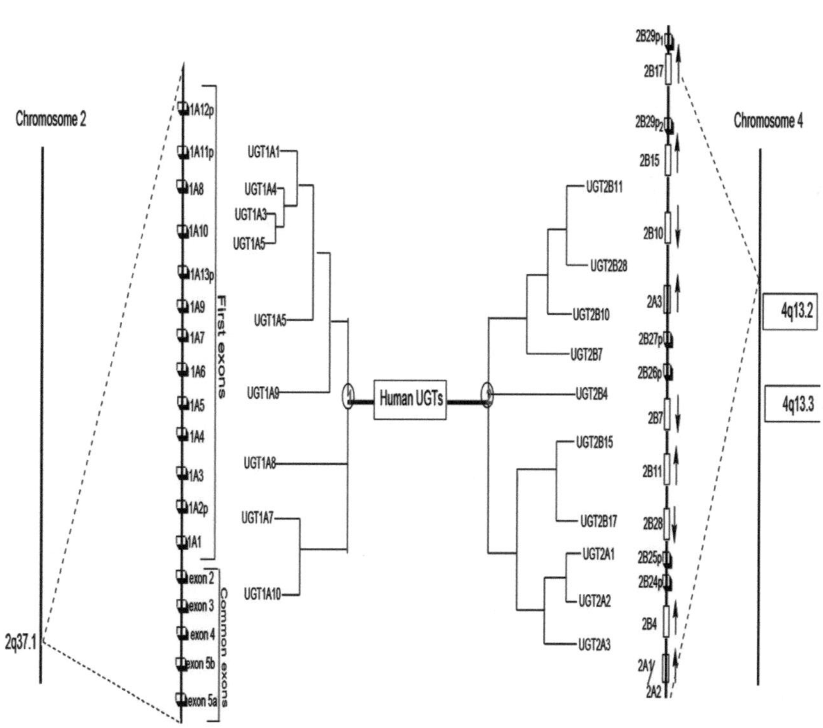

Figure 1. Schema representing the genetic polymorphic pattern of human UGT1A & UGT2B genes.

Lampe et al. evaluated the rate of recurrence of the UGT2B4, UGT2B7 and UGT2B15 polymorphisms in Caucasian and Asian individuals. For all polymorphisms, the genotype and allele frequencies were considerably different in both populations. The distribution of the genotypes also differed by ethnic group. All Asians were homozygous for common allele, and incidence of wild-type allele is two times higher in them as compared to Caucasians [56].

Navarro et al. investigated the effect of UGT1A6 and UGT2B15 genotypes on paracetamol glucuronidation in a controlled feeding trial. 1000 mg paracetamol was administered to healthy volunteers orally, and saliva and urine samples were collected for determining the concentration of paracetamol and its metabolites. The concentration of unchanged paracetamol is higher in men as compared to women who had more paracetamol glucuronide. The percentage of unchanged paracetamol is higher in individuals with homozygous common allele relative to heterozygote and homozygous variants. The UGT2B15 gene considerably affected the paracetamol glucuronidation while the involvement of UGT1A6 in paracetamol glucuronidation was moderate [61].

Mutlib et al. demonstrated the importance of UGT1A and UGT2B15 genotypes: 1A1, 1A6, 1A9 and 2B15 on paracetamol glucuronidation. It was observed that UGT1A1 and UGT2B15 contribution was highest in conjugating paracetamol [62]. The polymorphic variations in UGT1A and UGT2B genes are presented in **Figure 1**.

14. UDP-glucuronosyltransferase 3

The third family of UGT superfamily is UGT3A that consists of two genes: UGT3A1 and UGT3A2. It is situated in a 115 kb piece of chromosome number 5p13. Each gene of this family includes seven unique exons that are just about 30 kb size and encodes 523 amino acids of protein. At protein level, both genes are 80% similar which shows larger conservation of sequence in UGT3A than that found in UGT1A and UGT2B families [63].

15. UDP-glucuronosyltransferase 8

The fourth family of UGT superfamily is UGT8 gene family. This family is composed of a single gene which contains five exons and is situated on chromosome number four (4q26) together with genes that encode other phase II enzymes. The UGT8 gene is greatly conserved and does not involve in the biotransformation of drugs. This is due to its partial expression in the brain where exposure to xenobiotics is restricted [51].

16. Genotype-dependent functional polymorphism

In the human population, individual-to-individual variations exist genetically in UGT activity and are phenotypically divided as rapid or slow glucuronidator. On the basis of

UDP-glucuronosyltransferase activity, humans are divided into bimodal and trimodal distributions. In bimodal distribution, humans are categorized as fast and slow glucuronidators or fast, intermediate and slow glucuronidators in trimodal distribution. UGT1A and UGT2B subfamilies exhibit overlapping but different substrate specificities and variable levels of expression in different organs [16, 36, 64, 65].

An increasing integer of functional single-nucleotide polymorphisms (SNPs) is identified in humans at UGT1A gene locus with a potential relevance for drug therapy. A single-nucleotide polymorphism or a combination of multiple nucleotide substitutions and insertion or deletion is responsible for allelic variants of UGT (UGT1A and UGT2B) [66]. The most common isoforms of UGT associated with drug metabolism are UGT1A1, 1A6, 1A9 and UGT2B4, UGT2B15. Many studies have described associations between specific phenotypes for UGT polymorphic enzyme and susceptibility to cancer, particularly lung and bladder, breast cancer, Parkinson's disease and the autoimmune disease systemic lupus erythematosus. These associations may be due to differences in the ability of enzyme phenotypes to activate or detoxify chemical toxins or, alternatively, to linkage disequilibrium where a particular allele coding for another gene with a direct role in determining disease susceptibility shows genetic linkage with an allelic variant of the xenobiotic-metabolizing enzyme [67].

Genetic polymorphisms lead to truncated and shorter gene which efficiently diminishes enzymatic activity and even a single mutation alone can account for decrease or increase in enzymatic regulation. On the other hand, increased and elevated enzymatic activity may be due to elevated mRNA stability [59]. The expression and activity of UGT increase during childhood and adolescence. Many cis factors (polymorphism) and trans-factors including transcription factors (TFs) and nuclear receptors (NRs), miRNA targeting and other epigenetic regulating factors play an important role in the regulation of UGT enzyme expression. In the liver, transcription levels of UGTs determine their activity. The tissue specific and ligand-activated TFs and NRs play a chief role in the expression of UGTs by binding to cis-regulatory elements. The ontogeny of drug-metabolizing enzymes is analogous by the maturation of organ systems among children and has intense effects on drug disposition [68].

In the beginning, UGT1A and UGT2B families assumed to be evolved as consequences of their neutralizing function against noxious chemical at the hepatic and gastrointestinal barrier. Regulation of UGTs may have developed along with some other drug-metabolizing enzymes (DMEs) in the course of animal and plant competition [69]. The families expanded in different ways on different chromosomes, but similar exon-intron structures encode a protein family with similar functional architecture despite the amino acid sequence diversity [70]. UGTs performed their functions at pre-systemic, systemic level and locally in cells.

Glucuronidation by UGT provides a critical detoxification pathway for exogenous compounds and drugs from several therapeutic classes, including analgesic and non-steroidal anti-inflammatory agents, anticonvulsants, antipsychotics, anti-viral agents and benzodiazepines [27, 28, 71].

17. Role of UGT isoforms in metabolism

Some substrates and drugs are fairly selective for a particular UGT enzyme as the endogenous molecule; bilirubin is particularly glucuronidated by UGT1A1 enzyme. However, the bulk of substrates (small and hydrophobic molecules) are often metabolized by several UGT isoforms [72], thus making it complex to recognize which UGT enzyme is primarily accountable for the glucuronidation of compounds. The accessibility of individual cDNA has made it possible to study the function of each UGT enzyme, even though the quantitative variations in the rate of reaction might be present based on their expression [28]. Moreover, there are facts and figures which designate that UDP-glucuronosyltransferase enzymes are linked as homo and hetero-oligomers *in vitro* and *in vivo*. Oligomerization may be necessary for the activity of the UGT enzymes and sometimes it may even vary the rate of the biotransformation [65, 72]. Formation and disposition of glucuronides in cells and even in the whole organisms are under control of several factors. However, the activity of isoform-specific substrate *in vitro* associates very well with activity *in vivo* and is appropriate for the anticipation of metabolic detoxification *in vivo* [73, 74]. The functional significance of numerous UGT isoforms is ambiguous for many reasons: substrate specificity of isoform is weak displaying overlapping substrate specificity and substrate conjugating regions of UGT enzymes have not been recognized [75].

Lampe et al. found that individuals possessing homozygous variant allele of UGT1A1 and UGT1A6 isoform presented abnormality in the conjugation of a variety of drugs. In Tankanitlert's study, the combined effect of UGT1A1 and UGT1A6 genes was investigated in thalassemic patients. Thalassemic patients were grouped into three categories. It was figured out that there is no difference in glucuronidation capacity of patients with homozygous wild-type allele and those who were heterozygous, but rate of glucuronidation is lower in patients with variant alleles signifying that variant alleles are a potent modifier of acetaminophen glucuronidation [76].

In the human population, wide variations are found in their glucuronidation capacity of drugs. The extent of variations can range from 3-fold to more than 100-fold, considering the studied drug. Many genetic and environmental factors act discretely and in combination to produce broad inter-individual differences. Phenotype-like glucuronidation capacity of UGT is not separated from genotype but somewhat displays continuous and overlapping changes due to multiple interacting environmental and genetic factors [77].

In general population, polymorphisms in phase I and phase II drug-metabolizing enzymes lead to differences in enzyme expression level. This variability in enzyme expression is due to the presence of genetic polymorphisms and mutations in the wild-type gene, resulting in impaired or reduced activity of the enzyme. Individuals having mutated enzymes may differ from normal individuals in their vulnerability to certain diseases. Some specific phenotypes for these polymorphic enzymes are related to increased vulnerability to cancer, predominantly lung, bladder cancer and Parkinson's disease. This altered enzyme activation or certain chemicals including constituents of tobacco, xenobiotics and neurotoxin initiate these diseases [78].

Biotransformation is a key process in the body that finds out the pharmacokinetics of an administered drug. Several factors, which control the level of biotransformation, include physiological state of the patient, genetics and co-administered drugs, and these may cause the toxic or sub-therapeutic concentration of drugs. The large inter-individual variability is gradually accumulating in glucuronidation due to underlying genetic mechanisms but a few polymorphisms have been described in UGTs with probable clinical relevance. The polymorphisms can lead to altered drug clearance with a clinically relevant phenotype. However, the proof *in vivo* for such a link is very weak [36].

18. UGT SNPs and disease

Human UDP-glucuronosyltransferase enzyme was appeared to be polymorphic genetically. Genetic polymorphisms in this enzyme are unlikely to participate in toxicity of drugs since the isozymes illustrate broad overlapping specificity and tissue distribution [79]. Polymorphisms lead to varying degree of transcriptional as well as functional variations that might reduce the activity of UGT enzyme and consequently affected individuals present some sort of pathology. The polymorphisms in UGT1A and UGT2B gene families were also suggested to change the risk of diseases either due to reduced inactivation of hormone or as a result of decreased detoxification of carcinogenic chemicals and production of their reactive conjugates [64].

The variant alleles of UGT1A1 gene result in some syndromes associated with the diminishing bilirubin conjugation capacity of UGT1A1 isoform. Kadakol et al. summarized the data of approximately 50 polymorphisms of UGT1A1 gene contributing to Crigler-Najjar syndrome type I and II. Crigler-Najjar syndrome type 1, also known as non-hemolytic jaundice, is entirely deficient of UGT1A1 activity due to which bilirubin exerts toxic effects on brain [80]. One of the widespread diseases caused by inactivity of UGT1A1 gene is Gilbert's syndrome. More than 10% of the population suffered from this localized chaos was differentiated by sporadic unconjugated hyperbilirubinemia. This syndrome is associated with polymorphism in the promoter region of UGT1A1 enzyme [45]. In patients with Gilbert's syndrome, when irinotecan drug was administered, it resulted in increased toxicity of an active metabolite of SN–38 because in these patients, UGT1A1 gene is not functional as it is responsible for the formation of inactive glucuronide of irinotecan [81].

Several studies assessed the function and differential expression of the UGT1A isoforms in the colon [82], liver [83], pancreas [84] and kidney cancers [85]. The inquiry of a case-controlled study exposed that individuals carrying variant alleles of UGT1A gene were at increased risk of having colorectal cancer [86]. In two independent studies, it was investigated that polymorphisms in promoter and coding regions of UGT1A isoforms were correlated with the toxicity of irinotecan drug in Japanese cancer patients and with neutropenia [66, 87].

Yilmaz et al. examined the association between mRNA expression of UGT (1A3 and 1A7) isoforms and pancreatic cancer. Healthy and tumour samples were collected from pancreatic patients. The mRNA expression of both isoforms of UGT1A gene was notably higher in pancreatic cancer tissue than normal healthy tissue, and this high expression was also linked with tumour size and its progression [88].

Cengiz et al. reported that expression of UGT1A genes was different in healthy normal and tumour cells of patients suffering from stomach cancer. This differential expression might affect the growth and progression of a variety of cancers [89]. Several authors studied the role of UGTs in breast cancer risk and incidence in different populations. They focused on the expression of isoforms of UGT1A gene by using cell lines of breast cancer and concluded that women with mutations in UGT1A1 enzyme were at higher risk of developing breast cancer due to its reduced activity but no relationship was observed between estrogen receptor status and UGT1A1 genotype [44, 90].

Bigler et al. examined the function of UGT1A6 polymorphisms in healthy controls and patients of colon adenoma in the context of aspirin use. A conflicting association was found between aspirin users' colon adenoma patients and the UGT1A6 variants [82]. Several studies have explored the relationship between polymorphisms of UGT1A7 gene and colorectal, hepatocellular carcinoma and lung cancer in Japanese [91, 92], Chinese [83], Caucasian [93], French [94] and Koreans [95] with reduced incidence of common wild-type allele [96].

19. Risk assessment with SNPs

Uridine disphospho glucuronosyltransferase (UGT1A and UGT2B) enzyme contribute to the removal of miscellaneous drugs, environmental chemicals and endogenous compounds [27, 28]. The majority of human uridine disphospho glucuronosyltransferase enzymes metabolize aliphatic alcohol and phenol compounds of low molecular mass. Most of UGT genes contain single-nucleotide polymorphisms (SNPs) those altered drug metabolism, excretion and drug function and have been found to be associated with Crigler-Najjar syndrome type 1 and 2, hyperbilirubinemia and Gilbert's syndrome. It is believed that SNPs in regulatory regions have the highest impact on phenotype [97].

MacLeod et al. observed that the individuals with elevated level of androgens might be at higher risk of prostate cancer due to presence of lower activity allele [98]. An independent case-control study verified that the patients of prostate cancer with homozygous variant allele had lower enzymatic activity [99]. A positive association has been reported between prostate cancer risk and low-activity UGT2B15 allele or a complete UGT2B17 deleted gene [99, 100]. The UGT2B15 gene is recognized to be greatly expressed in cell lines of prostate cancer [58, 101], and a noteworthy involvement was found between the UGT2B15 homozygous variant genotype and cancer recurrence [102]. The UGT2B15*2 variant allele appeared to be a risk factor for the incidence and poor subsistence of patients of breast cancer. It was reported in breast cancer patients who had mutations in more than one drug-metabolizing enzymes as one UGT2B15*2 allele and also the SULT1A1*2 allele had mainly reduced survival rates of five years.

In humans, uridine diphospho glucuronosyltransferase 2B (UGT2B) proteins facilitate the elimination of testosterone hormone in form of glucuronide metabolites. Grant et al. evaluated the association between UGT2B15 and UGT2B17 genes of UGT2B family relative to plasma levels of androgens and development of cancer in Whites and Blacks. An association was determined between copy number variant of the UGT2B17 gene and plasma androgen levels in Whites, but surprisingly, no association was found in Blacks [103].

A number of glucuronides are known to acquire pharmacologically useful and harmful activities. Morphine is mainly cleared from the body by glucuronidation pathway and possessed two binding domains [38]. The morphine-3-glucuronide (M-3-G) is the main glucuronide and is a powerful inhibitor of morphine [31, 104]. The deposition of M-3-G reduces the effectiveness of morphine and exerts excitatory effects on the central nervous system [105]. Decreased glucuronidation of morphine to morphine-6-glucuronide *in vivo* was associated with polymorphisms in UGT2B7 gene [106].

Navarro et al. [61] evaluated the impact of UGT1A6 gene and dietary inducers on urinary excretion of aspirin in Caucasians and Asians. They undertook this study on healthy 264 men and 264 women aged between 21 and 45 years. These healthy volunteers were administered 650 mg aspirin, and their urine samples were collected at predetermined time intervals. Considerable variation was found in excretion pattern of aspirin between sexes and ethnicities. Asians excreted more aspirin, salicylic acid acyl-glucuronide and salicylic acid phenolic glucuronide as compared to Caucasians. Diet might manipulate the excretion of aspirin but effects were due to binding of glycine endogenous molecule rather than glucuronic acid. In another study, the glucuronidation of aspirin was undertaken in relevance to UGT isoforms: 1A1, 1A3, 1A4, 1A6, 1A7, 1A8, 1A9, 1A10, 2B4, 2B7, 2B15 and 2B17. It was analysed that all UGT isoforms conjugated aspirin except UGT1A4 and UGT2B17 [107].

Two polymorphisms in exon 1 region of UGT1A6 gene resulted in amino acid substitutions, and these substitutions were likely to be related to reduce enzyme activity towards numerous phenolic compounds [108]. UGT2B15 gene catalyses the metabolism of multiple substrates, thus enhancing their clearance from the body [60].

20. Conclusion

Many polymorphisms have been reported for UGT1A and UGT2B genes and new polymorphisms are continuously evolving. These polymorphisms affect the phenotype and extent of variation depends on the nature of the polymorphisms and their position in the gene. Knowledge about genetic polymorphisms underlying the extensive inter-individual differences in glucuronidation process is progressively gathering but only a small number of polymorphisms in UDP-glucuronosyltransferase enzyme have been reported with possible clinical significance. Patients possessing different genetic polymorphisms illustrated lower or even diminished glucuronidation of a wide range of drugs from almost all therapeutic classes. The incidence of polymorphisms is variable in different populations of the world for various isoforms of UGT1A and UGT2B.

Classification of UGT implicated in phenotyping reaction of a compound depends upon the activity of UGT, the expression and the incidence of glucuronidation rate. But the ever-increasing accessibility of agonists and antagonists probes for individual UGTs provides the dependable prospect for glucuronidation phenotyping. Moreover, many factors affect the functions and activities of UGT proteins *in vivo* such as age (i.e. neonatal period), consumption of alcohol, smoking of cigarette, diet and nutritional habits, pathological condition, ethnicity, hormonal factors and polymorphisms of genes (i.e. occurrence or frequency). The techniques required for glucuronidation phenotype of UGT enzymes have been developed extensively with the discovery and differentiation of specific and selective probes (substrates and inhibitors), accessibility of recombinant UGT enzymes and optimization of incubation states necessary for measuring glucuronidation of drugs.

The tissue-specific expression of each UGT1A and UGT2B isoforms is the subject of genetic polymorphisms, and these individual isoforms can be induced and inhibited by drugs. The individual isoforms differed from each other in sense of substrate specificity and selectivity, the incidence of genetic polymorphisms and gene functions that resulted in broad inter-individual variability in metabolic clearance. It is apparent that polymorphisms in the coding and regulatory segments of all UGT enzymes are likely to be altered their functions and expression. In addition, induction of metabolism may increase the clearance of therapeutic agents, leading to sub-therapeutic exposures and lack of pharmacological effect. Alternatively, inhibition of metabolism may reduce the clearance of drugs and lead to supratherapeutic exposures, resulting in undesired side effects or toxicity.

Variation in DNA sequence results in SNPs, and analysis of SNPs in diseases allows investigation of the influence of genetic polymorphisms on disease vulnerability, drug resistance and eventually the health care. The study of SNPs provides a potent resource for establishing a relationship between a phenotype and regions of the DNA. Genetic polymorphism are sources of variations at all levels. Genetic polymorphism of genes encoding phase I and phase II enzymes describes inter-individual variability in the biotransformation of xenobiotics.

Author details

Huma Mehboob[1]*, Imtiaz Mahmood Tahir[2]*, Tahira Iqbal[3], Naheed Akhter[2], Naveed Munir[4], Muhammad Riaz[5]

*Address all correspondence to: moona_farooqi21@yahoo.com ; imtiazmls@hotmail.com

1 Department of Biochemistry, Government College Women University, Faisalabad, Pakistan

2 College of Allied Health Professionals, Directorate of Medical Sciences, Government College University, Faisalabad, Pakistan

3 Department of Biochemistry, University of Agriculture, Faisalabad, Pakistan

4 Department of Biochemistry, Government College University, Faisalabad, Pakistan

5 Department of Allied Health Sciences, Sargodha Medical College, University of Sargodha, Sargodha, Pakistan

References

[1] Hess P, Cooper D. Impact of pharmacogenomics on the clinical laboratory. Molecular Diagnosis. 1999;**4**(4):289-298

[2] Balram C, Zhou Q, Cheung YB, Lee EJ. CYP3A5* 3 and* 6 single nucleotide polymorphisms in three distinct Asian populations. European Journal of Clinical Pharmacology. 2003;**59**(2):123-126

[3] Chowbay B, Zhou S, Lee E. An interethnic comparison of polymorphisms of the genes encoding Drug-Metabolizing enzymes and drug transporters: Experience in Singapore. Drug Metabolism Reviews. 2005;**37**(2):327-378

[4] Tate SK, Goldstein DB. Will tomorrow's medicines work for everyone? Nature Genetics. 2004;**36**:S34-S42

[5] Ma Q, Lu AYH. Pharmacogenetics, pharmacogenomics, and individualized medicine. Pharmacological Reviews. 2011;**63**(2):437-459

[6] Cascorbi I. Genetic basis of toxic reactions to drugs and chemicals. Toxicology Letters. 2006;**162**(1):16-28

[7] Westphal GA, Schnuch A, Schulz TG, Reich K, Aberer W, Brasch J, et al. Homozygous gene deletions of the glutathione S-transferases M1 and T1 are associated with thimerosal sensitization. International Archives of Occupational and Environmental Health. 2000;**73(**6):384-388

[8] Satoh N, Akiba T, Yokoshima S, Fukuyama T. A practical synthesis of (−)-Oseltamivir. Angewandte Chemie. 2007;**119**(30):5836-5338

[9] Meyer UA. Pharmacogenetics and adverse drug reactions. The Lancet. 2000;**356**(9242): 1667-1671

[10] Shenfield GM. Genetic polymorphisms, drug metabolism and drug concentrations. The Clinical Biochemist Reviews. 2004;**25**(4):203

[11] Matimba A, Del-Favero J, Van Broeckhoven C, Masimirembwa C. Novel variants of major drug-metabolising enzyme genes in diverse African populations and their predicted functional effects. Human Genomics. 2009;**3**(2):169

[12] Koo SH, Lee EJD. Pharmacogenetics approach to therapeutics. Clinical and Experimental Pharmacology and Physiology. 2006;**33**(5-6):525-532

[13] Meyer UA, Zanger UM. Molecular mechanisms of genetic polymorphisms of drug metabolism. Annual Review of Pharmacology and Toxicology. 1997;**37**(1):269-296

[14] Desai AA, Innocenti F, Ratain MJ. UGT pharmacogenomics: Implications for cancer risk and cancer therapeutics. Pharmacogenetics and Genomics. 2003;**13**(8):517-523

[15] Ahn S-J, Dermauw W, Wybouw N, Heckel DG, Van Leeuwen T. Bacterial origin of a diverse family of UDP-glycosyltransferase genes in the *Tetranychus urticae* genome. Insect Biochemistry and Molecular Biology. 2014;**50**:43-57

[16] Tukey RH, Strassburg CP. Human UDP-glucuronosyltransferases: Metabolism, expression, and disease. Annual Review of Pharmacology and Toxicology. 2000;**40**(1):581-616

[17] Mackenzie PI, Bock KW, Burchell B, Guillemette C, Ikushiro S-I, Iyanagi T, et al. Nomenclature update for the mammalian UDP glycosyltransferase (UGT) gene superfamily. Pharmacogenetics and Genomics. 2005;**15**(10):677-685

[18] Turgeon D, Carrier J-Sb, Lévesque É, Hum DW, Bélanger A. Relative enzymatic activity, protein stability, and tissue distribution of human steroid-metabolizing UGT2B subfamily members 1. Endocrinology. 2001;**142**(2):778-787

[19] Mackenzie PI, Owens IS. Cleavage of nascent UDP glucuronosyltransferase from rat liver by dog pancreatic microsomes. Biochemical and Biophysical Research Communications. 1984;**122**(3):1441-1449

[20] Mackenzie PI, Owens IS, Burchell B, Bock KW, Bairoch A, Belanger A, et al. The UDP glycosyltransferase gene superfamily: Recommended nomenclature update based on evolutionary divergence. Pharmacogenetics and Genomics. 1997;**7**(4):255-269

[21] Mackenzie PI, Rogers A, Treloar J, Jorgensen BR, Miners JO, Meech R. Identification of UDP glycosyltransferase 3A1 as a UDP N-acetylglucosaminyltransferase. Journal of Biological Chemistry. 2008;**283**(52):36205-36210

[22] Izukawa T, Nakajima M, Fujiwara R, Yamanaka H, Fukami T, Takamiya M, et al. Quantitative analysis of UDP-glucuronosyltransferase (UGT) 1A and UGT2B expression levels in human livers. Drug Metabolism and Disposition. 2009;**37**(8):1759-1768

[23] Ohno S, Nakajin S. Determination of mRNA expression of human UDP-glucuronosyltransferases and application for localization in various human tissues by real-time reverse transcriptase-polymerase chain reaction. Drug Metabolism and Disposition. 2009;**37**(1):32-40

[24] Knights KM, Miners JO. Renal UDP-glucuronosyltransferases and the glucuronidation of xenobiotics and endogenous mediators. Drug Metabolism Reviews. 2010;**42**(1):63-73

[25] Zhang X. Expression of cytochrome P450 and other biotransformation genes in fetal and adult human nasal mucosa. Drug Metabolism and Disposition. 2005;**33**(10):1423-1428

[26] MacKenzie PI, Rogers A, Elliot DJ, Chau N, Hulin J-A, Miners JO, et al. The novel UDP glycosyltransferase 3A2: Cloning, catalytic properties, and tissue distribution. Molecular Pharmacology. 2011;**79**(3):472-478

[27] Miners JO, Mackenzie PI. Drug glucuronidation in humans. Pharmacology & Therapeutics. 1991;**51**(3):347-369

[28] Kiang TK, Ensom MH, Chang TK. UDP-glucuronosyltransferases and clinical drug-drug interactions. Pharmacology & Therapeutics. 2005;**106**(1):97-132

[29] Shipkova M, Wieland E. Glucuronidation in therapeutic drug monitoring. Clinica Chimica Acta. 2005;**358**(1):2-23

[30] Lau GS, Critchley J. The estimation of paracetamol and its major metabolites in both plasma and urine by a single high-performance liquid chromatography assay. Journal of Pharmaceutical and Biomedical Analysis. 1994;**12**(12):1563-1572

[31] Smith MT, Watt JA, Cramond T. Morphine-3-glucuronide-a potent antagonist of morphine analgesia. Life Sciences. 1990;**47**(6):579-585

[32] Ekhart C, Rodenhuis S, Smits PH, Beijnen JH, Huitema AD. An overview of the relations between polymorphisms in drug metabolising enzymes and drug transporters and survival after cancer drug treatment. Cancer Treatment Reviews. 2009;**35**(1):18-31

[33] Cantilena LR, Katki AG, Klecker RW, Collins JM. Metabolism by N-acetyltransferase 1 in vitro and in healthy volunteers: A prototype for targeted inhibition. The Journal of Clinical Pharmacology. 2004;**44**(12):1405-1411

[34] Grant DM, Tang BK, Kalow W. A simple test for acetylator phenotype using caffeine. British Journal of Clinical Pharmacology. 1984;**17**(4):459-464

[35] Männistö PT, Kaakkola S. Catechol-O-methyltransferase (COMT): Biochemistry, molecular biology, pharmacology, and clinical efficacy of the new selective COMT inhibitors. Pharmacological Reviews. 1999;**51**(4):593-628

[36] Wells PG, Mackenzie PI, Chowdhury JR, Guillemette C, Gregory PA, Ishii Y, et al. Glucuronidation and the UDP-glucuronosyltransferases in health and disease. Drug Metabolism and Disposition. 2004;**32**(3):281-290

[37] Miners JO, Smith PA, Sorich MJ, McKinnon RA, Mackenzie PI. Predicting human drug glucuronidation parameters: Application of in vitro and in silico modeling approaches. Annual Review of Pharmacology and Toxicology. 2004;**44**:1-25

[38] Ritter JK. Roles of glucuronidation and UDP-glucuronosyltransferases in xenobiotic bioactivation reactions. Chemico-Biological Interactions. 2000;**129**(1-2):171-193

[39] Gong Q-H, Cho JW, Huang T, Potter C, Gholami N, Basu NK, et al. Thirteen UDPglucuronosyltransferase genes are encoded at the human UGT1 gene complex locus. Pharmacogenetics and Genomics. 2001;**11**(4):357-368

[40] Girard H, Lévesque E, Bellemare J, Journault K, Caillier B, Guillemette C. Genetic diversity at the UGT1 locus is amplified by a novel 3′ alternative splicing mechanism leading to nine additional UGT1A proteins that act as regulators of glucuronidation activity. Pharmacogenetics and Genomics. 2007;**17**(12):1077-1089

[41] Bellemare J, Rouleau M, Harvey M, Guillemette C. Modulation of the human glucuronosyltransferase UGT1A pathway by splice isoform polypeptides is mediated through protein-protein interactions. Journal of Biological Chemistry. 2010;**285**(6): 3600-3607

[42] Bosma PJ, Chowdhury JR, Bakker C, Gantla S, de Boer A, Oostra BA, et al. The genetic basis of the reduced expression of bilirubin UDP-glucuronosyltransferase 1 in Gilbert's syndrome. New England Journal of Medicine. 1995;**333**(18):1171-1175

[43] Beutler E, Gelbart T, Demina A. Racial variability in the UDP-glucuronosyltransferase 1 (UGT1A1) promoter: A balanced polymorphism for regulation of bilirubin metabolism? Proceedings of the National Academy of Sciences. 1998;**95**(14):8170-8174

[44] Guillemette C, Millikan RC, Newman B, Housman DE. Genetic polymorphisms in uridine diphospho-glucuronosyltransferase 1A1 and association with breast cancer among African Americans. Cancer Research. 2000;**60**(4):950-956

[45] Monaghan G, Ryan M, Hume R, Burchell B, Seddon R. Genetic variation in bilirubin UDP-glucuronosyltransferase gene promoter and Gilbert's syndrome. The Lancet. 1996;**347**(9001):578-581

[46] Tahir IM, Iqbal T, Saleem S, Mehboob H, Akhter N, Riaz M. Effect of acetaminophen on sulfamethazine acetylation in male volunteers. International Journal of Immunopathology and Pharmacology. 2016;**29**(1):17-22

[47] Bridger S, Henderson K, Glucksman E, Ellis AJ, Henry JA, Williams R. Lesson of the week: Deaths from low dose paracetamol poisoning. British Medical Journal. 1998; **316**(7146):1724-1725

[48] Court MH, Freytsis M, Wang X, Peter I, Guillemette C, Hazarika S, et al. The UDP-Glucuronosyltransferase (UGT) 1A polymorphism c.2042C>G (rs8330) is associated with increased human liver acetaminophen glucuronidation, increased UGT1A Exon 5a/5b splice variant mRNA ratio, and decreased risk of unintentional Acetaminophen-Induced acute liver failure. Journal of Pharmacology and Experimental Therapeutics. 2013;**345**(2):297-307

[49] Bock K, Wiltfang J, Blume R, Ullrich D, Bircher J. Paracetamol as a test drug to determine glucuronide formation in man. Effects of inducers and of smoking. European Journal of Clinical Pharmacology. 1987;**31**(6):677-683

[50] Gupta E, Mick R, Ramirez J, Wang X, Lestingi TM, Vokes EE, et al. Pharmacokinetic and pharmacodynamic evaluation of the topoisomerase inhibitor irinotecan in cancer patients. Journal of Clinical Oncology. 1997;**15**(4):1502-1510

[51] Meech R, Miners JO, Lewis BC, Mackenzie PI. The glycosidation of xenobiotics and endogenous compounds: Versatility and redundancy in the UDP glycosyltransferase superfamily. Pharmacology & Therapeutics. 2012;**134**(2):200-218

[52] Hirohashi T, Suzuki H, Takikawa H, Sugiyama Y. ATP-dependent transport of bile salts by rat multidrug resistance-associated protein 3 (Mrp3). Journal of Biological Chemistry. 2000;**275**(4):2905-2910

[53] Monaghan G, Burchell B, Boxer M. Structure of the human UGT2B4 gene encoding a bile acid UDP-glucuronosyltransferase. Mammalian Genome. 1997;**8**(9):692-694

[54] Lévesque É, Beaulieu M, Hum DW, Bélanger A. Characterization and substrate specificity of UGT2B4 (E458): A UDP-glucuronosyltransferase encoded by a polymorphic gene. Pharmacogenetics and Genomics. 1999;**9**(2):207-216

[55] Riedy M, Wang J-Y, Miller AP, Buckler A, Hall J, Guida M. Genomic organization of the UGT2b gene cluster on human chromosome 4q13. Pharmacogenetics and Genomics. 2000;**10**(3):251-260

[56] Lampe JW, Bigler J, Bush AC, Potter JD. Prevalence of polymorphisms in the human UDP-glucuronosyltransferase 2B family: UGT2B4 (D458E), UGT2B7 (H268Y), and UGT2B15 (D85Y). Cancer Epidemiology and Prevention Biomarkers. 2000;**9**(3):329-333

[57] Levesque E, Beaulieu M, GreeN MD, Tephly TR, Belanger A, Hum DW. Isolation and characterization of UGT2B15 (Y85): A UDP glucuronosyltransferase encoded by a polymorphic gene. Pharmacogenetics and Genomics. 1997;**7**(4):317-325

[58] Levesque E. Effect of interleukins on UGT2B15 and UGT2B17 steroid uridine diphosphate-glucuronosyltransferase expression and activity in the LNCaP cell line. Endocrinology. 1998;**139**(5):2375-2381

[59] Court MH. Stereoselective conjugation of oxazepam by human UDP-glucuronosyltransferases (UGTs): S-Oxazepam is glucuronidated by UGT2B15, while R-oxazepam is glucuronidated by UGT2B7 and UGT1A9. Drug Metabolism and Disposition. 2002; **30**(11):1257-1265

[60] Green MD, Oturu EM, Tephly TR. Stable expression of a human liver UDP-glucuronosyltransferase (UGT2B15) with activity toward steroid and xenobiotic substrates. Drug Metabolism and Disposition. 1994;**22**(5):799-805

[61] Navarro SL, Chen Y, Li L, Li SS, Chang JL, Schwarz Y, et al. UGT1A6 and UGT2B15 polymorphisms and acetaminophen conjugation in response to a randomized, controlled diet of select fruits and vegetables. Drug Metabolism and Disposition. 2011;**39**(9):1650-1657

[62] Mutlib AE, Goosen TC, Bauman JN, Williams JA, Kulkarni S, Kostrubsky S. Kinetics of acetaminophen glucuronidation by UDP-glucuronosyltransferases 1A1, 1A6, 1A9 and 2B15. Potential implications in acetaminophen-induced hepatotoxicity. Chemical Research in Toxicology. 2006;**19**(5):701-709

[63] Meech R, Mackenzie PI. UGT3A: Novel UDP-glycosyltransferases of the UGT superfamily. Drug Metabolism Reviews. 2010;**42**(1):45-54

[64] Guillemette C. Pharmacogenomics of human UDP-glucuronosyltransferase enzymes. The Pharmacogenomics Journal. 2003;**3**(3):136-158

[65] Ouzzine M, Barré L, Netter P, Magdalou J, Fournel-Gigleux S. The human UDP-glucuronosyltransferases: Structural aspects and drug glucuronidation. Drug Metabolism Reviews. 2003;**35**(4):287-303

[66] Innocenti F, Undevia SD, Iyer L, Xian Chen P, Das S, Kocherginsky M, et al. Genetic variants in the UDP-glucuronosyltransferase 1A1 gene predict the risk of severe neutropenia of irinotecan. Journal of Clinical Oncology. 2004;**22**(8):1382-1388

[67] Daly AK, Cholerton S, Armstrong M, Idle JR. Genotyping for polymorphisms in xenobiotic metabolism as a predictor of disease susceptibility. Environmental Health Perspectives. 1994;**102**(Suppl 9):55

[68] Neumann E, Mehboob H, Ramírez J, Mirkov S, Zhang M, Liu W. Age-dependent hepatic UDP-glucuronosyltransferase gene expression and activity in children. Frontiers in Pharmacology. 2016;**7**:437

[69] Bock KW. Vertebrate UDP-glucuronosyltransferases: Functional and evolutionary aspects. Biochemical Pharmacology. 2003;**66**(5):691-696

[70] Burchell B, Brierley CH, Rance D. Specificity of human UDP-glucuronosyltransferases and xenobiotic glucuronidation. Life Sciences. 1995;**57**(20):1819-1831

[71] Sorich MJ, McKinnon RA, Miners JO, Smith PA. The importance of local chemical structure for chemical metabolism by human uridine 5′-diphosphate–glucuronosyltransferase. Journal of Chemical Information and Modeling. 2006;**46**(6):2692-2697

[72] Lin JH, Wong BK. Complexities of glucuronidation affecting in vitro-in vivo extrapolation. Current Drug Metabolism. 2002;**3**(6):623-646

[73] Mistry M, Houston JB. Glucuronidation in vitro and in vivo. Comparison of intestinal and hepatic conjugation of morphine, naloxone, and buprenorphine. Drug Metabolism and Disposition. 1987;**15**(5):710-717

[74] Soars MG. In vitro analysis of human drug glucuronidation and prediction of in vivo metabolic clearance. Journal of Pharmacology and Experimental Therapeutics. 2002;**301**(1):382-390

[75] Miners JO, McKinnon RA, Mackenzie PI. Genetic polymorphisms of UDP-glucuronosyltransferases and their functional significance. Toxicology. 2002;**181-182**:453-456

[76] Lampe JW, Bigler J, Horner NK, Potter JD. UDP-glucuronosyltransferase (UGT1A1* 28 and UGT1A6* 2) polymorphisms in Caucasians and Asians: Relationships to serum bilirubin concentrations. Pharmacogenetics and Genomics. 1999;**9**(3):341-350

[77] Vesell ES, Gaylor DW. Limitations of probit plots in pharmacogenetics: Requirement of genetic analyses to test hypotheses based on graphical methods. Pharmacogenetics and Genomics. 1995;**5**(1):18-23

[78] Daly AK, Armstrong M, Monkman SC, Idle ME, Idle JR. Genetic and metabolic criteria for the assignment of debrisoquine 4-hydroxylation (cytochrome P4502D6) phenotypes. Pharmacogenetics. 1991;**1**(1):33-41

[79] Burchell B. Genetic variation of human UDP-glucuronosyltransferase. American Journal of PharmacoGenomics. 2003;**3**(1):37-52

[80] Kadakol A, Ghosh SS, Sappal BS, Sharma G, Chowdhury JR, Chowdhury NR. Genetic lesions of bilirubin uridine-diphosphoglucuronate glucuronosyltransferase (UGT1A1) causing Crigler-Najjar and Gilbert syndromes: Correlation of genotype to phenotype. Human Mutation. 2000;**16**(4):297

[81] Wasserman E, Myara A, Lokiec F, Goldwasser F, Trivin F, Mahjoubi M, et al. Severe CPT-11 toxicity in patients with Gilbert's syndrome: Two case reports. Annals of Oncology. 1997;**8**(10):1049-1051

[82] Bigler J, Whitton J, Lampe JW, Fosdick L, Bostick RM, Potter JD. CYP2C9 and UGT1A6 genotypes modulate the protective effect of aspirin on colon adenoma risk. Cancer Research. 2001;**61**(9):3566-3569

[83] Tseng C-S, Tang K-S, Lo H-W, Ker C-G, Teng H-C, Huang C-S. UDP-glucuronosyltransferase 1A7 genetic polymorphisms are associated with hepatocellular carcinoma risk and onset age. American Journal of Gastroenterology. 2005;**100**(8):1758-1763

[84] Piepoli A. Lack of association between UGT1A7, UGT1A9, ARP, SPINK1 and CFTR gene polymorphisms and pancreatic cancer in Italian patients. World Journal of Gastroenterology. 2006;**12**(39):6343

[85] Rouleau M, Roberge J, Bellemare J, Guillemette C. Dual roles for splice variants of the glucuronidation pathway as regulators of cellular metabolism. Molecular Pharmacology. 2014;**85**(1):29-36

[86] Tang K-S. Link between colorectal cancer and polymorphisms in the uridine-diphosphoglucuronosyltransferase 1A7 and 1A1 genes. World Journal of Gastroenterology. 2005;**11**(21):3250

[87] Ando Y, Saka H, Ando M, Sawa T, Muro K, Ueoka H, et al. Polymorphisms of UDP-glucuronosyltransferase gene and irinotecan toxicity: A pharmacogenetic analysis. Cancer Research. 2000;**60**(24):6921-6926

[88] Yilmaz L, Borazan E, Aytekin T, Baskonus I, Aytekin A, Oztuzcu S, et al. Increased UGT1A3 and UGT1A7 expression is associated with pancreatic cancer. Asian Pacific Journal of Cancer Prevention. 2015;**16**(4):1651-1655

[89] Cengiz B, Yumrutas O, Bozgeyik E, Borazan E, Igci YZ, Bozgeyik I, et al. Differential expression of the UGT1A family of genes in stomach cancer tissues. Tumor Biology. 2015;**36**(8):5831-5837

[90] Adegoke OJ, Shu XO, Gao Y-T, Cai Q, Breyer J, Smith J, et al. Genetic polymorphisms in uridine diphospho-glucuronosyltransferase 1A1 (UGT1A1) and risk of breast cancer. Breast Cancer Research and Treatment. 2004;**85**(3):239-245

[91] Araki J, Kobayashi Y, Iwasa M, Urawa N, Gabazza EC, Taguchi O, et al. Polymorphism of UDP-glucuronosyltransferase 1A7 gene: A possible new risk factor for lung cancer. European Journal of Cancer. 2005;**41**(15):2360-2365

[92] Wang Y. UDP-glucuronosyltransferase 1A7 genetic polymorphisms are associated with hepatocellular carcinoma in Japanese oatients with Hepatitis C virus infection. Clinical Cancer Research. 2004;**10**(7):2441-2446

[93] Strassburg C, Vogel A, Kneip S, Tukey R, Manns M. Polymorphisms of the human UDP-glucuronosyltransferase (UGT) 1A7 gene in colorectal cancer. Gut. 2002;**50**(6):851-856

[94] Stücker I, Loriot M-A, N'Koutchou G, Cénée S, Bodin L, Mulot C, et al. UDP-glucuronosyltransferase UGT1A7 genetic polymorphisms in hepatocellular carcinoma: A differential impact according to seropositivity of HBV or HCV markers? BMC Cancer. 2007;**7**(1):214

[95] Kong SY, Ki CS, Yoo BC, Kim JW. UGT1A7 haplotype is associated with an increased risk of hepatocellular carcinoma in hepatitis B carriers. Cancer Science. 2008;**99**(2):340-344

[96] Ehmer U, Vogel A, Schütte JK, Krone B, Manns MP, Strassburg CP. Variation of hepatic glucuronidation: Novel functional polymorphisms of the UDP-glucuronosyltransferase UGT1A4. Hepatology. 2004;**39**(4):970-977

[97] Miners JO, Mackenzie PI, Knights KM. The prediction of drug-glucuronidation parameters in humans: UDP-glucuronosyltransferase enzyme-selective substrate and inhibitor probes for reaction phenotyping and in vitro–in vivo extrapolation of drug clearance and drug-drug interaction potential. Drug Metabolism Reviews. 2010;**42**(1):196-208

[98] MacLeod SL, Nowell S, Plaxco J, Lang NP. An allele-specific polymerase chain reaction method for the determination of the D85Y polymorphism in the human UDPGlucuronosyltransferase 2B15 gene in a case-control study of prostate cancer. Annals of Surgical Oncology. 2000;**7**(10):777-782

[99] Chouinard S, Yueh M-F, Tukey RH, Giton F, Fiet J, Pelletier G, et al. Inactivation by UDP-glucuronosyltransferase enzymes: The end of androgen signaling. The Journal of Steroid Biochemistry and Molecular Biology. 2008;**109**(3):247-253

[100] Nadeau G, Bellemare J, Audet-Walsh E, Flageole C, Huang S-P, Bao B-Y, et al. Deletions of the androgen-metabolizing UGT2B genes have an effect on circulating steroid levels and biochemical recurrence after radical prostatectomy in localized prostate cancer. The Journal of Clinical Endocrinology & Metabolism. 2011;**96**(9):E1550-E1557

[101] Bélanger A, Pelletier G, Labrie F, Barbier O, Chouinard S. Inactivation of androgens by UDP-glucuronosyltransferase enzymes in humans. Trends in Endocrinology & Metabolism. 2003;**14**(10):473-479

[102] Park J, Chen LAN, Shade K, Lazarus P, Seigne J, Patterson S, et al. ASP85TYR polymorphism in the UDP-glucuronosyltransferase (UGT) 2B15 gene and the risk of prostate cancer. The Journal of Urology. 2004;**171**(6):2484-2488

[103] Grant DJ, Hoyo C, Oliver SD, Gerber L, Shuler K, Calloway E, et al. Association of uridine diphosphate-glucuronosyltransferase 2B gene variants with serum glucuronide levels and prostate cancer risk. Genetic Testing and Molecular Biomarkers. 2013;**17**(1):3-9

[104] Smith M. Neuroexcitatory effects of morphine and hydromorphone: Evidence implicating the 3-glucuronide metabolites. Clinical and Experimental Pharmacology and Physiology. 2000;**27**(7):524-528

[105] Faura CC, Olaso JM, Cabanes CG, Horga JF. Lack of morphi-ne-6-glucuronide antinociception after morphine treatment is morphine-3-glucuronide involved? Pain. 1996;**65**(1):25-30

[106] Sawyer MB, Innocenti F, Das S, Cheng C, Ramírez J, Pantle-Fisher FH, et al. A pharmacogenetic study of uridine diphosphate–glucuronosyltransferase 2B7 in patients receiving morphine. Clinical Pharmacology & Therapeutics. 2003;**73**(6):566-574

[107] Kuehl GE, Bigler J, Potter JD, Lampe JW. Glucuronidation of the aspirin metabolite salicylic acid by expressed UDP-glucuronosyltransferases and human liver microsomes. Drug Metabolism and Disposition. 2006;**34**(2):199-202

[108] Ciotti M, Marrone A, Potter C, Owens IS. Genetic polymorphism in the human UGT1A6 (planar phenol) UDP-glucuronosyltransferase: Pharmacological implications. Pharmacogenetics and Genomics. 1997;**7**(6):485-495

Chapter 9

Recent Advances in Hypertrophic Cardiomyopathy: A System Review

Yamin Liu, Zhao Li, Xiaofan Guo, Xiong Jing, Xueli Zhang, Hua Shao, Yufan Guan and Maria R. Abraham

Additional information is available at the end of the chapter

http://dx.doi.org/10.5772/intechopen.69620

Abstract

Hypertrophic cardiomyopathy (HCM) is a common genetic cardiovascular disease present in 1 in 500 of the general population, leading to the most frequent cause of sudden death in young people (including trained athletes), heart failure, and stroke. HCM is an autosomal dominant inheritance, which is associated with a large number of mutations in genes encoding proteins of the cardiac sarcomere. Over the last 20 years, the recognition, diagnosis, and treatment of HCM have been improved dramatically. And moreover, recent advancement in genomic medicine, the growing amount of data from genotype-phenotype correlation studies, and new pathways for HCM help the progress in understanding the diagnosis, mechanism, and treatment of HCM. In this chapter, we aim to outline the symptoms, complications, and diagnosis of HCM; update pathogenic variants (including miRNAs); review the treatment of HCM; and discuss current treatment and efforts to study HCM using induced pluripotent stem cell–derived cardiomyocytes and gene editing technologies. The authors ultimately hope that this chapter will stimulate further research, drive novel discoveries, and contribute to the precision medicine in diagnosis and therapy for HCM.

Keywords: cardiac sarcomere, gene, hypertrophic cardiomyopathy, microRNA, pharmacology

1. Introduction

Hypertrophic cardiomyopathy (HCM) is a heterogeneous cardiac disease with a diverse clinical presentation and course, presenting in all age groups from infancy to the very elderly, which was first described in 1868, its functional consequences in 1957, left ventricular (LV) asymmetric and especially septal hypertrophy in 1958, and its familial nature in 1960 [1, 2]. HCM is a global disease, affecting 1 in every 500 people [3]. And, the existing epidemiological studies might have underestimated the prevalence of HCM because majority of the original prevalence studies enrolled unrelated adults only and employed a diagnostic criterion of maximal wall thickness (MWT) ≥15 mm, or both, thereby resulting in under-recognition of early, familial disease [1, 4]. Enhanced recognition of HCM is important, allowing more timely diagnosis and the implementation of appropriate treatment options for many patients.

HCM is characterized by left ventricular hypertrophy with histological features of myocyte hypertrophy, myofibrillar disarray, and interstitial fibrosis [5]. The thickened and stiff ventricle reduces the compliance of the heart muscle, decreases preload, and leads to the most frequent cause of sudden death in young people (including trained athletes), heart failure, and stroke [6].

Since its first description in the 1950s, much progress has been made in elucidating the extremely heterogeneous genetic, morphogenic, diagnosis, and patient management. The goals of this chapter are to outline the symptoms, complication, and diagnosis of HCM; update published pathogenic variants; and discuss current treatment and efforts to study HCM by using induced pluripotent stem cell-derived cardiomyocytes, next-generation sequencing, and gene editing technologies.

2. Symptoms and complications

HCM is a common inherited cardiomyopathy with a diverse clinical presentation. Most patients with HCM are asymptomatic and have a normal life span but some develop symptoms. The most frequent symptoms of HCM included chest pain, dizziness, shortness of breath, palpitations, fatigue, and inability to perform vigorous exercise. Another devastating manifestation of HCM is sudden cardiac death (SCD) [7].

Furthermore, HCM is related with disease complications that may be profound, with the potential to result in disease progression or premature death [8, 9]. Atrial fibrillation (AF) is the most common sustained arrhythmia in HCM. Paroxysmal episodes or chronic AF ultimately occur in 20–25% of HCM patients, increase in incidence with age, and are linked to left atrial enlargement [10]. AF is a precursor of stroke (incidence, about 1% annually; prevalence, 6%), which is associated with death as well as disability most frequently in the elderly, and progressive heart failure, particularly for patients who have AF before 50 years old and accompanied basal outflow obstruction [11, 12].

Heart failure is another severe complication of HCM. Symptoms of chronic heart failure are frequent; however, the clinical profile of advanced heart failure varies between patients. In some, the thickened and stiff ventricle reduces the compliance of the heart muscle, decreases preload, and contributes to diastolic heart failure [6]. On the other end of the spectrum, typical DCM cases show chamber volume dilatation and thin walls, which reduces contractile force and causes systolic heart failure [13].

Myocardial ischemia: the other common pathologic features of HCM are the thickened and narrowed intramural coronary arteries and myocardial fibrosis by increased collagen deposition, leading to symptoms related to myocardial ischemia [14].

3. Diagnosis

Accurate diagnosis is vital for the management of HCM patients. Echocardiography is the primary method of diagnosis of HCM by determination of left ventricular hypertrophy (LVH) [15], left ventricular outflow tract gradients [16], systolic and diastolic function, as well as mitral valve anatomy and function. Cardiac magnetic resonance imaging (MRI) is becoming more widely used in diagnosis of HCM by determining the extent and location of LVH and the anatomic abnormalities of the mitral valve and papillary muscles [17]. Besides, genetic testing that is now commercially available is currently used most effectively in the identification of affected relatives in families known to have HCM.

3.1. Echocardiography

Echocardiography (echo) was first used to aid diagnosis in HCM in 1969 [18]. Forty years later, echo is central to diagnosis and monitoring of HCM. Diagnostic criteria of HCM by echo: in an adult, HCM is defined by a wall thickness ≥15 mm in one or more LV myocardial segments. However, in some cases, genetic and nongenetic disorders may present with a lesser degrees of wall thickening (13–14 mm); for these patients, the diagnosis of HCM requires evaluation of other factors including electrocardiogram (ECG) abnormalities, laboratory tests, and MRI, as well as family history [19]. For children, HCM diagnosis requires an LV wall thickness more than two standard deviations greater than the predicted mean (z-score > 2, where a z-score is defined as the number of standard deviations from the population mean) [19, 20].

HCM typically can be classified in three categories (**Table 1**), "nonobstructive," "labile," or "obstructive at rest" depending on their degree of left ventricular outflow tract obstruction (LVOTO), which result from a hypertrophied interventricular septum and/or abnormal mitral valve morphology. About one-third of patients will have obstruction at rest (peak gradient >30 mm Hg), and one-third will have labile obstruction (peak gradient >30 mm Hg only

Hemodynamic state	Conditions	Outflow gradients*
No obstruction	Rest	<30 mm Hg
	Physiologically provoked	<30 mm Hg
Labile obstruction	Rest	<30 mm Hg
	Physiologically provoked	≥30 mm Hg
Basal obstruction	Rest	≥30 mm Hg

*Gradients are the peak instantaneous continuous wave Doppler gradient.

Table 1. Definition of dynamic left ventricular outflow tract obstruction [2].

during provocation, which includes the Valsalva maneuver, administration of a potent inhaled vasodilator, such as amyl nitrite, and exercise treadmill testing [7]. Another one-third will have no obstruction under provocation or resting conditions (peak gradient <30 mm Hg). It is clinically important to distinguish between the obstructive and nonobstructive forms of HCM because management strategies are largely dependent on the presence or absence of symptoms caused by obstruction.

3.2. Cardiovascular magnetic resonance

Magnetic resonance imaging (MRI) and computed tomography imaging are being used increasingly to evaluate patients with HCM. Cardiovascular magnetic resonance (CMR), with its superior spatial resolution as well as tomographic imaging capability, has provided the opportunity to more accurately characterize the diverse phenotypic expression of HCM [21]. CMR is mainly used in the following situations: (1) the patients are suspected with HCM, but the echocardiogram is inconclusive, mostly because of suboptimal imaging from poor acoustic windows or when hypertrophy is localized to regions of the LV myocardium not well visualized by echocardiography [22]. (2) Hypertrophy confined to the apex (i.e., apical HCM) may be difficult to visualize with echocardiography but is evident with CMR [23]. (3) CMR can more readily detect the presence of apical aneurysms, which are potential implications for management with ICDs and/or anticoagulation; then CMR may identify high-risk status on the basis of massive hypertrophy [24].

4. Hypertrophic cardiomyopathy-associated genes

Hypertrophic cardiomyopathy is a common genetic cardiovascular disease. Genetic disorders account for 60–70% of HCM etiology. Since the identification of the first locus for familial HCM and the first mutation in MYH7-encoded beta-myosin heavy chain 20 years ago [25], over 1500 causal mutations associated with HCM encode sarcomeric proteins have been revealed [26]. According to gene susceptibility, HCM can be divided to "myofilament (sarcomeric) HCM," "Z-disk HCM," and "calcium-handling HCM," with "myofilament (sarcomeric) HCM" being the most common genetic form of HCM, account for 50% of all HCM cases [13]. Recently, large genotype-phenotype analysis correlation studies established implications for septal morphology, disease onset, and prognosis of certain sarcomeric genes, which may further facilitate commercialized genetic testing. On the other hand, unexplained left ventricular hypertrophies that mimic HCM appear in some syndromic diseases. These diseases are usually called phenocopies and may contain rare variants in metabolism genes. These mutations alter myocardial metabolism, resulting in increased wall thickness, cardiac storage abnormalities, and conduction irregularities second to multiple systematic disorders. The information of HCM susceptibility genes and HCM phenocopies are listed in **Tables 2** and **3** [13, 27, 28].

Although more than 1500 mutations linked to hypertrophic cardiomyopathy, most of which are unique to individual families and less evident for pathogenicity. There are four sarcomeric

Gene	Chromosomal position[a]	Protein	HCM-associated mutations	Location or function[b]
ACTA1	1q42.13–q42.2	Actin, alpha 1	1	Sarcomere, skeletal muscle
ACTC1	15q11–q14	Actin, alpha, cardiac muscle 1	25	Actin, alpha, cardiac muscle 1
ACTN2	1q42–q43	Actinin, alpha 2	5	Z-disk
ANKRD1	10q23.33	Ankyrin repeat domain 1	3	Z-disk and nucleus (transcription factor)
BRAF	7q34	v-Raf murine sarcoma viral oncogene homolog B1	1	
COA5	2q11.2	Cytochrome c oxidase assembly factor 5	1	Mitochondrial
CALM3	19q13.2–q13.3	Calmodulin 3 (phosphorylase kinase, delta)	1	Calcium sensor and signal transducer
CALR3	19p13.11	Calreticulin 3	2	endoplasmic reticulum chaperone
CASQ2	1p13.3–p11	Calsequestrin 2	1	Sarcoplasmic reticulum; calcium storage
CASQ2	1p13.3–p11	Calsequestrin 2	1	Sarcoplasmic reticulum; calcium storage
CAV3	3p25	Caveolin 3	1	Plasma membrane
COX15	10q24	Cytochrome c oxidase assembly homolog 15	2	Mitochondrial respiratory chain
CSRP3	11p15.1	Cysteine and glycine-rich protein 3	15	Z-disk
DES	2q35	Desmin	1	Intermediate lament
FHL1	Xq26	Four and a half LiM domains 1	3	Biomechanical stress sensor
FHOD3	18q12	Formin homology 2 domain containing 3	1	Actin-organizing protein
FXN	9q13–q21.1	Frataxin	1	Mitochondrial iron transport and respiration
GLA	Xq22	Galactosidase, alpha	765	Lysosome
JPH2	20q13.12	Junctophilin 2	6	Junctional membrane complexes; calcium signaling
KLF10	8q22.2	Kruppel-like factor 10	6	Transcriptional repressor; inhibits cell growth
MAP2K1	15q22.1–q22.33	Mitogen-activated protein kinase kinase 1	1	MAP kinase kinase; signal transduction
MAP2K2	19p13.3	Mitogen-activated protein kinase kinase 2	1	MAP kinase kinase; signal transduction
MRPL3	3q21–q23	Mitochondrial ribosomal protein L3	1	Mitochondrial ribosomal protein

Gene	Chromosomal position[a]	Protein	HCM-associated mutations	Location or function[b]
MTO1	6q13	Mitochondrial tRNA translation optimization 1	2	Mitochondrial tRNA modi cation
MYBPC3	11p11.2	Myosin-binding protein C, cardiac	506	Sarcomere
MYH6	14q12	Alpha-myosin heavy chain	3	Sarcomere
MYH7	14q12	Beta-myosin heavy chain	491	Sarcomere
MYL2	12q23–q24.3	ventricular myosin regulatory light chain	20	Sarcomere
MYL3	3p21.3–p21.2	Myosin light chain 3	16	Sarcomere
MYLK2	20q13.31	Myosin light chain kinase 2	2	Calcium/calmodulin-dependent kinase
MYO6	6q13	Myosin VI	1	Actin-based reverse-direction motor protein
MYOM1	18p11.31	Myomesin 1	1	Sarcomere
MYOZ2	4q26–q27	Myozenin 2	2	Z-disk
MYPN	10q21.3	Myopalladin	8	Z-disk
NDUFAF1	15q11.2–q21.3	NADH dehydrogenase (ubiquinone) complex I, assembly factor 1	2	Mitochondrial chaperone
NDUFV2	18p11.31–p11.2	NADH dehydrogenase (ubiquinone) avoprotein 2	1	Mitochondrial respiratory chain
NEXN	1p31.1	Nexilin	2	Z-disk
OBSCN	1q42.13	Obscurin	1	Sarcomere
PDLIM3	4q35	PDZ and LiM domain 3	1	Z-disk
PRKAG2	7q36.1	5′-AMP-activated protein kinase subunit gamma-2	7	energy sensor protein kinase
PLN	6q22.1	Phospholamban	7	Sarcoplasmic reticulum; regulates Ca^{2+} -ATPase
RAF1	3p25	v-Raf-1 murine leukemia viral oncogene homolog 1	1	Serine/threonine-protein kinase; signal transduction
SLC25A3	12q23	Solute carrier family 25, member 3	1	Phosphate carrier protein (cytosol to mitochondria)
SLC25A4	4q35	Solute carrier family 25, member 4	2	Adenine nucleotide translocator (cytosol/ mitochondria)
SOS1	2p22–p21	Son of sevenless homolog 1	1	Guanine nucleotide exchange factor for RAS proteins; signal transduction
SRI	7q21.1	Sorcin	2	Calcium-binding; modulates

Gene	Chromosomal position[a]	Protein	HCM-associated mutations	Location or function[b]
TCAP	17q12	Telethonin	7	Z-disk
TNNC1	3p21.3–p14.3	Troponin C	14	Sarcomere
TNNI3	19q13.4	Troponin I	70	Sarcomere
TNNT2	1q32	Troponin T	90	Sarcomere
TPM1	15q22.1	Alpha-tropomyosin	38	Sarcomere
TRIM63	1p34–p33	Tripartite motif-containing 63	3	Sarcomere; regulates protein degradation
TTN	2q31	Titin	6	Sarcomere
VCL	10q22.1–q23	Vinculin	1	Sarcomere

[a]Human genome mutation database (http://www.hgmd.cf.ac.uk/ac/index.php).

[b]National Center for Biotechnology information (http://ncbi.nlm.nih.gov/). Abbreviations: HCM, hypertrophic cardiomyopathy;tRNA, transfer RNA; AMP, adenosine monophosphate; ATP, adenosine triphosphate.

Table 2. HCM susceptibility genes [28].

Gene	Locus	Protein	Syndrome
TAZ	Xq28	Tafazzin (G4.5)	Barth syndrome/LVNC
DTNA	18q12	Alpha-dystrobrevin	Barth syndrome/LVNC
PRKAG2	7q35–q36.36	AMP-activated protein kinase	WPW/HCM
LAMP2	Xq24	Lysosome-associated membrane protein 2	Danon's syndrome/WPW
GAA	17q25.2–q25.3	Alpha-1,4-glucosidase deficiency	Pompe's disease
GLA	Xq22	Alpha-galactosidase A	Fabry's disease
AGL	1p21	Amylo-1,6-glucosidase	Forbes disease
FXN	9q13	Frataxin	Friedrich's ataxia
PTPN11	12q24.1	Protein tyrosine phosphatase, nonreceptor type 11, SHP-2	Noonan's syndrome, LEOPARD syndrome
RAF1	3p25	V-RAF-1 murine leukemia viral oncogene homolog 1	Noonan's syndrome, LEOPARD syndrome
KRAS	12p12.1	v-Ki-ras2 Kirsten rat sarcoma viral oncogene homolog	Noonan's syndrome
SOS1	2p22–p21	Son of sevenless homolog 1	Noonan's syndrome

AMP, adenosine monophosphate; HCM, hypertrophic cardiomyopathy; LEOPARD, mnemonic for syndrome with clinical characteristics of lentigines, electrocardiographic conduction abnormalities, ocular hypertelorism, pulmonary hypertension, abnormal genitalia, retarded growth, deafness; LVNC, left ventricular noncompaction; WPW, Wolff-Parkinson-White syndrome

Table 3. HCM phenocopies [29].

genes that carry the majority of HCM-related mutations and encode the proteins: myosin heavy chain (*MYH7*) and myosin-binding protein C3 (MYBPC3) are most common, together account for 75–80% of sarcomere mutations in HCM, while an additional 10% come from cardiac troponin T type 2 (*TNNT2*) and cardiac troponin I type 3 (TNNI3) (**Figure 1**) [3].

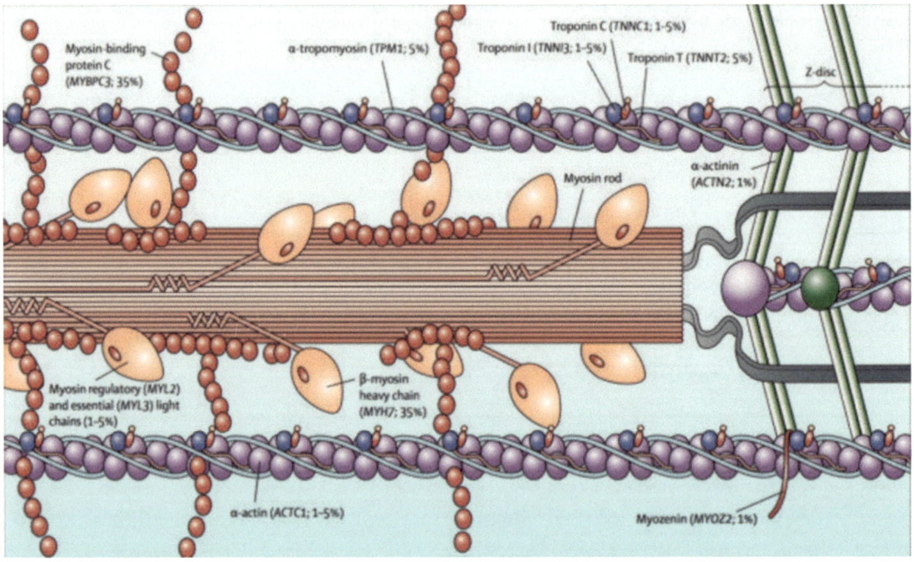

Figure 1. Locations of genes within the cardiac sarcomere known to cause hypertrophic cardiomyopathy [3].

5. Hypertrophic cardiomyopathy-associated miRNA

Despite extensive exploration of many genes, potential genetic associations remain to be found in approximately 30% of HCM patients. The recent newly developed field that has won extensive attention is microRNAs (miRNAs) in cardiovascular biology. miRNAs are noncoding RNAs with a length of approximately 22 ribonucleic acid molecules that bind mRNAs and regulate their expression through posttranslational repression or mRNA cleavage and degradation [30, 31]. It is estimated that the human genome contains more than 1000 miRNAs, which regulate at least 30–60% of protein-coding genes [32]. Multiple studies revealed that single or combined function of miRNAs is directly involved in the pathophysiology of cardiac hypertrophy, fibrosis, and electrical remodeling in vivo and in vitro [33]. The biological functions regulated by miRNAs affecting HCM are listed below (**Table 4** and **Figure 2**). Since miRNAs play a more and more important role in the development of HCM, they are being studied for potential diagnostic biomarkers and a promising therapeutics for HCM.

The schematic shows the miRNAs and their targets involving in cellular hypertrophy, gene switching, electrical remodeling, as well as fibrosis during cardiac hypertrophy. An upward

miRNA	Target	Biological effect	References
miR-340	Dystrophin	Cardiac eccentric	[34]
		Cardiac hypertrophy	
		Heart failure	
miR-133	RhoA	Cardiac hypertrophy	[35, 36]
	Cdc42	Heart failure	
	Nelf-A/WHSC2		
	HCN2		
miR-1	IGF-1	Cardiac hypertrophy	[35, 37, 38]
	calmodulin	Dilated cardiomyopathies	
	Mef2a	Heart failure	
	RasGAP		
	Cdk-9		
miR-208	Thrap1	Cardiac hypertrophy	[39]
	Myostatin		
miR-21	sprouty1	Cardiac hypertrophy	[40]
		Cardiac fibrosis	
miR-23a	MuRF1	Cardiac hypertrophy	[41]
miR-195		Cardiac hypertrophy	[42]
		Heart failure	
miR-99a	mTOR	Cardiac hypertrophy	[43]
	FGFR3	Heart failure	
miR-199a	NFAT	Cardiac hypertrophy	[44]
		Cardiac fibrosis	
		Heart failure	
miR-30	CTGF	Cardiac fibrosis	[35]
miR-29		Cardiac hypertrophy	[45]
		Cardiac fibrosis	

Thrap1, thyroid hormone receptor-associated protein 1; MuRF1, myostatin, muscle-specific ring finger protein 1; RasGAP, Ras GTPase-activating protein; Cdk9, cyclin-dependent kinase 9; Mef2a, calmodulin, myocyte enhancer factor 2A; IGF1, insulin-like growth factor 1; CTGF, connective tissue growth factor; HCN2, hyperpolarization-activated, cyclic nucleotide-gated K þ 2; FGFR3, fibroblast growth factor receptor 3; NFAT, nuclear factor of activated T-cells

Table 4. MiRNA in cardiac hypertrophy.

or a downward arrow is used to represent the upregulation or downregulation of a specific miRNA, respectively. All listed targets have been validated: Thrap1, thyroid hormone receptor-associated protein 1; MuRF1, myostatin, muscle-specific ring finger protein 1; RasGAP, Ras

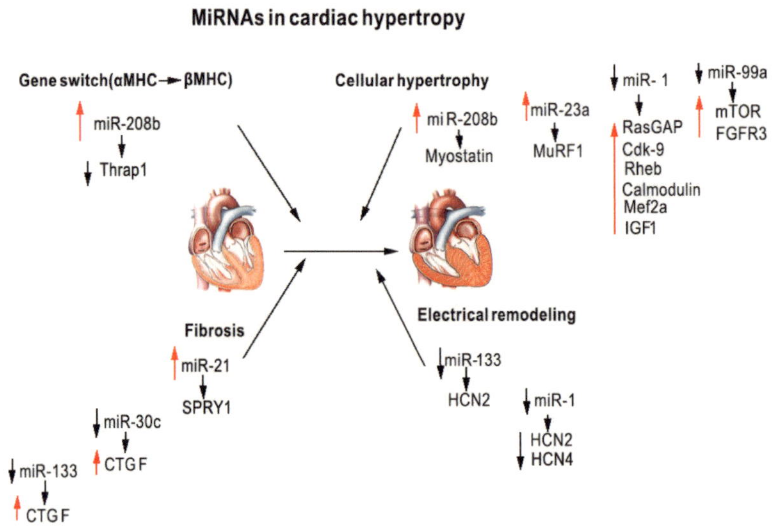

Figure 2. MiRNAs in hypertrophic cardiomyopathy.

GTPase-activating protein; Cdk9, cyclin-dependent kinase 9; Rheb, Ras homolog enriched in the brain; Mef2a, calmodulin, myocyte enhancer factor 2A; IGF1, insulin-like growth factor 1; SPRY1, sprouty 1; CTGF, connective tissue growth factor; HCN2/4, hyperpolarization-activated, cyclic nucleotide-gated K þ 2/4; and FGFR3, fibroblast growth factor receptor 3.

6. Treatment of HCM

As is typical for many forms of CVD, many current therapeutic strategies for HCM try to alleviate symptoms and prevent complications. Although once considered rare and terminal with annual mortality rates of up to 6%, HCM has now emerged as a very treatable form of heart disease [46]. Due to contemporary management strategies and treatment interventions, including ICDs for SD prevention, a variety of available surgical HCM mortality rates have dropped to 0.5% per year [47].

6.1. Pharmacology management

It has been clearly demonstrated that left ventricular outflow tract obstruction at rest in HCM patients is a strong, independent predictor of progression to severe symptoms of heart failure and of death [48]. Considering the mechanisms underlying myocardial contraction (calcium ions binding to troponin C and excitation-contraction coupling), a number of medical regimens have been used in these patients with the goal of lessening or eliminating the LVOT gradient through negative inotropy [7].

Pharmacological therapy of HCM consists of β-blockers and calcium channel blockers. β-Blockers and calcium channel blockers are used to improve diastolic function in patients with HCM. Small and mostly retrospective studies suggest that oral propranolol can abolish or reduce resting and provocable LVOTO and provide symptomatic benefit [49, 50]. Donald et al.'s study showed that β-blocker abolished the increase in gradient caused by isoproterenol and, more importantly, halved the increase in gradient caused by exercise [51]. In a 5-year follow-up, a study demonstrated that propranolol significantly improved the HCM patient's syndrome (dyspnea, angina, palpitations, dizziness, and syncope) by 58–100% [52].

Calcium channel blockade is used to HCM patients since it might ameliorate the hypercontractility characteristic of HCM. Verapamil, which has the best profile of the calcium antagonists, has been widely used in the treatment of HCM. A double-blind, placebo-controlled crossover trial studied oral propranolol, verapamil, and placebo, to 19 patients with HCM (17 with hypertrophic obstructive cardiomyopathy). Most patients derived symptomatic benefit from drug therapy, especially with verapamil [53]. In a recent study, the calcium channel blocker diltiazem was used to treat 38 HCM patients carrying *MYBPC3* mutation; results showed that diltiazem is safe and may improve early LV remodeling in HCM [54].

Another medicine used in hypertrophic obstructive cardiomyopathy (HOCM) patients is disopyramide, which is an effective negative inotropic agent by mediating sodium-calcium exchange [55]. Pollick et al. administered intravenous disopyramide to 43 patients with HOCM. The LVOT gradient was abolished or reduced; the effect was greater than that seen previously for either propranolol or verapamil [56]. By virtue of its atrial antiarrhythmic properties, disopyramide may be of particular benefit in HOCM patients with atrial fibrillation. Then, the ESC guideline recommended disopyramide, as Class IA anti-arrhythmic drug, which may be added to a maximum tolerated dose (usually 400–600 mg/day), if β-blockers alone are ineffective [19]. It can improve exercise tolerance and functional capacity as well as abolish basal LV outflow pressure gradients without proarrhythmic effects or an increased risk of sudden cardiac death.

6.2. Invasive treatment of LVOTO

Invasive treatment should be considered in patients with an LVOTO. The American and European colleges of cardiology recommend invasive treatment to (1) patients with labile obstruction and peak LVOT pressure gradients ≥50 mm Hg during exercise or provocation and resting gradients >30 mm Hg and (2) patients with moderate-to-severe symptoms (New York Heart Association (NYHA) functional classes III–IV) refractory to medical therapy [7, 19]. Two common surgical procedures performed in about 3% of obstructive HCM patients are septal myectomy and alcohol septal ablation [28].

6.2.1. Ventricular septal myectomy

Since the time of the first myectomy through the aortic root by Cleland in Great Britain in November 1958 [57], ventricular septal myectomy (Morrow procedure) is the most commonly performed surgical procedure used to treat LVOTO [58]. In a 10-year follow-up in 185 patients, the patients with hypertrophic cardiomyopathy (HCM) were treated with septal myotomy-myomectomy (MM) with a significant reduction in left ventricular outflow gradient at rest, which improves exercise capacity and symptoms. Long-term symptomatic benefit is achieved in 70–80% of patients with a long-term survival compared to that of the general population [59]. Notably, operative mortality at surgical centers is now low, reduced to less than 1%.

6.2.2. *Alcohol septal ablation*

Percutaneous alcohol septal ablation is an alternative to surgical myectomy, which is a selective injection of alcohol into a septal perforator artery to create a localized septal scar. There are no randomized trials comparing surgery and septal alcohol ablation (SAA), but several meta-analyses have shown that SAA procedures improve functional status with a similar surgery in terms of gradient reduction, symptom improvement, and exercise capacity [60]. The main nonfatal complications are AV block in 7–20% of patients and a procedural mortality of about 2% [3]. Alcohol ablation has been recommended as a selective alternative for older patients, those with comorbidities, or patients with an absolute reluctance toward surgery.

6.2.3. *Implant cardiac defibrillator*

In addition to myectomy, the implantable cardioverter-defibrillator (ICD) has proven to be effective in terminating life-threatening ventricular tachyarrhythmia in HCM, altering the natural course of the disease and prolonging life [61, 62]. The indications for ICD placement are (1) positive family history of several sudden cardiac deaths in a distant family member, (2) nonsustained ventricular tachycardia on Holter monitoring, (3) LVH >30 mm, (4) prior unexplained syncope during exercise or at rest, and (5) an abnormal blood pressure response during exercise, which can be described as progressive decrease in the systolic value by 20 mm Hg after an initial increase or an increase in systolic blood pressure of <20 mm Hg from the baseline value or a [2, 63, 64]. The decision for placement of primary prevention of ICD in HCM often involves a large measure of individual clinical judgment, particularly when the evidence for risk is ambiguous.

7. Recent advances toward precision medicine for HCM

7.1. iPSC-CMs

Induced pluripotent stem cells (also known as iPS cells or iPSCs) are a type of embryonic stemlike cells that can be generated directly from adult cells [65–67]. The emergence of patient-derived induced pluripotent stem cells (iPSCs), which can be differentiated into functional cardiomyocytes (CMs) in vitro, may provide an exciting new approach to understand disease mechanisms underpinning inherited heart diseases (**Figure 3**) [26, 68].

iPSC-CMs derived from a patient with HCM caused by the MYH7 mutation p.Arg442Gly and mutation p.Arg663His have demonstrated the pathogenic effects [69, 70]. HCM iPSC-CMs exhibited structural abnormalities consistent with the HCM phenotype. Similar calcium-handling abnormalities were identified, consistent with observations made from animal models [70]. These studies explored the possible patient-specific and mutation-specific disease mechanism of HCM and demonstrated the potential of using HCM iPSC-CMs for future development of therapeutic strategies.

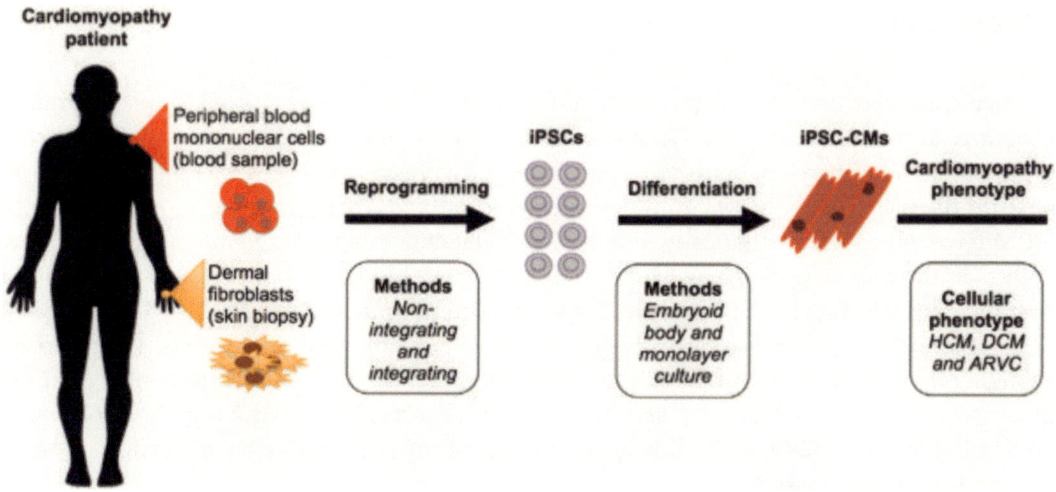

Figure 3. Generation of iPSCs from patients and then the differentiation to cardiomyocytes and then to their use in different cardiomyopaties. HCM, hypertrophic cardiomyopathy; DCM, dilated cardiomyopathy; ARVC, arrhythmogenic right ventricular cardiomyopathy.

In vivo direct cardiac reprogramming of somatic cells into cardiomyocytes is a potential offshoot of current reprogramming techniques but has not yet been tested in humans [71]. For HCM in particular, the possibility of converting cardiac fibroblasts into functional cardiomyocytes could theoretically ameliorate hypertrophy and improve diastolic function.

Although still in a nascent stage, direct cardiac reprogramming has undergone great advances and attracted considerable attention, these techniques could offer a renewable source of cardiomyocytes and deliver medicine individually tailored to each patient [72].

7.2. Gene editing technology

Gene editing is rapidly progressing from being a research/screening tool to one that promises important applications downstream in drug development and cell therapy. As primarily inherited cardiomyopathies, HCM is perhaps the strongest candidate for gene editing technologies [73, 74]. Recently, genome modification technologies, such as TALEN (transcription activator-like effector nucleases), ZFN (zinc finger nucleases), as well as CRISPR/Cas9 nuclease (clustered regularly interspaced short palindromic repeats/Cas9 nuclease systems), allow for specific editing of individual gene mutations [74, 75].

This CRISPR/Cas9 system makes it possible to efficiently, easily, and cheaply modify the genome, which is the current front-runner of these gene modification technologies [76]. To date, the CRISPR/Cas9 system has been used to successfully engineer cardiomyopathy into in zebra fish and mice models and is currently being applied to larger animals such as pigs and nonhuman primates [77]. This new technology promises to provide researchers with more accurate model for studying and treating HCM [78].

8. Conclusion

Hypertrophic cardiomyopathy (HCM) is a global and is considered one of the most common genetic cardiovascular diseases. Genetic variants, molecular mechanisms, and clinical phenotypes of HCM vary on a patient-by-patient basis. Fifty years ago, HCM was thought to be an obscure disease. Today, however, our understanding and ability to diagnose patients with HCM have improved dramatically, due to improvements in screening and detection of gene defects in the human genome as well as iPSC-CM model in HCM patients and gene editing technology (including CRISPR/Cas9). However, currently, treatments for HCM are directed at symptomatic relief, preventing sudden death. The future goal of research is focused on changing the natural course of the disease and preventing its phenotypic expression. Working group from clinical, translational, and basic science aspects should work together to develop novel treatments to HCM. Then, finally, with the effort of all groups, we will reach the goal of the precision medicine of HCM.

Author details

Yamin Liu[1,2]*, Zhao Li[3], Xiaofan Guo[3], Xiong Jing[4], Xueli Zhang[1], Hua Shao[1], Yufan Guan[2] and Maria R. Abraham[2]

*Address all correspondence to: liuyamincn@hotmail.com

1 Department of Pharmacy, Zhongda Hospital, School of Medicine, Southeast University, Nanjing, China

2 Department of Cardiology, School of Medicine, Johns Hopkins University, MD, USA

3 Department of Cardiology, The First Hospital of China Medical University, Shenyang, Liaoning, China

4 Department of Pharmacology, Nanjing Medical University, Nanjing, China

References

[1] Sen-Chowdhry S, Jacoby D, Moon JC, McKenna WJ. Update on hypertrophic cardiomyopathy and a guide to the guidelines. Nature. Reviews. 2016;**13**(11):651-675

[2] Hensley N, Dietrich J, Nyhan D, Mitter N, Yee MS, Brady M. Hypertrophic cardiomyopathy: A review. Anesthesia and Analgesia. 2015;**120**(3):554-569

[3] Maron BJ, Maron MS. Hypertrophic cardiomyopathy. Lancet. 2013;**381**(9862):242-255

[4] Semsarian C, Ingles J, Maron MS, Maron BJ. New perspectives on the prevalence of hypertrophic cardiomyopathy. Journal of the American College of Cardiology. 2015;**65**(12): 1249-1254

[5] Towbin JA. Hypertrophic cardiomyopathy. Pacing and Clinical Electrophysiology. 2009; **32**Suppl 2:S23-31

[6] Jacoby DL, DePasquale EC, McKenna WJ. Hypertrophic cardiomyopathy: diagnosis, risk stratification and treatment. CMAJ. 2013;**185**(2):127-134

[7] American College of Cardiology Foundation/American Heart Association Task Force on Practice Guidelines, American Association for Thoracic Society, American Society of Echocardiography, American Society of Nuclear Cardiology, Heart Failure Society of America, Heart Rhythm Society, Society for Cardiovascular Angiography and Interventions, Society of Thoracic Surgeons, Gersh BJ, et al. 2011 ACCF/AHA guideline for the diagnosis and treatment of hypertrophic cardiomyopathy: executive summary: A report of the American College of Cardiology Foundation/American Heart Association Task Force on Practice Guidelines. The Journal of Thoracic and Cardiovascular Surgery. 2011;**142**(6):1303-1338

[8] Yang YJ, Fan CM, Yuan JQ, Zhang HB, Duan FJ, Wang ZM, Guo XY, Zhai SS, An SY, Hang F et al. Long-term survival after acute myocardial infarction in patients with hypertrophic cardiomyopathy. Clinical Cardiology. 2017;**40**(1):26-31

[9] Rodrigues JC, Rohan S, Ghosh Dastidar A, Harries I, Lawton CB, Ratcliffe LE, Burchell AE, Hart EC, Hamilton MC, Paton JF et al. Hypertensive heart disease versus hypertrophic cardiomyopathy: multi-parametric cardiovascular magnetic resonance discriminators when end-diastolic wall thickness >/= 15 mm. European Radiology. 2017;**27**(3):1125-1135

[10] Maron BJ, Casey SA, Poliac LC, Gohman TE, Almquist AK, Aeppli DM. Clinical course of hypertrophic cardiomyopathy in a regional United States cohort. JAMA. 1999;**281**(7):650-655

[11] Maron BJ. Hypertrophic cardiomyopathy: a systematic review. JAMA. 2002;**287**(10):1308-1320

[12] Maron BJ, Olivotto I, Bellone P, Conte MR, Cecchi F, Flygenring BP, Casey SA, Gohman TE, Bongioanni S, Spirito P. Clinical profile of stroke in 900 patients with hypertrophic cardiomyopathy. Journal of the American College of Cardiology. 2002;**39**(2):301-307

[13] Kraker J, Viswanathan SK, Knoll R, Sadayappan S. Recent advances in the molecular genetics of familial hypertrophic cardiomyopathy in south Asian descendants. Frontiers in Physiology. 2016;**7**:499

[14] Shirani J, Pick R, Roberts WC, Maron BJ. Morphology and significance of the left ventricular collagen network in young patients with hypertrophic cardiomyopathy and sudden cardiac death. Journal of the American College of Cardiology. 2000;**35**(1):36-44

[15] Devereux RB, Reichek N. Echocardiographic determination of left ventricular mass in man. Anatomic validation of the method. Circulation. 1977;**55**(4):613-618

[16] Maron MS, Olivotto I, Zenovich AG, Link MS, Pandian NG, Kuvin JT, Nistri S, Cecchi F, Udelson JE, Maron BJ. Hypertrophic cardiomyopathy is predominantly a disease of left ventricular outflow tract obstruction. Circulation 2006;**114**(21):2232-2239

[17] Heatlie GJ, Pointon K. Cardiac magnetic resonance imaging. Postgraduate Medical Journal. 2004;**80**(939):19-22

[18] Shah PM, Gramiak R, Kramer DH. Ultrasound localization of left ventricular outflow obstruction in hypertrophic obstructive cardiomyopathy. Circulation 1969;**40**(1):3-11

[19] Authors/Task Force Members, Elliott PM, Anastasakis A, Borger MA, Borggrefe M, Cecchi F, Charron P, Hagege AA, Lafont A, Limongelli G, et al. 2014 ESC guidelines on diagnosis and management of hypertrophic cardiomyopathy: The Task Force for the Diagnosis and Management of Hypertrophic Cardiomyopathy of the European Society of Cardiology (ESC). European Heart Journal. 2014;**35**(39):2733-2779

[20] Kampmann C, Wiethoff CM, Wenzel A, Stolz G, Betancor M, Wippermann CF, Huth RG, Habermehl P, Knuf M, Emschermann T, et al. Normal values of M mode echocardiographic measurements of more than 2000 healthy infants and children in central Europe. Heart (British Cardiac Society). 2000;**83**(6):667-672

[21] Maron MS. Clinical utility of cardiovascular magnetic resonance in hypertrophic cardiomyopathy. Journal of Cardiovascular Magnetic Resonance. 2012;**14**:13

[22] Maron MS, Maron BJ, Harrigan C, Buros J, Gibson CM, Olivotto I, Biller L, Lesser JR, Udelson JE, Manning WJ, et al. Hypertrophic cardiomyopathy phenotype revisited after 50 years with cardiovascular magnetic resonance. Journal of the American College of Cardiology. 2009;**54**(3):220-228

[23] Moon JC, Fisher NG, McKenna WJ, Pennell DJ. Detection of apical hypertrophic cardiomyopathy by cardiovascular magnetic resonance in patients with non-diagnostic echocardiography. Heart (British Cardiac Society). 2004;**90**(6):645-649

[24] Maron MS, Lesser JR, Maron BJ. Management implications of massive left ventricular hypertrophy in hypertrophic cardiomyopathy significantly underestimated by echocardiography but identified by cardiovascular magnetic resonance. The American Journal of Cardiology. 2010;**105**(12):1842-1843

[25] Jarcho JA, McKenna W, Pare JA, Solomon SD, Holcombe RF, Dickie S, Levi T, Donis-Keller H, Seidman JG, Seidman CE. Mapping a gene for familial hypertrophic cardiomyopathy to chromosome 14q1. The New England Journal of Medicine. 1989;**321**(20):1372-1378

[26] Ross SB, Fraser ST, Semsarian C. Induced pluripotent stem cells in the inherited cardiomyopathies: From disease mechanisms to novel therapies. Trends in Cardiovascular Medicine. 2016;**26**(8):663-672

[27] Landstrom AP, Ackerman MJ. Mutation type is not clinically useful in predicting prognosis in hypertrophic cardiomyopathy. Circulation. 2010;**122**(23):2441-2449; discussion 2450

[28] Roma-Rodrigues C, Fernandes AR. Genetics of hypertrophic cardiomyopathy: Advances and pitfalls in molecular diagnosis and therapy. The Application of Clinical Genetics. 2014;**7**:195-208

[29] Bos JM, Towbin JA, Ackerman MJ. Diagnostic, prognostic, and therapeutic implications of genetic testing for hypertrophic cardiomyopathy. Journal of the American College of Cardiology. 2009;**54**(3):201-211

[30] Bartel DP. MicroRNAs: Genomics, biogenesis, mechanism, and function. Cell. 2004;**116**(2): 281-297

[31] Papageorgiou N, Tslamandris S, Giolis A, Tousoulis D: MicroRNAs in Cardiovascular Disease: Perspectives and Reality. Cardiology in review 2016;**24**(3):110-118

[32] Zhao W, Zhao SP, Zhao YH. MicroRNA-143/-145 in cardiovascular diseases. BioMed Research International. 2015;**2015**:531740

[33] Condorelli G, Latronico MV, Cavarretta E. microRNAs in cardiovascular diseases: Current knowledge and the road ahead. Journal of the American College of Cardiology. 2014;**63**(21):2177-2187

[34] Zhou J, Gao J, Zhang X, Liu Y, Gu S, Zhang X, An X, Yan J, Xin Y, Su P. microRNA-340-5p functions downstream of cardiotrophin-1 to regulate cardiac eccentric hypertrophy and heart failure via target gene dystrophin. International Heart Journal. 2015;**56**(4):454-458 (electronic)

[35] Han M, Toli J, Abdellatif M. MicroRNAs in the cardiovascular system. Current Opinion in Cardiology. 2011;**26**(3):181-189

[36] Care A, Catalucci D, Felicetti F, Bonci D, Addario A, Gallo P, Bang ML, Segnalini P, Gu Y, Dalton ND et al. MicroRNA-133 controls cardiac hypertrophy. Nature Medicine. 2007;**13**(5):613-618

[37] Ikeda S, He A, Kong SW, Lu J, Bejar R, Bodyak N, Lee KH, Ma Q, Kang PM, Golub TR et al. MicroRNA-1 negatively regulates expression of the hypertrophy-associated calmodulin and Mef2a genes. Molecular and Cellular Biology. 2009;**29**(8):2193-2204

[38] Elia L, Contu R, Quintavalle M, Varrone F, Chimenti C, Russo MA, Cimino V, De Marinis L, Frustaci A, Catalucci D et al. Reciprocal regulation of microRNA-1 and insulin-like growth factor-1 signal transduction cascade in cardiac and skeletal muscle in physiological and pathological conditions. Circulation. 2009;**120**(23):2377-2385

[39] Callis TE, Pandya K, Seok HY, Tang RH, Tatsuguchi M, Huang ZP, Chen JF, Deng Z, Gunn B, Shumate J, et al. MicroRNA-208a is a regulator of cardiac hypertrophy and conduction in mice. The Journal of Clinical Investigation. 2009;**119**(9):2772-2786

[40] Thum T, Gross C, Fiedler J, Fischer T, Kissler S, Bussen M, Galuppo P, Just S, Rottbauer W, Frantz S, et al. MicroRNA-21 contributes to myocardial disease by stimulating MAP kinase signalling in fibroblasts. Nature. 2008;**456**(7224):980-984

[41] Sayed D, Hong C, Chen IY, Lypowy J, Abdellatif M. MicroRNAs play an essential role in the development of cardiac hypertrophy. Circulation Research. 2007;**100**(3):416-424

[42] van Rooij E, Sutherland LB, Liu N, Williams AH, McAnally J, Gerard RD, Richardson JA, Olson EN. A signature pattern of stress-responsive microRNAs that can evoke cardiac hypertrophy and heart failure. Proceedings of the National Academy of Sciences of the United States of America. 2006;**103**(48):18255-18260

[43] Li Q, Xie J, Wang B, Li R, Bai J, Ding L, Gu R, Wang L, Xu B. Overexpression of microRNA-99a attenuates cardiac hypertrophy. PLoS One. 2016;**11**(2):e0148480

[44] da Costa Martins PA, Salic K, Gladka MM, Armand AS, Leptidis S, el Azzouzi H, Hansen A, Coenen-de Roo CJ, Bierhuizen MF, van der Nagel R et al. MicroRNA-199b targets the nuclear kinase Dyrk1a in an auto-amplification loop promoting calcineurin/NFAT signalling. Nature Cell Biology. 2010;**12**(12):1220-1227

[45] Roncarati R, Viviani Anselmi C, Losi MA, Papa L, Cavarretta E, Da Costa Martins P, Contaldi C, Saccani Jotti G, Franzone A, Galastri L, et al. Circulating miR-29a, among other up-regulated microRNAs, is the only biomarker for both hypertrophy and fibrosis in patients with hypertrophic cardiomyopathy. Journal of the American College of Cardiology. 2014;**63**(9):920-927 (electronic)

[46] Maron BJ, Ommen SR, Semsarian C, Spirito P, Olivotto I, Maron MS. Hypertrophic cardiomyopathy: Present and future, with translation into contemporary cardiovascular medicine. Journal of the American College of Cardiology. 2014;**64**(1):83-99

[47] Maron BJ, Rowin EJ, Casey SA, Link MS, Lesser JR, Chan RH, Garberich RF, Udelson JE, Maron MS. Hypertrophic cardiomyopathy in adulthood associated with low cardiovascular mortality with contemporary management strategies. Journal of the American College of Cardiology. 2015;**65**(18):1915-1928

[48] Maron MS, Olivotto I, Betocchi S, Casey SA, Lesser JR, Losi MA, Cecchi F, Maron BJ. Effect of left ventricular outflow tract obstruction on clinical outcome in hypertrophic cardiomyopathy. The New England Journal of Medicine. 2003;**348**(4):295-303

[49] Adelman AG, Shah PM, Gramiak R, Wigle ED. Long-term propranolol therapy in muscular subaortic stenosis. British Heart Journal. 1970;**32**(6):804-811

[50] Fifer MA, Vlahakes GJ. Management of symptoms in hypertrophic cardiomyopathy. Circulation. 2008;**117**(3):429-439

[51] Harrison DC, Braunwald E, Glick G, Mason DT, Chidsey CA, Ross J, Jr. Effects of beta adrenergic blockade on the circulation with particular reference to observations in patients with hypertrophic subaortic stenosis. Circulation. 1964;**29**:84-98

[52] Frank MJ, Abdulla AM, Canedo MI, Saylors RE. Long-term medical management of hypertrophic obstructive cardiomyopathy. The American Journal of Cardiology. 1978;**42**(6):993-1001

[53] Gilligan DM, Chan WL, Joshi J, Clarke P, Fletcher A, Krikler S, Oakley CM. A double-blind, placebo-controlled crossover trial of nadolol and verapamil in mild and moderately symptomatic hypertrophic cardiomyopathy. Journal of the American College of Cardiology. 1993;**21**(7):1672-1679

[54] Ho CY, Lakdawala NK, Cirino AL, Lipshultz SE, Sparks E, Abbasi SA, Kwong RY, Antman EM, Semsarian C, Gonzalez A et al. Diltiazem treatment for pre-clinical hypertrophic cardiomyopathy sarcomere mutation carriers: a pilot randomized trial to modify disease expression. JACC: Heart Failure. 2015;**3**(2):180-188

[55] Kondo N, Mizukami M, Shibata S. Negative inotropic effects of disopyramide on guinea-pig papillary muscles. British Journal of Pharmacology. 1990;**101**(4):789-792

[56] Pollick C, Kimball B, Henderson M, Wigle ED. Disopyramide in hypertrophic cardiomyopathy. I. Hemodynamic assessment after intravenous administration. The American Journal of Cardiology. 1988;**62**(17):1248-1251

[57] Morrow AG, Brockenbrough EC. Surgical treatment of idiopathic hypertrophic subaortic stenosis: Technic and hemodynamic results of subaortic ventriculomyotomy. Annals of Surgery. 1961;**154**:181-189

[58] Morrow AG, Reitz BA, Epstein SE, Henry WL, Conkle DM, Itscoitz SB, Redwood DR. Operative treatment in hypertrophic subaortic stenosis. Techniques, and the results of pre and postoperative assessments in 83 patients. Circulation. 1975;**52**(1):88-102

[59] Krajcer Z, Leachman RD, Cooley DA, Coronado R. Septal myotomy-myomectomy versus mitral valve replacement in hypertrophic cardiomyopathy. Ten-year follow-up in 185 patients. Circulation. 1989;**80**(3 Pt 1):I57-64

[60] Sigwart U. Non-surgical myocardial reduction for hypertrophic obstructive cardiomyopathy. Lancet. 1995;**346**(8969):211-214

[61] Yin K, Ding L, Li Y, Hua W: Long-term follow-up of arrhythmogenic right ventricular cardiomyopathy patients with an implantable cardioverter-defibrillator for prevention of sudden cardiac death. Clinical cardiology 2017;**40**(4):216-221

[62] Amara N, Boveda S, Defaye P, Klug D, Treguer F, Amet D, Perier MC, Gras D, Algalarrondo V, Bouzeman A, et al. Implantable cardioverter-defibrillator therapy among patients with non-ischaemic vs. ischaemic cardiomyopathy for primary prevention of sudden cardiac death. Europace; 2017:1-8. Doi: 10.1093/europace/euw379

[63] Maron BJ, Spirito P, Shen WK, Haas TS, Formisano F, Link MS, Epstein AE, Almquist AK, Daubert JP, Lawrenz T et al. Implantable cardioverter-defibrillators and prevention of sudden cardiac death in hypertrophic cardiomyopathy. JAMA. 2007;**298**(4):405-412

[64] Jayatilleke I, Doolan A, Ingles J, McGuire M, Booth V, Richmond DR, Semsarian C. Long-term follow-up of implantable cardioverter defibrillator therapy for hypertrophic cardiomyopathy. The American Journal of Cardiology. 2004;**93**(9):1192-1194

[65] Quintanilla RH, Jr. Cellular characterization of human pluripotent stem cells. Methods in Molecular Biology (Clifton, NJ) 2013;**997**:179-190

[66] Hackett CH, Fortier LA. Embryonic stem cells and iPS cells: Sources and characteristics. The Veterinary Clinics of North America. Equine Practice. 2011;**27**(2):233-242

[67] Chou SJ, Yu WC, Chang YL, Chen WY, Chang WC, Chien Y, Yen JC, Liu YY, Chen SJ, Wang CY, et al. Energy utilization of induced pluripotent stem cell-derived cardiomyocyte in Fabry disease. International Journal of Cardiology. 2017;**232**:255-263

[68] Novak A, Barad L, Zeevi-Levin N, Shick R, Shtrichman R, Lorber A, Itskovitz-Eldor J, Binah O. Cardiomyocytes generated from CPVTD307H patients are arrhythmogenic in response to beta-adrenergic stimulation. Journal of Cellular and Molecular Medicine. 2012;**16**(3):468-482

[69] Lan F, Lee AS, Liang P, Sanchez-Freire V, Nguyen PK, Wang L, Han L, Yen M, Wang Y, Sun N, et al. Abnormal calcium handling properties underlie familial hypertrophic cardiomyopathy pathology in patient-specific induced pluripotent stem cells. Cell Stem Cell. 2013;**12**(1):101-113

[70] Han L, Li Y, Tchao J, Kaplan AD, Lin B, Li Y, Mich-Basso J, Lis A, Hassan N, London B, et al. Study familial hypertrophic cardiomyopathy using patient-specific induced pluripotent stem cells. Cardiovascular Research. 2014;**104**(2):258-269

[71] Sadahiro T, Yamanaka S, Ieda M. Direct cardiac reprogramming: Progress and challenges in basic biology and clinical applications. Circulation Research. 2015;**116**(8):1378-1391

[72] Chen O, Qian L. Direct cardiac reprogramming: Advances in cardiac regeneration. BioMed Research International. 2015;**2015**:580406

[73] Chadwick AC, Musunuru K. Genome editing for the study of cardiovascular diseases. Current Cardiology Reports. 2017;**19**(3):22

[74] Strong A, Musunuru K. Genome editing in cardiovascular diseases. Nature. Reviews. 2017;**14**(1):11-20

[75] Chen L, Tang L, Xiang H, Jin L, Li Q, Dong Y, Wang W, Zhang G. Advances in genome editing technology and its promising application in evolutionary and ecological studies. Gigascience. 2014;**3**:24

[76] Eyquem J, Mansilla-Soto J, Giavridis T, van der Stegen SJ, Hamieh M, Cunanan KM, Odak A, Gonen M, Sadelain M. Targeting a CAR to the TRAC locus with CRISPR/Cas9 enhances tumour rejection. Nature. 2017;**543**(7643):113-117

[77] Duncker DJ, Bakkers J, Brundel BJ, Robbins J, Tardiff JC, Carrier L. Animal and in silico models for the study of sarcomeric cardiomyopathies. Cardiovascular Research. 2015;**105**(4):439-448

[78] Waddington SN, Privolizzi R, Karda R, O'Neill HC. A broad overview and review of CRISPR-Cas technology and stem cells. Current Stem Cell Reports. 2016;**2**:9-20

Chapter 10

Genetic Polymorphisms and Ischemic Heart Disease

Francesco Fedele, Mariateresa Pucci and
Paolo Severino

Additional information is available at the end of the chapter

http://dx.doi.org/10.5772/intechopen.69621

Abstract

Although the progression in diagnostic tools, prevention strategies, and therapies, ischemic heart disease still represents the major cause of mortality and morbidity worldwide that globally represents an important problem for individuals and healthcare resources. By convention, ischemic heart disease is associated with the presence of an atherosclerotic plaque that is able to limit the flow in large-medium-sized coronary arteries. Nevertheless, several findings suggest a more complex pathophysiology of ischemic heart disease. At this time, there is no well-defined assessment of myocardial ischemia pathophysiology. Moreover, several data have identified genetic variations at different loci that are linked with ischemic heart disease susceptibility. This chapter aims to examine this complicated disease and to review the evidence on the genetic heritability acting with other factors in determining the presence of ischemic heart disease, due to either an obstruction in epicardial vessels or a dysfunction of coronary microcirculation.

Keywords: atherosclerosis, coronary artery disease, coronary microvascular disease, endothelial dysfunction, ion channel, ischemic heart disease, myocardial infarction, myocardial ischemia, risk factor, single-nucleotide polymorphism

1. Introduction

Nowadays, ischemic heart disease remains a major cause of death and disability worldwide for both men and women, although the evolution in prevention and therapy strategies [1]. By convention, ischemic heart disease is equated with atherosclerotic plaque due to flow-limiting obstruction in epicardial coronary arteries. Nevertheless, several findings suggest a more complex pathophysiology of this complex disease [2–8]. In fact, it has been showed that beyond the presence of epicardial atherosclerotic plaques, coronary microcirculation is crucial in the genesis of ischemic heart disease [9, 10]. In addition, in the last few years, a growing body of data is underlying the importance of heritability acting with other factors in order to determine the presence of ischemic heart disease, due to either an obstruction in epicardial vessels [11–13] or a dysfunction of coronary microcirculation [14, 15]. In fact, over the past decade, genome-wide association studies have identified several loci, explaining a part of the ischemic heart disease's heritability. Existing knowledge of genetic variants affecting risk of ischemic heart disease is largely based on genome-wide association studies analysis of common single-nucleotide polymorphisms.

Therefore, this chapter proposes an overview of the loci that have been identified as connected with ischemic heart disease genesis, from epicardial plaque to microvascular dysfunction.

2. Coronary artery disease

Coronary artery disease is defined by the presence of a plaque in the epicardial coronary arteries. Usually, the atherosclerotic plaque narrow coronary arteries, decreasing blood flow. In subjects with genetic susceptibility factors, coronary artery disease is determined by exposure to some risk factors. In the last years, several researches have enhanced our understanding of the risk factors as well as the genetic basis of coronary artery disease. Some of these factors relate to lifestyles, such as tobacco smoking, lack of physical activity, and dietary habits, and are thus modifiable. Other risk factors are also modifiable, such as elevated blood pressure, type 2 diabetes, and dyslipidemias, or non-modifiable, such as age, male gender, and genetic susceptibility.

To date, more than 50 loci have been identified for susceptibility of coronary artery disease, as described by the meta-analysis carried out by the CARDIoGRAMplusC4D Consortium, on almost 185,000 cases and controls [11]. Moreover, data from a meta-analysis of genome-wide association studies have also been carried out for conventional risk factors and biomarker for coronary artery disease, like dyslipidemia and blood pressure, diabetes mellitus, atherosclerosis, inflammation, coagulation, oxidation, and amino acid metabolism, identifying several genes for each respective factor [12].

2.1. Genetic polymorphisms and risk factors for coronary artery disease

2.1.1. Dyslipidemia

Lipid metabolism can be altered in different ways, leading to variations in plasma lipoprotein function and concentration. Through interaction with other cardiovascular risk factors, dyslipidemias may affect the development of coronary artery disease. Dyslipidemias may be related to the interaction between genetic predisposition and environmental factors. Up to the present time, 12 loci were significantly associated by genome-wide association studies with the concentrations of blood lipids and coronary artery disease. Among these, eight loci were associated with LDL concentration (ABCG5, ABCG8, ABO, APOB, APOE, LDLR, LPA PCSK9, and SORT1), two loci with triglyceride concentration (APOA5 and TRIB1), and one locus with HDL concentration

(ANKS1A). At another locus, there was a near-equivalent association for triglyceride and HDL (LPL). In severely obese patients, a single-nucleotide polymorphism within the ARPC3 Gene Promoter was associated with hypertriglyceridemia [16]. Moreover, among different ethnicities Lysosomal Acid Lipase A (LIPA), polymorphisms have been described as associated with susceptibility to premature coronary artery disease [17]. APOA5 polymorphisms, air pollution, and the development of coronary artery disease have been associated, although methylation studies are needed to examine epigenetic factors associated with those single-nucleotide polymorphisms. Another interesting correlation is between TNNT1 variations, HDL levels, and coronary artery disease [15]. Finally, it has been suggested that Numb gene haplotypes, the regulating factor for intestinal cholesterol absorption and plasma cholesterol level, are related to coronary artery disease in Han Chinese [18].

2.1.2. Arterial hypertension

The relationship between blood pressure values and cardiovascular fatal events has been determined in several studies [19]. Numerous rare, monogenic forms of hypertension have been described, where a single gene mutation explains the pathogenesis of hypertension [20]. On the other side, essential hypertension is a heterogeneous disease with a multifactorial etiology. Genetic approaches raised the understanding of pathways underlying individual variations in blood pressure. Primary analyses evaluated associations between 2.5 million genotyped or imputed single-nucleotide polymorphisms (single-nucleotide polymorphisms) and SBP and DBP. Several genome-wide association studies and their meta-analyses point to a total of 29 single-nucleotide polymorphisms, which are associated with systolic and/or diastolic blood pressure [21]. In particular, latest genome-wide association studies data described four coronary artery disease risk loci (CYP17A1- NT5C2, SH2B3, ZC3HC1, GUCY1A3, and FES) associated with systolic and diastolic blood pressure [11, 21]. Moreover, endothelial nitric oxide synthase (eNOS) single-nucleotide polymorphism G894T significantly increases hypertension risk and coronary artery disease [22]. Selective expression of the Rho GTPase-activating protein ARHGAP42 in vascular smooth muscle cells regulates arterial blood pressure, as it inhibits RhoA-dependent contractility [23]. Furthermore, PDE3A, PRDM6, IGFBP3, and KCNK3 genes regulate vascular smooth muscle cells [24]. Particularly, PDE3A is phosphodiesterase acting in cyclic GMP metabolism [25], whereas KCNK3 has been related to pulmonary hypertension [26]. Other genes related to renal function have been described as acting in blood pressure regulation: ARHGAP24 influences podocyte formation [27], OSR1 influences renal mass and function [28], and SLC22A7 encodes for a renal solute transporter [29]; DNA methylation is probably involved in the regulatory pathway linking common single-nucleotide polymorphisms with blood pressure, according to data from experimental models of hypertension [30].

The single-nucleotide polymorphism Gly460Trp has been associated with hypertension and salt sensitivity [31] and an increased risk for coronary heart disease or peripheral vascular disease [32] and stroke [33]. An individual with this single-nucleotide polymorphism is a responder to diuretics better than wild-type homozygotes [31] in terms mostly of reduction of cardiovascular risk [34].

2.1.3. Diabetes mellitus

Diabetes mellitus has an increasing prevalence worldwide: 360 million people had diabetes in 2011, of which more than 95% type 2 diabetes. Diabetes mellitus is a complex, chronic disease requiring multifactorial risk-reduction strategies beyond glycemic control. Diabetes mellitus and cardiovascular disease develop with metabolic abnormalities causing dysfunction in the vasculature. Mortality and morbidity in people with diabetes are related to cardiovascular disease. Diabetes is a condition defined by an elevated level of blood glucose, and it can be classified into general categories: type 1 diabetes (due to b-cell destruction) and type 2 diabetes (due to a progressive loss of insulin secretion on the background of insulin resistance).

Usually, type 2 diabetes mellitus is more frequent with obesity, lack of physical activity, in women with prior gestational diabetes, in association with hypertension or dyslipidemia, and in certain ethnic groups. Insulin resistance plays an important role in the pathophysiology of type 2 diabetes mellitus and coronary artery disease: both genetic and environmental factors collaborate to its development. In fact, more than 90% of people with type 2 diabetes mellitus are obese [35]. Nevertheless, type 2 diabetes mellitus is often associated with a strong genetic predisposition, more so than type 1 diabetes. However, the genetics of type 2 diabetes is poorly understood. Classically, both the single-nucleotide polymorphism Pro12Ala in the peroxisome proliferator-activated receptor gamma (PPARG) gene [36] and the single-nucleotide polymorphism Glu23Lys in KCNJ11 gene [37] are common polymorphisms connected with influence risk of diabetes mellitus [38]. In particular, single-nucleotide polymorphisms for KCNJ11 have been described as involved in the susceptibility of ischemic heart disease, including coronary artery disease and CM (see below). Moreover, transcription factor 7-like 2 (TCF7L2) gene is involved in diabetes mellitus susceptibility [39]. Some single-nucleotide polymorphisms of the gene associated with fat mass and obesity (FTO) [40] have an impact on body mass index (BMI). Other single-nucleotide polymorphisms of the gene within or adjacent to hematopoietically expressed homeobox (HHEX)/insulin degrading enzyme (IDE), CDK5 regulatory subunit associated protein 1-like 1 (CDKAL1), insulin-like growth factor 2 mRNA-binding protein 2 (IGF2BP2), cyclin-dependent kinase inhibitors 2a, b (CDKN2A and CDKN2B), and solute carrier family 30, member 8 (SLC30A8) have an effect on insulin secretion [41–43].

Several other loci are implicated in diabetes mellitus as PPARG [44] and KCNJ11 [45] and for HNF1B (TCF2) [46] and WFS1 [47]. However, recent data suggest a possible role of other genes [48]: Notch homologue 2, Drosophila (NOTCH2) that is known to be involved in pancreatic development. Mapping within or adjacent to ADAM metallopeptidase with thrombospondin type 1 motif 9 (ADAMTS9), calcium/calmodulin-dependent protein kinase 1D (CAMK1D), compared with another zinc finger gene 1 (JAZF1), tetraspanin 8 (TSPAN8)/leucine-rich repeat containing G-protein coupled (LGR5), and thyroid adenoma associated (THADA), the mechanisms involved remain unclear [38].

2.1.4. Atherosclerosis

Cardiovascular disease due to atherosclerosis of the arterial vessel wall and to thrombosis is the foremost cause of premature mortality and of disability-adjusted life years (DALYs) in Europe and is also increasingly common in developing countries. Atherosclerotic lesions (i.e., atheroma) are asymmetric focal thickenings of the innermost layer of the artery, the intima. The pathophysiology of atherosclerosis suggests an inflammatory disease characterized by arterial plaque rich in cholesterol, inflammatory cell infiltrates, and connective tissue [49]. Data from clinical researches, studies in animal models, and cell culture experiments found important evidences to the pathogenesis of atherosclerosis. Several types of research demonstrated an association of IL6R-related gene pathways with atherosclerosis and coronary artery disease [50].

In patients with established coronary artery disease, it has been showed that the −174 C allele of the IL-6 gene increases the risk for progression of coronary plaques [14]. Moreover, patients with the Cox-2 GG single-nucleotide polymorphism have a higher risk of coronary artery disease while the Cox-2 (−765G>C) polymorphism is associated with lower interleukin-6 levels [51]. Moreover, multiple single-nucleotide polymorphisms as FGB-FGA-FGG, NLRP3, IL1RN, and IRF1-SCL22A5 show a strong association with fibrinogen expression and function [52]. Analogously the plaque composition has been associated with specific genes: matrix metalloproteinase genes (MMP1, 9, 12, 14) and the co-stimulatory ligands CD80 and CD86 [53] are associated with vulnerable plaques. Moreover, indoleamine 2, 3-dioxygenase 1 (IDO1) and integrin alpha V expression levels seem to be higher in vulnerable than in stable plaques [53].

In atherosclerotic plaques, there is an overexpression of CB2 gene (CNR2), that is an inflammatory marker, compared with normal arteries, whereas stable and vulnerable plaques displayed similar CNR2 levels [53]. Lectin-like oxidized low-density lipoprotein receptor 1 (LOX-1) is the main scavenger receptor for oxidized low-density lipoprotein (ox-LDL) in endothelial cells. The single-nucleotide polymorphism c.501G>C determines a single amino acid change (K>N at codon 167) reduces ox-LDL binding and uptake. Ox-LDL activated extracellular signal-regulated kinases 1 and 2 (ERK 1/2) is inhibited [54–56].

3. Coronary microvascular disease

The coronary microcirculation is often considered an underwater world beyond the epicardial arteries, often inaccessible for routine investigation, unachievable for targeted treatment. However, microcirculation is crucial in the cross talk between perfusion to myocardial demand. Pathway for coronary metabolic dilation is determining genetic associations in genes encoding for coronary blood flow regulators (i.e., ion channels, nitric oxide synthase, SERCA pump, and so on) with the susceptibility for microcirculation dysfunction and ischemic heart disease [57].

Recently, a study comparing the prevalence of single-nucleotide polymorphisms in genes encoding coronary ion channels between patients with coronary artery disease or microvascular dysfunction and those with both anatomically and functionally normal coronary arteries suggested the possibility of associations between single-nucleotide polymorphisms and ischemic heart disease in term of coronary artery disease and microvascular dysfunction [57]. In fact, data show that specific single-nucleotide polymorphisms detected in NOS3 gene encoding for endothelial nitric oxide synthase (eNOS), as well as in KCNJ8 encoding for the inward rectifying subunit of ATP-sensitive potassium channel (Kir6.2) and SCN5A encoding for voltage-dependent Na+ channel (Nav1.5) were found to be correlated with ischemic heart disease and microvascular dysfunction [58]. Specifically, the single-nucleotide polymorphisms rs5215_GG, rs5218_CT, and rs5219_AA for Kir6.2/KCJ11 could reduce susceptibility to ischemic heart disease; the single-nucleotide polymorphism rs5219_AA of Kir6.2/KCNJ11 may suggest a protecting role against coronary microvascular dysfunction; the rs1805124_GG genotype of Nav1.5/SCN5A seems to play a role in coronary artery disease. In the same study, also eNOS/NOS3 gene was investigated, demonstrating that rs1799983 polymorphism for this gene seems to be an independent risk factor for microvascular dysfunction [57]. The Transient Receptor Potential Ankyrin 1 (TRPA1) has been evaluated in vasodilation using KO mice [59]. On the other side, smooth muscle Kv7 channels have been associated with the control of vascular reactivity and vasorelaxant responses in coronary circulation [60]. To date, five subtypes of Kv7 channels encoded by KCNQ genes have been identified [61]. Kv7.1 and Kv7.4 were expressed at higher levels compared to Kv7.2, Kv7.3, and Kv7.5 in coronary arteries [62].

Regarding nitric oxide synthase, the allele "a" of intron 4a/b (eNOS4) has been described as a risk factor for patients with microvascular endothelial dysfunction and slow coronary flow [63].

Microvascular angina has been also associated with CYP2C19 variants that may affect coronary microvascular dysfunction [64]. Moreover, recent data in the female population showed that the specific CYP2C19 poor metabolizer genotype can lead to coronary microvascular disorders via inflammation [65].

Nuclear factor (erythroid-derived 2)-like-2 (NRF2) is an antioxidant and cell protective transcription factor that controls antioxidant defenses. NRF2 suppression plays an essential role in the development of oxidant stress, endothelial dysfunction, and microvessel rarefaction [66]. Moreover, Nox4 has been described as a positive transcriptional regulator of cystathionine-γ-lyase (CSE) in endothelial cells. It regulates vascular tone via the modulation of gasotransmitter, hydrogen sulfide (H2S) production [67].

Hypoxia-inducible factor-1 (HIF-1) is a peptide regulator of genes such as heme oxygenase (HO)-1 expressed during hypoxia. HIF-1 activation induces HO-1 expression attenuating proinflammatory chemokine production by microvascular endothelium in vitro and in vivo [68]. The single-nucleotide polymorphism C242T causes p22 (phox) structural changes that inhibit endothelial Nox2 activation and oxidative response to tumor necrosis factor-α or high-glucose stimulation. The single-nucleotide polymorphism C242T has been proposed a protective factor against cardiovascular diseases [69]. Novel regions of genetic variations within vascular endothelial growth factor A (VEGFA) and CDKN2B antisense RNA1 (CDKN2B-AS1) genes have been associated with coronary microvascular dysfunction. Furthermore, there were sex-specific differences in single-nucleotide polymorphisms which are associated with microvascular dysfunction, in particular, myosin heavy chain 15 (MYH15), VEGFA, and NT5E. In the male, single-nucleotide polymorphisms for NT5E are associated with abnormal coronary flow reserve; however, mutations in NT5E are associated with arterial calcification [70]. NT5E gene encodes for CD73 that transforms adenosine monophosphate (AMP) to adenosine, supporting a role for this metabolic pathway in inhibiting vascular calcification [70, 71]. In fact, lack of CD73 leads to a reduction in extracellular adenosine levels, causing vascular calcification [72].

In a meta-analysis of genome-wide association studies, data identified four novel loci on chromosomes 19q13, 6q24, 12q24, and 5q14 that were associated with retinal venular caliber. The retinal vasculature is comparable with human microcirculation. Retinal venular caliber has been shown to predict a range of subclinical [73] and clinical cardiovascular disease. RASIP1 gene (rs2287921, p = 1.61610225) on chromosome 19q13 is the most significant single-nucleotide polymorphism associated with retinal venular caliber, and the single-nucleotide polymorphisms were located in or adjacent to VTA1 and NMBR genes on chromosome 6q24. VTA1 gene encodes for a protein involved in trafficking of the multivesicular body. The signals for the association on chromosome 12q24 were spread across a large one Mb LD block, including genes such as SH2B3, ATXN2, and PTPN11. The most significant single-nucleotide polymorphisms at the 5q14 locus were located closest to MEF2C that plays an important role in cardiogenesis, epithelial cell survival, and maintenance of blood vessel integrity [74].

Finally, sarcomere gene mutations are associated with adverse remodeling of the microcirculation in hypertrophic cardiomyopathy [75, 76]. In fact, patients with hypertrophic cardiomyopathy with sarcomere myofilament mutations are characterized by more severe impairment of microvascular function and increased prevalence of myocardial fibrosis, compared with genotype-negative individuals [75].

4. Sex differences

Gender difference deserves a separate section. Scientific interest in ischemic heart disease in women has grown significantly over the past decades, mostly on clinical aspects. In fact, ischemic heart disease differs in term of pathogenesis, symptoms, and prognosis between males and females. Several studies show that different single-nucleotide polymorphisms of different genes can be involved. Single-nucleotide polymorphisms within genes of MYH15, linked to the maintenance of tonic force in vascular smooth muscle cells, VEGFA, involved in cell proliferation, migration, and angiogenic potential and NT5E which contributes to overall microvessel stiffness were associated with microvascular dysfunction in men [63, 77]. Studies on polymorphisms at the cholesteryl ester transfer protein (CETP) locus showed that women displayed a higher HDL-C than men and an equally high incidence of coronary heart disease in B2 homozygotes as in other genotypes [78]. Thus, in type 2 diabetic patients, the B polymorphism seems to exert a modulating role in males only. This may contribute to the loss of macrovascular protection in type 2 diabetic females [78].

Moreover, the specific CYP2C19 poor metabolizer has been described as a risk factor for coronary microvascular disorders via inflammation exclusively in the female population [65]. Usually, in fertile female exhibits a protection in ischemic injury compared to age-related men, a phenomenon designated as sex-specific cardioprotection. PKC-mediated regulation of sarcolemmal ATP-dependent K [sarcK(ATP)] channels may account for the gender difference in cardioprotection upon both PKC and sarcK(ATP). It involves PKC-dependent sarcolemma increase with a major expression of sarcK(ATP) in female [77]. Microcirculation dysfunction can also be associated with cardiac hypertrophy, which can be related to the expression of Kvβ1.1, particularly in females. In an animal model, Kvβ1 KO female mice have a growing myosin heavy chain α expression in myocytes. Changes in molecular and cell signaling pathways clearly point toward a distinct electrical and structural remodeling consistent with cardiac hypertrophy in the Kvβ1.1 KO female mice [79].

5. Conclusions

Ischemic heart disease is a common disease that globally represents an important problem for individuals and healthcare resources. An enhanced understanding of its pathophysiology is needed. By convention, ischemic heart disease is associated with the presence of an atherosclerotic plaque that is able to limit the flow in large-medium sized coronary arteries. Multiple different mechanisms are responsible for symptoms suggesting ischemic heart disease without apparent flow-limiting obstruction on angiography. In fact, both coronary artery disease and coronary microvascular disease can be responsible for an impaired cross talk between myocardial demand and oxygen supply. Interestingly, discordance between epicardial coronary function and microvascular function has generated recent interest. Finding no obstructive epicardial stenosis, but reduced microvascular function, indicating coronary microvascular disease, is associated with a negative prognosis [80].

In contrast, preserved microvascular function in the presence of flow-limiting epicardial stenosis has been associated with a long-term clinical outcome. In fact, several findings suggest a complex pathophysiology of ischemic heart disease. Both genetic and lifestyle factors contribute to the individual-level risk of ischemic heart disease, both coronary artery disease and coronary microvascular disease. Genetic susceptibility is determined by several single-nucleotide polymorphisms of genes encoding for both elements involved in the coronary homeostasis as well as for major risk factors for cardiovascular events (i.e., hypertension, diabetes, dyslipidemia). Genetic susceptibility is independent of healthy lifestyle behaviors and can be associated with an increased risk of coronary events, although a healthy lifestyle is associated with event risk reductions in rates.

Nowadays, associative hypothesis between single-nucleotide polymorphisms and ischemic heart disease has been numerous in literature, and, in some case, researches show speculative data with no provided plausible causal mechanism. Large-scale studies in human populations, genome-wide association studies, and meta-analysis, together with genetic technologies improvements, are helping the comprehension of genetic susceptibility of ischemic heart disease over the last decade. Moreover, a functional understanding of the discovered genetic associations with ischemic heart disease could help in the development of novel therapeutic strategies. However, we are still distant to the fully knowledge of the pathophysiology of this complex disease and the real role of heritability.

Conflict of interest

No conflict of interest to declare, no relationship with industry.

Author details

Francesco Fedele*, Mariateresa Pucci and Paolo Severino

*Address all correspondence to: francesco.fedele@uniroma1.it

Department of Cardiovascular, Respiratory, Nephrology, Anesthesiology and Geriatric Sciences, Sapienza University, Rome, Italy

References

[1] Moran AE, Forouzanfar MH, Roth GA, et al. Temporal trends in ischemic heart disease mortality in 21 world regions, 1980 to 2010: The Global burden of disease 2010 study. Circulation. 2014;**129**:1483-1489. DOI: 10.1161/CIRCULATIONAHA.113.004042

[2] Tiefenbacher CP, Chilian WM. Heterogeneity of coronary vasomotion. Basic Research in Cardiology. 1998;**93**:446-454

[3] Wolin MS, Ahmad M, Gupte SA. Oxidant and redox signaling in vascular oxygen sensing mechanisms: Basic concepts, current controversies, and potential importance of cytosolic NADPH. American Journal of Physiology. Lung Cellular and Molecular Physiology. 2005;**289**:159-173. DOI: 10.1152/ajplung.00060.2005

[4] Tune JD. Withdrawal of vasoconstrictor influences in local metabolic coronary vasodilation. The American Journal of Physiology-Heart and Circulatory Physiology. 2006; **291**:2044-2046. DOI: 10.1152/ajpheart.00653.2006

[5] Dzeja PP, Bast P, Pucar D, et al. Defective metabolic signaling in adenylate kinase AK1 gene knock-out hearts compromises post-ischemic coronary reflow. The Journal of Biological Chemistry. 2007;**282**:31366-31372. DOI: 10.1074/jbc.M705268200

[6] Ottaviani G, Lavezzi AM, Rossi L, Matturri L. Proliferating cell nuclear antigen (PCNA) and apoptosis in hyperacute and acute myocardial infarction. European Journal of Histochemistry. 1999;**43**:7-14

[7] Wong B, Kruse G, Kutikova L, et al. Cardiovascular disease risk associated with familial hypercholesterolemia: A systematic review of the literature. Clinical Therapeutics. 2016;**38**:1696-1709. DOI: 10.1016/j.clinthera.2016.05.006

[8] Feldman RD. Heart disease in women: Unappreciated challenges, GPER as a new target. International Journal of Molecular Sciences. 2016;**18**:17(5). DOI: 10.3390/ijms17050760

[9] Komaru T, Kanatsuka H, Shirato K. Coronary microcirculation: Physiology and pharmacology. Pharmacology & Therapeutics. 2000;**86**:217-261. DOI: http://dx.doi.org/10.1016/S0163-7258(00)00057-7

[10] Chilian WM. Coronary microcirculation in health and disease. Summary of an NHLBI workshop. Circulation. 1997;**95**:522-528. DOI: https://doi.org/10.1161/01.CIR.95.2.522

[11] Deloukas P, Kanoni S, Willenborg C, for the CARDIoGRAMplusC4D Consortium. Large-scale association analysis identifies new risk loci for coronary artery disease. Nature Genetics. 2013;**45**:25-33. DOI: 10.1038/ng.2480

[12] Nikpay M, Goel A, Won HH. A comprehensive 1,000 genomes-based genome-wide association meta-analysis of coronary artery disease. Nature Genetics. 2015;**47**:1121-1130. DOI: 10.1038/ng.3396

[13] Webb TR, Erdmann J, Stirrups KE, et al. Systematic evaluation of pleiotropy identifies 6 further loci associated with coronary artery disease. Journal of the American College of Cardiology. 2017;**21**(69):823-836. DOI: 10.1016/j.jacc.2016.11.056

[14] Toutouzas K, Klettas D, Anousakis-Vlachochristou N, et al. The –174 G>C interleukin-6 gene polymorphism is associated with angiographic progression of coronary artery disease in a 4-year period. Hellenic Journal of Cardiology. 2017;**14**:S1109-9666(16)30361-X. DOI: 10.1016/j.hjc.2017.02.002

[15] Guay SP, Légaré C, Brisson D, et al. Epigenetic and genetic variations at the TNNT1 gene locus are associated with HDL-C levels and coronary artery disease. Epigenomics. 2016;**8**(3):359-371. DOI: 10.2217/epi.15.120

[16] de Toro-Martín J, Guénard F, Tchernof A, et al. A CpG-SNP Located within the ARPC3 gene promoter is associated with hypertriglyceridemia in severely obese patients. Annals of Nutrition and Metabolism. 2016;**68**:203-212. DOI: 10.1159/000445358

[17] Vargas-Alarcón G, Posadas-Romero C, Villarreal-Molina T, et al. Single nucleotide polymorphisms within LIPA (Lysosomal Acid Lipase A) gene are associated with susceptibility to premature coronary artery disease. A replication in the genetic of atherosclerotic disease (GEA) Mexican study. PLoS One. 2013;**8**(9):e74703. DOI: 10.1371/journal.pone.0074703

[18] Abudoukelimu M, Fu ZY, Maimaiti A, et al. The association of cholesterol absorption gene Numb polymorphism with coronary artery disease among Han Chinese and Uighur Chinese in Xinjiang, China. Lipids in Health and Disease. 2015;**14**:120. DOI: 10.1186/s12944-015-0102-6

[19] Lewington S, Clarke R, Qizilbash N, Peto R, Collins R. Age-specific relevance of usual blood pressure to vascular mortality: A meta-analysis of individual data for one million adults in 61 prospective studies. Lancet. 2002;**360**:1903-1913. DOI: http://dx.doi.org/10.1016/S0140-6736(02)11911-8

[20] Lifton RP, Gharavi AG, Geller DS. Molecular mechanisms of human hypertension. Cell. 2001;**104**:545-556. DOI: http://dx.doi.org/10.1016/S0092-8674(01)00241-0

[21] International Consortium For Blood Pressure Genome-Wide Association Studies. Genetic variants in novel pathways influence blood pressure and cardiovascular disease risk. Nature. 2011;**478**:103-109. DOI: 10.1038/nature10405

[22] ALrefai AA, Habib MS, Yaseen RI, Gabr MK, Habeeb RM. Association of endothelial nitric oxide synthase (eNOS) gene G894T polymorphism with hypertension risk and complications. Molecular and Cellular Biochemistry. 2016;**421**:103-110. DOI: 10.1007/s11010-016-2790-2

[23] Bai X, Mangum KD, Dee RA, et al. Blood pressure-associated polymorphism controls ARHGAP42 expression via serum response factor DNA binding. Journal of Clinical Investigation. 2017;**127**:670-680. DOI: 10.1172/JCI88899

[24] Kato N, Loh M, Takeuchi F, et al. Trans-ancestry genome-wide association study identifies 12 genetic loci influencing blood pressure and implicates a role for DNA methylation. Nature Genetics. 2015;**47**:1282-1293. DOI: 10.1038/ng.3405

[25] Beca S, et al. Phosphodiesterase type 3A regulates basal myocardial contractility through interacting with sarcoplasmic reticulum calcium ATPase type 2a signaling complexes in mouse heart. Circulation Research. 2013;**112**:289-297. DOI: 10.1161/CIRCRESAHA.111.300003

[26] Ma L, et al. A novel channelopathy in pulmonary arterial hypertension. The New England Journal of Medicine. 2013;**369**:351-361. DOI: 10.1056/NEJMc1311060#SA2

[27] Akilesh S, et al. Arhgap24 inactivates Rac1 in mouse podocytes, and a mutant form is associated with familial focal segmental glomerulosclerosis. Journal of Clinical Investigation. 2011;**121**:4127-4137. DOI: 10.1172/JCI46458

[28] Zhang Z, et al. A variant OSR1 allele which disturbs OSR1 mRNA expression in renal progenitor cells is associated with reduction of newborn kidney size and function. Human Molecular Genetics. 2011;**20**:4167-4174. DOI: 10.1093/hmg/ddr341

[29] Cheng Y, Vapurcuyan A, Shahidullah M, Aleksunes LM, Pelis RM. Expression of organic anion transporter 2 in the human kidney and its potential role in the tubular secretion of guanine-containing antiviral drugs. Drug Metabolism & Disposition. 2012;**40**:617-624. DOI: 10.1124/dmd.111.042036

[30] Flister MJ, et al. Identifying multiple causative genes at a single GWAS locus. Genome Research. 2013;**23**:1996-2002. DOI: 10.1101/gr.160283.113

[31] Barlassina C, Schork NJ, Manunta P, et al. Synergistic effect of alpha-adducin and ACE genes causes blood pressure changes with body sodium and volume expansion. Kidney International. 2000;**57**:1083-1090. DOI: http://dx.doi.org/10.1046/j.1523-1755.2000.00935.x

[32] Morrison AC, Bray MS, Folsom AR, Boerwinkle E. ADD1 460 W allele associated with cardiovascular disease in hypertensive individuals. Hypertension. 2002;**39**:1053-1057. DOI: https://doi.org/10.1161/01.HYP.0000019128.94483.3A

[33] Zafarmand MH, Van der Schouw YT, Grobbee DE, de Leeuw PW, Bots ML. AlphaAdducin Gly460Trp variant increases the risk of stroke in hypertensive Dutch women. Hypertension. 2008;**51**:1665-1670. DOI: 10.1161/HYPERTENSIONAHA

[34] Sitia S, Tomasoni L, Atzeni F, et al. From endothelial dysfunction to atherosclerosis. Autoimmunity Reviews. 2010;**9**:830-834. DOI: 10.1016/j.autrev.2010.07.016

[35] Hossain P, Kawar B, El Nahas M. Obesity and diabetes in the developing world: A growing challenge. The New England Journal of Medicine. 2007;**356**:213-215. DOI: 10.1056/NEJMp068177

[36] Altshuler D, et al. The common PPARg Pro12Ala polymorphism is associated with decreased risk of type 2 diabetes. Nature Genetics. 2000;**26**:76-80. DOI: 10.1038/79216

[37] Gloyn AL, et al. Large scale association studies of variants in genes encoding the pancreatic b-cell K-ATP channel subunits Kir6.2 (KCNJ11) and SUR1 (ABCC8) confirm that the KCNJ11 E23K variant is associated with increased risk of type 2 diabetes. Diabetes. 2003;**52**:568-572. DOI: https://doi.org/10.2337/diabetes.52.2.568

[38] Prokopenko I, McCarthy MI, Lindgren CM. Type 2 diabetes: New genes, new understanding. Trends in Genetics. 2008;**24**:613-621. DOI: 0.1016/j.tig.2008.09.004

[39] Grant SFA, et al. Variant of transcription factor 7-like 2 (TCF7L2) gene confers risk of type 2 diabetes. Nature Genetics. 2006;**38**:320-323. DOI: 10.1038/ng1732

[40] Frayling TM, et al. A common variant in the FTO gene is associated with body mass index and predisposes to childhood and adult obesity. Science. 2007;**316**:889-894. DOI: 10.1126/science.1141634

[41] Grarup N, et al. Studies of association of variants near the HHEX, CDKN2A/B, and IGF2BP2 genes with type 2 diabetes and impaired insulin release in 10,705 Danish subjects: Validation and extension of genome-wide association studies. Diabetes. 2007;**56**:3105-3111. DOI: 10.2337/db07-0856

[42] Pascoe L, et al. Common variants of the novel type 2 diabetes genes, CDKAL1 and HHEX/IDE, are associated with decreased pancreatic b-cell function. Diabetes. 2007;**56**:3101-3104. DOI: 10.2337/db07-0634

[43] Grarup N, et al. Association testing of novel type 2 diabetes risk alleles in the JAZF1, CDC123/CAMK1D, TSPAN8, THADA, ADAMTS9, and NOTCH2 loci with insulin release, insulin sensitivity and obesity in a population-based sample of 4,516 glucose-tolerant middle-aged Danes. Diabetes. 2008;**57**:2534-2540. DOI: 10.2337/db08-0436

[44] Barroso I, et al. Dominant negative mutations in human PPARg associated with severe insulin resistance, diabetes mellitus and hypertension. Nature. 1999;**402**:880-883. DOI: 10.1038/47254

[45] Gloyn AL, et al. Activating mutations in the gene encoding the ATP-sensitive potassium-channel subunit Kir6.2 and permanent neonatal diabetes. The New England Journal of Medicine. 2004;**350**:1838-1849

[46] Maestro MA, et al. Distinct roles of HNF1beta, HNF1alpha, and HNF4alpha in regulating pancreas development, beta-cell function and growth. Endocrine Development. 2007;**12**:33-45. DOI: 10.1159/0000109603

[47] Domenech E, et al. Wolfram/DIDMOAD syndrome, a heterogenic and molecularly complex neurodegenerative disease. Pediatric Endocrinology Reviews. 2006;**3**:249-257

[48] Zeggini E, et al. Meta-analysis of genome-wide association data and large-scale replication identifies additional susceptibility loci for type 2 diabetes. Nature Genetics. 2008;**40**:638-645. DOI: 10.1038/ng.120

[49] Hansson GK, Hermansson A. The immune system in atherosclerosis. Nature Immunology. 2011;**12**:204-212. DOI: 10.1038/ni.2001

[50] IL6R Genetics Consortium Emerging Risk Factors Collaboration. Interleukin-6 receptor pathways in coronary heart disease: A collaborative meta-analysis of 82 studies. Lancet. 2012;**379**:1205-1213. DOI: 10.1016/S0140-6736(11)61931-4

[51] Ol KK, Agachan B, Gormus U, Toptas B, Isbir T. Cox-2 gene polymorphism and IL-6 levels in coronary artery disease. Genetics and Molecular Research. 2011;**10**:810-816. DOI: 10.4238/vol10-2gmr967

[52] Christina LW, Leslie AL, Brendan JK. Association of genomic loci from a cardiovascular gene SNP array with fibrinogen levels in European Americans and African-Americans from six cohort studies: The Candidate Gene Association Resource (CARe). Blood. 2011;**117**:268-275. DOI: 10.1182/blood-2010-06-289546

[53] Meletta R, Slavik R, Mu L, et al. Cannabinoid receptor type 2 (CB2) as one of the candidate genes in human carotid plaque imaging: Evaluation of the novel radiotracer [^{11}C] RS-016 targeting CB2 in atherosclerosis. Nuclear Medicine and Biology. 2017;**47**:31-43. DOI: 10.1016/j.nucmedbio.2017.01.001

[54] Tur J, Chapalamadugu KC, Padawer T, et al. Deletion of Kvβ1.1 subunit leads to electrical and haemodynamic changes causing cardiac hypertrophy in female murine hearts. Experimental Physiology. 2016;**101**:494-508. DOI: 10.1113/EP085405

[55] Mollace V, Gliozzi M, Musolino V, et al. Oxidized LDL attenuates protective autophagy and induces apoptotic cell death of endothelial cells: Role of oxidative stress and LOX-1 receptor expression. International Journal of Cardiology. 2015;**184**:152-158. DOI: 10.1016/j.ijcard.2015.02.007

[56] Biocca S, Falconi M, Filesi I, et al. Functional analysis and molecular dynamics simulation of LOX-1 K167N polymorphism reveal alteration of receptor activity. PLoS One. 2009;**4**:e4648. DOI: 10.1371/journal.pone.0004648

[57] Fedele F, Mancone M, Chilian WM, et al. Role of genetic polymorphisms of ion channels in the pathophysiology of coronary microvascular dysfunction and ischemic heart disease. Basic Research in Cardiology. 2013;**108**:387. DOI: 10.1007/s00395-013-0387-4

[58] Fedele F, Severino P, Bruno N, et al. Role of ion channels in coronary microcirculation: A review of the literature. Future Cardiology. 2013;**9**:897-905. DOI: 10.2217/fca.13.65

[59] Pozsgai G, Bodkin JV, Graepel R, Bevan S, Andersson DA, Brain SD. Evidence for the pathophysiological relevance of TRPA1 receptors in the cardiovascular system in vivo. Cardiovascular Research. 2010;**87**:760-768. DOI: 10.1093/cvr/cvq118

[60] Zhong XZ, Harhun MI, Olesen SP, Ohya S, Moffatt JD, et al. Participation of KCNQ (Kv7) potassium channels in myogenic control of cerebral arterial diameter. The Journal of Physiology. 2010;**588**:3277-3293. DOI: 10.1113/jphysiol.2010.192823

[61] Gutman GA, Chandy KG, Grissmer S, Lazdunski M, McKinnon D, et al. International union of pharmacology. LIII. Nomenclature and molecular relationships of voltage-gated potassium channels. Pharmacological Reviews. 2005;**57**:473-508. DOI: 10.1124/pr.57.4.10

[62] Lee S, Yang Y, Tanner MA, Li M, Hill MA. Heterogeneity in Kv7 channel function in the cerebral and coronary circulation. Microcirculation. 2015;**22**:109-121. DOI: 10.1111/micc.12183

[63] Ekmekci A, Güngör B, Özcan KS, et al. Evaluation of coronary microvascular function and nitric oxide synthase intron 4a/b polymorphism in patients with coronary slow flow. Coronary Artery Disease. 2013;**24**:461-467. DOI: 10.1097/MCA.0b013e328363258c

[64] Akasaka T, Sueta D, Arima Y, et al. Association of CYP2C19 variants and epoxyeicosatrienoic acids on patients with microvascular angina. The American Journal of Physiology-Heart and Circulatory Physiology. 2016;**311**:H1409-H1415. DOI: 10.1152/ajpheart.00473.2016

[65] Akasaka T, Hokimoto S, Sueta D, et al. Sex differences in the impact of CYP2C19 polymorphisms and low-grade inflammation on coronary microvascular disorder. The American Journal of Physiology-Heart and Circulatory Physiology. 2016;**310**:H1494-H1500. DOI: 10.1152/ajpheart.00911.2015

[66] Priestley JR, Kautenburg KE, Casati MC, et al. The NRF2 knockout rat: A new animal model to study endothelial dysfunction, oxidant stress, and microvascular rarefaction. The American Journal of Physiology-Heart and Circulatory Physiology. 2016;**310**:H478-H487. DOI: 10.1152/ajpheart.00586.2015

[67] Mistry RK, Murray TV, Prysyazhna O, et al. Transcriptional regulation of cystathionine-γ-lyase in endothelial cells by NADPH oxidase 4-dependent signaling. The Journal of Biological Chemistry. 2016;**291**:1774-1788. DOI: 10.1074/jbc.M115.685578

[68] Ockaili R, Natarajan R, Salloum F, et al. HIF-1 activation attenuates postischemic myocardial injury: Role for heme oxygenase-1 in modulating microvascular chemokine generation. The American Journal of Physiology-Heart and Circulatory Physiology. 2005;**289**:H542-548. DOI: 10.1152/ajpheart.00089.2005

[69] Meijles DN, Fan LM, Ghazaly MM, Howlin B, Krönke M, Brooks G, Li JM. p22phox C242T single-nucleotide polymorphism inhibits inflammatory oxidative damage to endothelial cells and vessels. Circulation. 2016;**133**:2391-2403. DOI: 10.1161/CIRCULATIONAHA.116.021993

[70] St Hilaire C, Ziegler SG, Markello TC, et al. NT5E mutations and arterial calcifications. The New England Journal of Medicine. 2011;**364**:432-442. DOI: 10.1056/NEJMc1102515#SA1

[71] Markello TC, Pak LK, St Hilaire C, et al. Vascular pathology of medial arterial calcifications in NT5E deficiency: Implications for the role of adenosine in pseudoxanthoma elasticum. Molecular Genetics and Metabolism. 2011;**103**:44-50. DOI: 10.1016/j.ymgme.2011.01.018

[72] Yoshino S, Cilluffo R, Best PJ, Atkinson EJ, et al. Single nucleotide polymorphisms associated with abnormal coronary microvascular function. Coronary Artery Disease. 2014;**25**:281-289. DOI: 10.1097/MCA.0000000000000104

[73] Sim X1, Jensen RA, Ikram MK, Cotch MF, et al. Genetic loci for retinal arteriolar microcirculation. PLoS One. 2013;**8**:e65804. DOI: 10.1371/journal.pone.0065804

[74] Ikram MK, Sim X, Jensen RA, et al. Four novel Loci (19q13, 6q24, 12q24, and 5q14) influence the microcirculation in vivo. PLoS Genetics. 2010;**6**:e1001184. DOI: 10.1371/journal.pgen.1001184

[75] Olivotto I, Girolami F, Sciagra` R, et al. Microvascular function is selectively impaired in patients with hypertrophic cardiomyopathy and sarcomere myofilament gene mutations. Journal of the American College of Cardiology. 2011;**58**:839-848. DOI: 10.1016/j.jacc.2011.05.018

[76] Spoladore R, Fisicaro A, Faccini A, Camici PG. Coronary microvascular dysfunction in primary cardiomyopathies. Heart. 2014;**100**:806-813. DOI: 10.1136/heartjnl-2013-304291

[77] Leopold JA. Microvascular dysfunction: Genetic polymorphisms suggest sex-specific differences in disease phenotype. Coronary Artery Disease. 2014;**25**:275-276. DOI: 10.1097/MCA.0000000000000122

[78] Fisher SA. Vascular smooth muscle phenotypic diversity and function. Physiological Genomics. 2010;**42A**:169-187. DOI: 10.1152/physiolgenomics.00111.2010

[79] Edwards AG, Rees ML, Gioscia RA, Zachman DK, Lynch JM, Browder JC, Chicco AJ, Moore RL. PKC-permitted elevation of sarcolemmal KATP concentration may explain female-specific resistance to myocardial infarction. The Journal of Physiology. 2009;**587**:5723-5737. DOI: 10.1113/jphysiol.2009.181040

[80] van de Hoef TP, van Lavieren MA, Damman P, et al. Physiological basis and long-term clinical outcome of discordance between fractional flow reserve and coronary flow velocity reserve in coronary stenoses of intermediate severity. Circulation: Cardiovascular Interventions. 2014;**7**:301-331. DOI: 10.1161/CIRCINTERVENTIONS.113.001049

Chapter 11

Hepcidin: SNP-Like Polymorphisms Present in Iron Metabolism and Clinical Complications of Iron Accumulation and Deficiency

Cadiele Oliana Reichert, Joel da Cunha,
Débora Levy, Luciana Morganti Ferreira Maselli,
Sérgio Paulo Bydlowski and Celso Spada

Additional information is available at the end of the chapter

http://dx.doi.org/10.5772/intechopen.69507

Abstract

The metabolism of iron is regulated by the peptide hormone hepcidin. Genetic alterations in the proteins involved in the signalling pathway and hepcidin transcription cause damage to the organism. Mutations and polymorphisms in the hepcidin antimicrobial peptide(HAMP), HFE, HJV, ferroportin and matriptase-2 genes influence serum hepcidin concentration. Genetic deficiency of hepcidin increases iron overload in tissues, leading to haemochromatosis. However, genetics changes in the TMPRSS6 gene promote an increase in serum hepcidin, with the development of severe anaemia and resistance to iron treatment, as observed in IRIDA. Making the flow and efflux of extracellular and intracellular iron is impossible. To date, no drug that works by inhibiting or enhancing hepcidin transcription is available, largely because of the cytotoxicity described *in vitro* models. The proposed therapeutic targets are still in the early stages of clinical trials, some are good candidates, such as heparin derivatives and mini-hepcidins.

Keywords: anaemia, ferroportin gene, HAMP gene, haemojuvelin gene, haemochromatosis hepcidin, HFE gene, IRIDA, iron homeostasis, polymorphism, TMPRSS6 gene, transferrin gene

1. Introduction

Disorders related to iron metabolism involve genetic alterations between hepcidin and the modulation pathway of the HAMP gene causing damage to the organism, and iron overload or deficiency may occur [1–3]. Intracellular iron excess, hyperferremia, contributes to the formation of reactive oxygen species (ROS), damaging cell membranes and tissues, especially cardiac, endocrine and hepatic tissue, which are the clinical alterations observed in hereditary haemochromatosis [4]. However, iron deficiency due to genetic alterations, with an increased synthesis of hepcidin, reduces the synthesis of haemoglobin, limiting the formation of erythroid precursors and reduction of iron stores, with the development of anaemia [5, 6]. Hepcidin inhibits food absorption of iron in the duodenum, by blocking the release of iron recycled by macrophages and controlling the movement of iron stores contained in hepatocytes [7]. Thus, systemic iron stores, high concentration of plasma transferrin, erythropoietic activity, inflammatory mediators and hypoxia modulate the synthesis of hepcidin [8]. Plasma iron content is the main factor for transcription of hepcidin mRNA into hepatic tissue. When serum iron decreases, there is also a decrease in hepcidin transcription in the liver [9, 10].

The *HAMP* gene encodes hepcidin [1]. Studies have shown that changes in this gene or in genes that act on iron metabolism, by regulating the expression of hepcidin, influence the pathogenesis of hereditary diseases. Juvenile hereditary haemochromatosis originates from a polymorphism present in the HAMP gene, where deficiency occurs in the synthesis of hepcidin, with accumulation of iron in tissues [11–13]. Other factors, not related to genetic alterations, influence the serum concentration of hepcidin, such as viral infections and bacterins, vitamins A, D, C and E, hormones, stress of the endoplasmic reticulum, among others [14].

2. Hepcidin

The hepcidin molecule ('hep' hepatic origin, 'cidin' antimicrobial activity) was described in the year 2000, being characterized as a new anti-microbial peptide acting in part on innate immunity, such as β-defensin. Initially called liver-expressed antimicrobial peptide 1 (LEAP-1), it was isolated from human blood ultrafiltrates and urine in their active form, as a cysteine-rich peptide synthesized in the liver [1, 2]. Adipocytes, macrophages, lymphocytes, neutrophils, pancreatic β-cells and renal cells also produce hepcidin [15–19].

Physiologically active hepcidin originates from a pre-prohepcidin, containing 84 amino acids, which after proteolytic cleavage gives rise to pro-hepcidin that is composed of 64 amino acids. Pro-hepcidin is biologically inactive and is cleaved subsequently by the enzyme furin in a specific NH2 region, to provide biologically active source hepcidin, composed of eight cysteine residues bound by four bisulfite bridges and containing 25 amino acids [1, 2, 18]. The active molecule of hepcidin degrades in the N-terminal portion by giving molecules of −20, −22 and −24 amino acids, being this region, essential for the connection to cause ferroportina to occur. The smaller peptides show a progressive loss of regulation of ferroportin, with accumulation of intracellular ferritin [20].

2.1. Iron metabolism

Senescent erythrocyte recycling provides about 90–95% of iron required for physiological functions and for erythropoiesis. Enterocytes present in the duodenum and the proximal portion of the jejunum absorb about 1–2 mg of iron from the feed, which maintains the iron stores [21–23]. In the cytoplasmic membrane of enterocytes, apical ferric reductase enzymes are present, such as cytochrome b duodenal enzyme (dCytB). The dCytB promotes the reduction of ferric iron (Fe^{3+}) to its ferrous state (Fe^{2+}) and consequent mobilization of ferrous iron through the divalent metal transporter (DMT-1). The haem iron, coming from diet, is internalized by the haem carrier protein 1 (HCP-1) into the cells, where it is stored as ferritin [24, 25]. When serum iron concentration is low, mobilization of iron stores by the ferroportin to the extracellular medium occurs. The released iron is in its ferrous state and for binding to serum transferrin to occur, it must be oxidized to its ferric state, only the Fe^{3+} binds to transferrin. This oxidation reaction occurs through the action of oxidase enzymes: Hephaestin is present in enterocytes, ceruloplasmin, hepatocytes, plasma and zyklopen in the placenta. Then occurs the release of iron into the tissues [26–28].

Iron recycling by macrophages occurs through phagocytosis of senescent erythrocytes, haemoglobin phagocytosis and haem group of the intravascular haemolysis. When the haem group is internalized by the macrophage, it undergoes the action of the enzyme haem oxygenase (HO) and releases ferrous iron, which can be exported to the extra-cellular medium by ferroportin or stored as ferritin [29]. The highest concentration of iron in the body is stored as ferritin or haemosiderin in the liver, spleen, duodenum, bone marrow and other organs. The ferritin molecule is composed of 24 subunits with a spherical 'shell' shape, which accommodates about 4000 iron atoms. Ferroportin mediates the efflux of iron stores, being negatively regulated by hepcidin [30, 31].

2.2. Ferroportin

Ferroportin is a transmembrane protein composed of monomer dimers present in hepatocytes, enterocytes, macrophages, spleen and bone marrow, which regulates the amount of iron present in the extracellular and intracellular medium. By means of stimuli originated by elevated levels of serum iron, the hepcidin mRNA increase occurs [32]. Binding of the mature hepcidin peptide to ferroportin leads to binding of the tyrosine kinase Jak2 to each ferroportin monomer. After the binding of Jak2 to ferroportin, the autophosphorylation of Jak2 occurs, which then phosphorylates the ferroportin. Phosphorylated ferroportin binds to hepcidin, and both are internalized by cavity coated with clathrin within the cell. Once internalized, the phosphates are removed and ferroportin is ubiquitinated in amino acid lysine 253. The ubiquitination is necessary for the entry of ferroportin in multivesicular bodies, which by fusion with lysosomes provides the degradation of ferroportin. A mutation at residue 253 does not preclude the internalization of ferroportin, but decreases its degradation [33].

2.3. Gene regulation hepcidin

The HAMP gene located on chromosome 19q13 transcribes hepcidin mRNA. Factors modulate the transcription pathway of this gene, hypoxia, iron concentration, erythropoiesis, inflammation, anaemia, among others. These factors activate two major pathways that act directly on the gene. The first signalling pathway occurs through the induction of the pathway related to bone morphogenetic proteins (BMPs) and the second Janus kinase/signal transducer and activator of transcription (JAK/ STAT) signalling pathway is related to inflammation [2].

The protein (HFE) protein acts on the regulation of hepcidin transcription through its interaction with the transferrin receptor (TfR). HFE is displaced from TfR1 by high concentrations of the transferrin-iron complex [Tf-Fe^{3+}] to promote its interaction with the transferrin 2 receptor (TfR2). HFE and TfR2 bind the BMP co-receptor haemojuvelin (HJV) and activate HAMP gene transcription via the BMP/Son of the mothers against decapentaplegic(SMAD) [34]. This interaction induces phosphorylation of the activated BMP receptor, promoting an intracellular signalling cascade, by binding to a threonine/serine kinase type I and type II receptor complex [35]. Activated type II receptor activates type I receptor, which then transmits the signal to the SMAD regulatory receiver (R-SMAD), phosphorylating SMAD-1, SMAD-5 and SMAD-8. In this way, the formation of a transcription complex involving the SMAD-4 factor occurs. The activated complex moves to the nucleus in order to regulate gene transcription [36]. SMAD-4 and matriptase-2 protein act as suppressor of BMP/SMAD pathway activation. Matriptase-2 interacts with HJV and causes fragmentation [6, 37].

The regulation of the HAMP gene through the JAK/STAT pathway begins when specific ligands act on the JAKs generating a multimerization of their subunits. Erythropoietin and growth hormone associate with the receptor forming a homodimer, whereas inflammatory cytokines and interferons form a heterodimer [38]. Interleukin-6 (IL-6) binds to its receptor, which is formed by two subunits, one alpha subunit (IL-6-R) and another beta subunit (gp130). When IL-6 binds to IL-6-R, a dimerization of gp130 occurs which recruits the cytoplasmic JAK to phosphorylate the gp130 protein. After phosphorylation, STAT proteins (STAT-1 and STAT-3) bind to gp130 and autophosphorylate, then migrate to the nucleus, binding to gene-specific transcription sites, promoting increased transcription of hepcidin mRNA into hepatocytes [39, 40].

2.4. Genetic alterations with iron overload

Genetic alterations in the HFE gene have always been associated with haemochromatosis, a situation in which iron accumulation occurs in the body with the development of cirrhosis, hepatocarcinoma, diabetes and heart failure. The main hypothesis for the development of haemochromatosis, is the interaction of HFE protein and β2-microglobulin. These two proteins together form a complex with the transferrin-1 receptor (β_2M-HFE-TfR1), located in the crypt of the duodenal enterocytes, which regulates the iron absorption of the diet. The interaction between these three proteins affects the processes of iron utilisation, i.e. on the intensity of erythropoiesis and liver metabolism of iron. Genetic changes in the formation of this complex give rise to the clinical picture observed in haemochromatosis. However, after the description of hepcidin in iron metabolism, this initial theory was altered [41, 42].

New genes involved in iron metabolism have been reported, and now the hereditary haemochromatosis term encompasses two types, HFE haemochromatosis, which is characterized by presenting changes in the HFE gene, this being the most frequent in the caucasian population. In the second type, known as non-HFE haemochromatosis, other genes involved in metabolism are described, which by polymorphic genetic alterations or mutation generate the phenotype of iron overload. Non-HFE haemochromatosis, the HJV gene, the HAMP gene, the TFR gene and the ferroportin gene are present with variable clinical characteristics among the diseases, but all have altered levels of hepcidin. Genetic alterations in ferritin and ceruloplasmin also promote accumulation of iron in the body with hyperferritinemia, but these diseases are of recessive genetic inheritance and rare in the population [40, 12]. The accumulation of iron in the body compromises the function of several organs. In some severe cases of the disease, where diagnosis and treatment started very late, hepatic failure and development of cirrhosis, cardiac problems, changes in metabolic hormones with the development of diabetes, pituitary gland involvement, gonads, joints, hyperpigmentation of the skin, abdominal pain, testicular atrophy [43].

The diagnosis of haemochromatosis involves clinical features, biochemical measurements and genetic testing. Liver biopsy is performed in specific cases [44]. Elevated levels of serum ferritin (FS) and transferrin-iron saturation (TS) and liver enzymes are markers that help to identify patients with haemochromatosis. Serum ferritin levels greater than 200 μg/L in women and 300 μg/L in men and transferrin saturation greater than 45% are indicative of haemochromatosis when associated with clinical symptoms. When serum ferritin and transferrin saturation are altered, it is necessary to perform a genetic mutation analysis of the HFE, HJV, HAMP, ferroportin and transferrin receptor genes to make the differential diagnosis between haemochromatosis 1, 2, 3 and 4 [45, 46].

2.4.1. HFE gene mutation

The most frequent change that leads to the origin of hereditary haemochromatosis type-1 is the polymorphism and mutations present in the HFE gene present in chromosome 6. The allelic frequency observed in the European population is 5–7% for homozygosis C282Y, which is found about 80–85% of patients presenting with the disease [46]. The single point mutation, 845G → A, in exon 4, in the HFE gene leads to the substitution of cysteine by tyrosine at position 282 in the haemochromatosis (HFE) protein, which is the most severe case of the disease. Another variant of the HFE gene is the allele 187C → G, in exon 2, where an aspartate is exchanged for a histidine in the HFE protein (H63D), this alteration is of minor clinical importance, being harmful when it appears in heterozygous C282Y/H63D. The S65C variant is less frequent. The third mutation of the HFE gene is the substitution of a serine for a cysteine at amino acid position 65, 193A → T, (S65C). The most serious clinical manifestations are heterozygosis, C282Y/S65C, etc. [47, 48].

The cysteine residue in the α3 domain of the HFE protein that is altered in variant A of the C282Y HFE gene is necessary, as it forms bisulphite bonds and interacts with β2-microgloblulin, increasing its expression on the cell surface. The H63D mutation is present in the α1 domain of the peptide bond of the HFE protein, causing it to decrease the affinity between HFE and the transferrin receptor [49, 50]. Another aggravating factor of this variant is that the activation of the BMP/SMAD pathway for the transcription of hepcidin in the HAMP gene does not occur, due to the inability of the HFE protein to bind to the transferrin receptor. Therefore, changes in this protein contributes to the systemic accumulation of iron, by preventing iron absorption from the diet and by inhibiting the transcription of hepcidin [51].

HFE gene polymorphisms are associated with other clinical manifestations [52]. The H63D genotype modified the association between lead and iron metabolism, so that increased lead in the blood is associated with a higher iron content in the body or a lower concentration of transferrin, favouring lead poisoning [53]. The H63D polymorphism is attributed to a greater propensity to develop disorders in porphyrin metabolism, insulin resistance and diabetes development, as well as being associated with increased aggressiveness of hepatocarcinoma and pancreatic cancer [54, 55]. The H63D variant is associated with the development of neurodegenerative diseases, due to stress generated in the endoplasmic reticulum and iron accumulation in individuals with β-thalassemea [56, 57].

Iron overload in haemochromatosis type 1 is rarely observed in children. In a study with 42 boys and 41 girls, aged approximately 12 years, both diagnosed with the H63D HFE heretozygen gene, the measurement biochemical parameters for iron, ferritin, transferrin saturation and total iron binding capacity. All values were statistically higher in the H63D HFE individuals, when compared to the control group. H63D-HFE boys presented higher iron content than the mean concentration found in girls. This fact can be explained by the loss of blood in menstruation [58].

Iron accumulation and oxidative stress have been associated with the development of neurodegenerative diseases. Studies describe that the C282Y and H63D HFE polymorphisms contribute to the pathogenesis of Parkinson's disease and Alzheimer's disease [59]. However, two meta-analysis studies indicate that these polymorphisms do not contribute to the development of these diseases [60, 61]. The C282Y genotype is related to propensity for the development of hepatocarcinoma, amyotrophic lateral sclerosis, non-fatty liver disease and venous ulceration, even in patients who do not show signs and symptoms of haemochromatosis [62–65]. Lifestyle, epigenetic factors, diet, alcoholism contribute to the development of iron overload in patients presenting the HFE gene C282Y, H63D and S65C polymorphisms. The diagnosis and early monitoring of iron overload indicators is necessary to reduce the damage caused by iron to the body [66].

2.4.2. HAMP gene mutation

Genetic alterations in the HAMP gene compromise hepcidin function. The HAMP gene on chromosome 19 contains exon 3, the final exon that encodes the active peptide, and which has the largest polymorphic region of the gene [1, 2, 18]. Polymorphisms present in the HAMP gene are less frequent than polymorphisms in the HFE gene. Currently, about 16 different types of Single Nucleotide Polymorphism (SNP) polymorphism are described, but only a few are of clinical importance, since they are present in haemochromatosis. The first genetic alteration in the HAMP gene was identified using microsatellite marker probes in a region of 2.7 cm in the 19q13. A homozygous region with two mutations was identified (93delG e 166C → T) in two families that presented iron overload in the first decades of life, characterizing juvenile haemochromatosis type 2B [67].

In the mutation minisense homozygosis c.233G>A occurs the exchange of amino acids in the biologically active peptide, with a homozygous substitution of amino acids in the coding region, C78, by a tyrosine, C78T. This mutation disturbs one of the eight cysteines that make the bisulfite bonds necessary for the binding of hepcidin to ferroportin, causing the accumulation and exaggerated absorption of iron [68]. The C70R mutation also causes malformation in one of the bisulfite bridges of hepcidin cysteines. The amino acid cysteine is exchanged for an arginine, this exchange of neutral amino acid by an acidic amino acid interrupts the formation of the bisulfite bridge between the third and the sixth cysteine in the mature hepcidin peptide [69].

The C → T transition at position 166 in exon 3 of the HAMP (166C-T) cDNA, changes an arginine at position 56 to a stop codon (R56X), 193A → T. The amino acid change of R56X occurs at a region of the mature peptide, at amino acid residues 55–59. This region is a cleavage site for the pro-hormone convertase enzyme to recognize and produce a pro-hepcidin of 64 amino acids. With the change in the peptide chain, the convertase enzyme generates a truncated pro-hepcidin without all the mature sequences. Thus, truncated hepcidin does not bind to ferroportin, causing iron overload from infancy. In contrast, the deletion of a guanine in exon 2 at position 93 of the cDNA (93delG) results in a mutated RNA, which after translation yields a mature peptide of 179 amino acids, which is unstable and inefficient [67, 70].

The deletion Met50del IVS2þ1 (−G) in frameshift of exon 2, is a four nucleotide ATGG deletion that causes a shift of reading frames, disrupting expression of the active peptide, which is encoded by exon 3. The mutation suppresses the last exon 2 codon (Met50) and the first base of the intron 2 binding site (IVS + 1 (−G)). This change increases the reading frame beyond the end of the normal transcript. Another mutation, G71D, alters the charge of amino acid 71, which is between the third and fourth cysteines, at amino acids residues 70 and 72 in leaf β of the peptide, preventing binding with ferroportin [71].

The HAMP-G71D variant in association with the HFE-H63D variant patients with sickle cell disease increases the iron overload [72]. In the Spanish population, the HAMP-G71D variant appearing 1/100 diagnosed cases of haemochromatosis, is not attributed to iron overload [73]. The transition polymorphism G → A at the +14 position of the 5′-UTR region results in a new initiation codon at the +14 position of the 5′-UTR, inducing a change in the reading frame, yielding a new abnormal protein. The transition generates an unstable protein, which is degraded shortly after the translation of the messenger RNA [74].

The TG haplotype of the HAMP gene, caused by the binding of polymorphisms nc-1010C > T and nc-582A > G, is more frequent in H63D HFE individuals, with serum ferritin levels above 300 μg/L [75]. The association of HAMP and HFE gene polymorphisms is frequent. In some cases, there is a mixed clinical condition, with onset of iron accumulation in childhood and severe organ involvement in adult life and vulnerability to infections. The variants C-153C > T and C, 582A > G, reduce the expression of hepcidin, but the mature peptide mechanism of action remains the same, without increasing ferritin and transferrin saturation [76].

Genetic alterations in the HAMP gene may cause a defective or truncated hepcidin, making its mechanism of action impossible. Iron accumulation, as well as increased ferritin enables the development and pathogenesis of certain diseases, such as type 2 diabetes mellitus, coronary disease, increases plasma viremia of HIV, HCV and HBV, generates reactive oxygen species that damage the tissues and cell membranes [77, 78]. The plasma concentration of hepcidin influences the development of neurodegenerative diseases, such as Parkinson's disease,

Alzheimer's disease, multiple sclerosis and in dyslipidemias, some authors attribute this fact, the constant production of IL-6 and the activation of the STAT/Janus kinase pathway [79].

2.4.3. Haemojuvelin gene mutation

The HJV gene or HFE2 encodes the haemojuvelin protein, present on chromosome 1q21. The haemojuvelin is expressed in the liver, heart and skeletal muscle. The haemojuvelin transcript has five isoforms, with the longest protein having 426 amino acids [80]. Haemojuvelin is a co-receptor of the BMP protein, analogous to the Repulsive Guidance Molecules (RGM) family, which binds to BMP receptors to increase SMAD phosphorylation [81, 82]. Genetic alterations in the HFE2 gene make it impossible to transcribe hepcidin. In this way, parenchymal and tissue iron accumulation occurs in the first decades of life and is classified as juvenile haemochromatosis type-2A [83].

Currently, there are 43 HIV mutations identified that cause juvenile haemochromatosis, G320V being the most frequent, with the exchange of a glutamate by a valine [80, 84]. In the Greek population, this polymorphism is frequent in homozygosis, and in the Canadian population, this SNP has been reported in heterozygosity with R326X. Hyperferritinemia and transferrin saturation occur above 45%. More severe cases are found in heterozygosity with the HFE gene, for the polymorphisms C282Y and H63D [85]. Heterozygous patients for G320V and C282Y/H63D have iron and ferritin content 6–8 times higher than patients homozygous for G320V [86, 87]. The severity of the disease can be attributed to the fact that two signalling pathways of the HAMP gene for hepcidin transcription are defective, with the activation of BMP [88–90]. Several different polymorphisms may be involved in iron overload Of hemochromatosis, making difficult the correct diagnosis and precocious. Since each change It presents different clinical characteristics and the need for differentiated treatments, since Iron overload is associated with increased risk of early-onset liver cancer [91–93].

2.4.4. Transferrina (TFR2) gene mutation

The gene encoding the transferrin receptor type 2 (TFR2) is located on chromosome 7. The transferrin receptor 2 is a member of the TFR family, homologous to TFR1. TFR2 in the liver is considered as an iron sensor and activator of the hepcidin pathway. TFR is expressed in the erythroid tissue, where it is a component of the Erythropoietin (EPO) receptor, necessary for effective erythropoiesis to occur. The homozygous nonsense mutation at the 7q22 locus of the TFR2 gene leads to a rare form of iron overload, hereditary haemochromatosis type 3 [94, 95]. Sequencing of the coding region in exon 6 of the gene detected a transversion C $\rightarrow$ G at position 750 of the cDNA sequence that substitutes a tyrosine (TAC) for a stop sign (TAG) at residue 250 of the transcript (Y250X), giving a defective receptor [94].

Type 3 haemochromatosis is considered as an intermediary between haemochromatosis HFE and haemochromatosis 2. The first signs of iron accumulation occur after 30 years, with heterozygosis for HFE, but some more severe cases, the onset of signs and symptoms begins in childhood. Cardiac disorders and endocrine dysfunctions are less frequent than in juvenile haemochromatosis, with low serum concentrations of hepcidin [96, 97]. TRF2 acts the transcription in the HAMP gene through its interaction with the HFE protein [98]. Defective formation in the HFE and TFr2 proteins causes an overload of iron [99, 100]. Some authors suggest that TFR2 is required for phosphorylation of BMP6 in response to iron levels, playing a prominent role in the signalling pathway of the HAMP gene and the HFE protein being a contributor to the transcription of the HAMP gene [101, 102].

2.4.5. Ferroportin gene mutation

On chromosome 2, the SLC40A1 gene is located. Alterations in this gene give rise to the disease of ferroportina, an autosomal dominant disease, with two forms, classic form or type A and the non-classic form or type B. It has a global geographic distribution with heterogeneous phenotypic, clinical and genetic characteristics. Although rare, type 4 haemochromatosis is the second major form of iron overload after haemochromatosis HFE. Patients present hyperferritinemia, normal or low transferrin saturation and increased iron load on the Kupffer cells, liver and spleen [103, 104].

The classical form of the disease is usually asymptomatic without tissue damage and without other complications in young life. With age, damage to the liver and pancreas may occur with the development of fibrosis and low haemoglobin concentration [105]. Mutations A77D, D157G, V162del, N174I, Q182H, Q248H and G323V are most frequent in the European, Asian, Indian, Australian and African populations [106, 107]. The genotype Q248H is associated with hyperferritinemia, being frequent in the African population [108, 109]. Classical mutations D157N, D181V, G80V, Q182H, R489K and V162del, alter the folding of ferroportin, damaging the export of iron, and with intracellular accumulation of ferritin in monocytes [107, 110].

The non-classical or B form of ferroportin is more rare and similar to haemochromatosis type 1. Mutations N144H, Y64N, C326Y/S, S338R, Y501C are related to this disease phenotype [107]. Genotypes Y64N, V72F and Y501C confer resistance to hepcidin. These mutations alter the thiol form at residue 326 of the protein, which is essential for the binding of hepcidin to ferroportin, resulting in more severe iron overload at an early age [109]. The S209L mutation described in the Chinese population showed resistance and hepcidin [110]. *In vitro* experiments have demonstrated that the N144D/T and Y64N mutations prevent the internalization of the hepcidin-ferroportin complex, avoiding the ubiquitination of ferroportin within the lysosomal endosomes [111]. The differential diagnosis between types of haemochromatosis type 4 should be made through molecular tests and the patients' clinic [112].

2.4.6. Hereditary a(hypo)ceruloplasminemia and hyperferritinemia

Ceruloplasmin exhibits ferroxidase activity, a condition in which ferrous iron is oxidized to ferric iron to bind to transferrin. Genetic alterations inhibit ferroxidase activity or preclude complete transcription of the enzyme [99]. Aceruloplasminemia is an autosomal recessive disease characterized by progressive neurodegeneration of the retina and basal ganglia associated with inherited mutations. The disease reaches the central nervous system, with increased lipid peroxidation and ataxia syndrome. Other parenchymal tissues, liver and pancreas are also affected [113, 114].

Changes in chromosome 3q24-q25, give rise to the truncated formation of a premature stop codon. The activity of ceruloplasmin ferroxidase is dependent on a trinuclear copper pool, which is encoded by exon 18. The Y356H, R701W and G876A variants are associated with impaired ferroxidase activity of the enzyme, as they generate proteins with altered iron binding sites and changes in the copper cluster. Studies show the association of these variants with Alzheimer's disease, Parkinson's disease and the development of type 1 diabetes with the appearance of signs and symptoms between 30 and 35 years old, with decreased iron content and increased ferritin (hyperferritinemia) [115–117].

Another hereditary alteration that causes hyperferritinemia, is mutation in the L-ferritin ferritin light chain (FTL) gene located on chromosome 19q13 [118]. The hereditary hyperferritinemia-cataract syndrome (HHCS) is caused by heterogeneous mutations in the iron responsive element (IRE) in the 5′ region of L-ferritin mRNA that reduce the binding affinity of iron-responsive proteins (IRPs) to IREs and decrease the negative control of L-ferritin. This leads to the constitutive positive regulation of the L-chain synthesis of ferritin that characterizes HHCS. Serum ferritin concentrations are high and constant and transferrin saturation is normal. Patients with HHCS do not develop iron overload. The deposition of L-ferritin in the ocular lens causes bilateral cataract at an early age [119]. The 51G-C mutation in the UTR region (ITR) of the FTL gene induces a base pair rearrangement in the lateral structure of the IRE, changing the IRE conformation. The phenotype presents with a moderate increase of serum ferritin, and the development of cataracts may occur throughout life in cases of homozygous [120, 121].

Neuroferritinopathy is a rare, late-onset movement disorder characterized by iron and ferritin accumulation in the brain, normal or low levels of serum ferritin and variable clinical characteristics. The mutations 458dupA, 460insA, A96T, 498insTC alter the conformation and structure of ferritin, resulting in long sequences (26–33 amino acids) that are added to the protein [122]. The insertion, 460insA, of an adenine after nucleotide 460 of the FTL gene alters 22 amino acid residues in the C-terminal region, adding four more amino acid residues after translation of the mRNA. This mutation alters the final conformation of the ferritin molecule as it disrupts the D and E helices. These helices are important because they structure hydrophobic channels for iron core formation in ferritin [123]. Several pathologies such as diabetes, Parkinsonism and dementia are associated with hyperferritinemia [124].

2.5. Genetic changes related to iron deficiency

Genetic changes related to iron deficiency anaemia involve polymorphisms and mutations in the TMPRSS6 gene, present in the chromosome 22 (22q12.3-13.1). This gene encodes the transmembrane protein matritase-2, which cleaves the haemojuvelin, preventing the activation of the BMP/SMAD pathway in the HAMP gene. Genetic alterations involving this gene characterize a phenotype of iron resistance. The iron-refractory iron deficiency anaemia (IRIDA) is an autosomal recessive disease characterized by microcytic and hypochromic congenital anaemia, low transferrin saturation, low iron concentration, elevated serum ferritin and excess hepcidin in serum, plasma and urine, without a therapeutic response to iron replacement and erythropoietin [125, 126]. Excess hepcidin in IRIDA may explain: (1) the development of systemic iron deficiency, preventing the absorption of iron into duodenal enterocytes and the movement of iron stores, (2) the inability to obtain a haematological response to oral therapies with iron and (3) slow and incomplete use of parent iron formulations, consisting of ferro-carbohydrate complexes that require macrophage processing to be available in erythropoiesis [125].

The polymorphisms of the SNPs type, the TMPRSS6 gene, with the greatest clinical impact are K225E, K253E, G228D, R446W, V736A and V795I. In the rs855791 polymorphism, a substitution of the amino acid alanine for a valine at position 736, in the serine protease domain of matriptase-2 (p.Ala736Val) occurs, is the most frequent, being responsible for the picture observed in IRIDA, with the T allele being associated with decreased iron reserves in men. Mice with Tmprss6–/– phenotype presented severe alopecia and severe iron deficiency anaemia with elevated serum levels of hepcidin and decreased expression of ferroportin [6, 127, 128].

The variant p.V736A influences the susceptibility to hepatic iron accumulation in patients with thalassemia, and the risk allele is 736 (A) [129]. The T287N variant contributes to a history of microcytic anaemia and increases in hepcidin levels due to the inactivation of haemojuvelin cleavage in soluble haemojuvelin, thereby preventing haemojuvelin and hepcidin [130, 131]. Thus, the BMP path remains enabled [132, 133]. The mutation c.1113G >A disrupts the splicing process of mRNA, causing decrease of plasma protein matriptase-2 [133]. The H448R variant and the A719T and V795I polymorphisms are attributed to partial response to treatment with oral iron replacement in iron deficiency anaemia. The lack of response to treatment with oral iron is attributed to high concentration of hepcidin [134].

2.6. Therapeutic targets

The serum concentration of hepcidin determines the pathological state of many diseases-related to iron metabolism, since the modulation of the hepcidin/ferroportin axis has been studied as one of the main therapeutic targets for the treatment of diseases related to serum iron content, among them, haemochromatosis. Currently, the treatment of the hereditary hyperferritinemia (HH) is based on iron chelators and phlebotomy in patients; however, these are not effective treatments, bringing damage to the patient over a long time [135]. However, a stimulus for increased production of hepcidin or a hepcidin analogue may aid in the treatment of hereditary haemochromatosis. On the other hand, IRIDA and iron deficiency anaemia stand out as the main iron-deficient diseases. In this sense, the use of hepcidin inhibitors or TMPRSS6 analogues is a good deal for the treatment of these diseases [136].

2.7. Hepcidin agonist

Hepcidin agonist drugs are being investigated for the treatment of diseases related to lack or partial deficiency of hepcidin. It is a therapeutic alternative for diseases related to iron overload. PR65, a prototype of hepcidin, had its structure developed based on the N-terminal portion of the hepcidin molecule, which contains the amino acid residues, DTHFPICIF, required to bind to ferroportin and promote its ubiquitination, but did not exhibit activity *in vivo*. After molecular improvement of the PR65 prototype, a mini-hepcidin was synthesized. PR65 was administered twice weekly, subcutaneously in rats *knockout* (*HAMP–/–*), which presented iron overload and haemochromatosis phenotype. Iron deficiency was observed in cardiac and hepatic tissue, intestinal adsorption and retention of iron in the spleen and duodenum. When high doses of PR65 were administered in rats, anaemia was observed in these animals. The mini-hepcidins may be used in the auxiliary treatment of β-thalassemia and in policitemia vera [137–140].

Another alternative for the treatment of iron overload is an inhibitor of TMPRSS6, to increase serum hepcidin levels [141]. The use of interfering RNA (siRNA) in suppression of the TMPRSS6 gene in rats with β-thalassemia increased the concentration of hepcidin [142, 143].

Another alternative in the study is the modulation of the BMP/SMAD pathway, with exogenous treatment of BMP6, stimulating the transcription of the HAMP gene [144].

2.7.1. *Hepcidin antagonists*

Inhibition of the JAK/STAT pathway is used as a therapeutic target in order to reduce the serum hepcidin content with the use of anti-IL-6 receptor antibodies. Studies in animals with anaemia using the antibody, tocilizumab, demonstrated that protein C-reactive (PCR) levels and anaemia improved significantly within 1 week of treatment [145–147]. Siltuximab and infliximab (anti-TNF-α) antibodies have shown good results in the treatment of chronic disease anaemia due to blockage of the JAK/STAT3 pathway, increase in haemoglobin (15 g/dL) and decrease in hepcidin [147, 148]. Inhibition of the STAT3 pathway was also observed using AG490 (Calbiochem), and the peptide PpYLKTK, curcumin [149, 150].

Another alternative for the serum decrease in hepcidin is the intravenous use of *Spiegel mer* lexaptepid. *Spiegelmers* are synthetic oligonucleotides binding to molecular targets. Currently, three oligonucleotides are in clinical study, NOX-E36 (anti-CCL2), NOX-A12 (anti-CXCL12) and NOX-H94 (anti-hepcidin). *Spiegelmer* NOX-H94 blocks the binding of hepcidin to ferroportin, preventing its proteolytic ubiquitination, and may be used in the treatment of IRIDA and in diseases with increased hepcidin and increased IL-6. Studies in monkeys have shown improvement in anaemia and increased serum iron concentration [151–154].

The LDN-193189 is an inhibitor of BMP type I receptor, attenuates BMP/SMAD signalling in hepatic tissue and reduces HAMP gene [155]. The administration of LDN193189 facilitated the movement of iron stores in rats with anaemia of inflammation, with increased haemoglobin, erythropoiesis and reticulocytosis [156, 157]. The inibition of hepcidin synthesis may occur by blocking the ALK2 (activin-like receptor), receptor the BMPs proteins [158]. TP-0184 is an inhibitor of the ALK2 receptor, and in pre-clinical phase studies, it has shown to be a negative regulator of hepcidin expression. The monoclonal antibodies ABT-207 and h5F9-AM8 that inhibit haemojuvelin has been demonstrated to be effective in decreasing the expression of hepcidin in rats. Another treatment alternative to inhibit HAMP gene transcription is the fusion between Hemojuvelin soluble (sHJV) with the Fc portion of an IgG, giving Hemojuvelin Fracion (sHJV.Fc), which binds to BMPr, inhibiting the BMP6/SMAD pathway [136, 159–161].

Fursultiamine and LY2928057 antibodies prevent the interaction between ferroportin-hepcidin by sequestering the Cys326-HS residue of ferroportin and blocking the internalization of ferroportin/hepcidin [136, 162]. Anti-hepcidin antibodies efficacy was confirmed in a model of anaemia of inflation induced by *Brucella abortus*, in which hepcidin neutralization occurred and anaemia improved. The humanized antibody, 12B9m, has been shown to be a potent inhibitor of hepcidin [163–165].

The first evidence of heparin's action in controlling hepcidin expression was demonstrated in HepG2 cells and in rats that were given pharmacological doses of heparin. In the study, hepatic hepcidin mRNA expression decreased, from the sequestration of the BMP-6 protein and subsequent phosphorylation of the SMAD1/5/8 complex with reduction of iron concentration in the spleen and increase of serum iron. From these results, structural modifications in the heparin molecule were performed in order to decrease its anticoagulant activity for the clinical use of hepcidin elevation diseases. Modified heparins, by oxidation/ reduction, heparins *glycol-split* (*GS-heparin*), or sulfation (*SS-heparin*), demonstrated in clinical trials with little or no toxicity, being potent inhibitors of hepcidin *in vitro* in HepG2 cells and primary hepatocytes, and *in vivo* in rats, without presenting anticoagulant activity [166–169].

Growth differentiation factor 15 (GDF15) was shown to negatively regulate hepcidin mRNA expression in humans [170]. The compound K7174 GDF15 increases synthesis and reduces hepcidin expression in HepG2 cells and in rats [171]. The erythroid Erythroferrone (ERFE) hormone presents suppression activity of hepcidin mRNA in rat model with β-thalassemia [172, 173]. The siRNAs, siHJV, siTRF2 and siHepcidin are the main apostasy for suppression of the HAMP gene with inhibition of hepcidin synthesis [174].

2.8. Conclusion

The homeostasis of iron metabolism involves several signalling pathways and gene regulations. Genetic alterations influence the development of several pathologies involving hepcidin. Currently, screening for the diagnosis and research of polymorphisms and mutations related to iron metabolism is scarce. Genetic diseases with iron overload are diagnosed very late, bringing damage to patients' health. Studies of allelic frequencies in the most diverse populations are still scarce, making it difficult to trace genetic polymorphisms and phenotypic changes. There are few therapeutic options for the treatment of genetic diseases related to iron metabolism, and are still in clinical research phase II and I. Although these diseases are rare, the diagnosis is underestimated and directly interferes with the treatment of the patient. Epigenetic alterations can affect non-pathogenic polymorphisms by making them harmful; therefore, a complete description of the possible interferents in the genetic polymorphisms and the probable changes that these polymorphisms offer to the human organism are necessary.

Conflict of interests

The authors state that there are no conflicts of interest.

Author details

Cadiele Oliana Reichert[1*], Joel da Cunha[1,2], Débora Levy[2], Luciana Morganti Ferreira Maselli[2,3], Sérgio Paulo Bydlowski[1,3] and Celso Spada[1]

*Address all correspondence to: kadielli@hotmail.com

1 Clinical Analysis Department, Health Sciences Center, Federal University of Santa Catarina (UFSC), Florianópolis, Brazil

2 Laboratory of Genetics and Molecular Hematology (LIM31), University of São Paulo School of Medicine (FMUSP), São Paulo, Brazil

3 Research Division, Pró-Sangue Hemocentro de São Paulo Foundation, São Paulo, Brazil

References

[1] Krause A, Neitz S, Mägert HJ, Schulz A, Forssmann WG, Schulz-Knappe P, et al. LEAP-1, a novel highly disulfide-bonded human peptide, exhibits antimicrobial activity. FEBS Letters. 2000;**480**(2-3):147-150

[2] Park CH, Valore EV, Waring AJ, Ganz T. Hepcidin, a urinary antimicrobial peptide synthesized in the liver. Journal of Biological Chemistry. 2001;**276**(11):7806-7810. DOI: 10.1074/jbc.M008922200

[3] Nemeth E, Ganz T. Anemia of inflammation. Hematology/Oncology Clinics of North America. 2014;**28**(4):671-681. DOI: 10.1016/j.hoc.2014.04.005

[4] Kaiser L, Davis JM, Patterson J, Johnson AL, Bohart G, Olivier NB, et al. Iron sufficient to cause hepatic fibrosis and ascites does not cause cardiac arrhythmias in the gerbil. Translational Research. 2009;**154**(4):202-213. DOI: 10.1016/j.trsl.2009.07.002

[5] Fleming MD. The regulation of hepcidin and its effects on systemic and cellular iron metabolism. Hematology American Society of Hematology Education Program. 2008; **2008**:151-158. DOI: 10.1182/asheducation-2008.1.151

[6] De Falco L, Sanchez M, Silvestri L, Kannengiesser C, Muckenthaler MU, Iolascon A, et al. Iron refractory iron deficiency anemia. Haematologica. 2013;**98**(6):845-853. DOI: 10.3324/haematol.2012.075515

[7] Ganz T. Hepcidin and its role in regulating systemic iron metabolism. Hematology American Society of Hematology Education Program. 2006;**2006**:29-35. 507. DOI: 10.1182/asheducation-2006.1.29

[8] Piperno A, Galimberti S, Mariani R, Pelucchi S, Ravasi G, Lombardi C, et al. Modulation of hepcidin production during hypoxia-induced erythropoiesis in humans in vivo: Data from the HIGHCARE project. Blood. 2011;**117**(10):2953-2959. DOI: 10.1182/blood-2010-08-299859

[9] Ramos E, Kautz L, Rodriguez R, Hansen M, Gabayan V, Ginzburg Y, et al.Evidence for distinct pathways of hepcidin regulation by acute and chronic iron loading in mice. Hepatology. 2011;**53**(4):1333-1341. DOI: 10.1002/hep.24178

[10] Pak M, Lopez MA, Gabayan V, Ganz T, Rivera S. Suppression of hepcidin during anemia requires erythropoietic activity. Blood. 2006;**108**(12):3730-3735. DOI: 10.1182/blood-2006-06-028787

[11] Ganz T. Hepcidin and iron regulation, 10 years later. Blood. 2011;**117**(17):4425-4433. DOI: 10.1182 /blood-2011-01-258467

[12] Pietrangelo A. Genetics, genetic testing, and management of hemochromatosis: 15 years since hepcidin. Gastroenterology. 2015;**149**(5):1240-1251. DOI: 10.1053/j.gastro.2015.06.045

[13] Gozzelino R, Arosio P. Iron homeostasis in health and disease. International Journal of Molecular Sciences. 2016;**17**(1):130. DOI: 10.3390/ijms17010130

[14] Drakesmith H, Prentice A. Viral infection and iron metabolism. Nature Reviews Microbiology. 2008;**6**(7):541-552. DOI: 10.1038/nrmicro1930

[15] Sow FB, Florence WC, Satoskar AR, Schlesinger LS, Zwilling BS, Lafuse WP. Expression and localization of hepcidin in macrophages: A role in host defense against tuberculosis. Journal of Leukocyte Biology. 2007;**82**(4):934-945. DOI: 10.1189/jlb.0407216

[16] Kulaksiz H, Fein E, Redecker P, Stremmel W, Adler G, Cetin Y. Pancreatic beta-cells express hepcidin, an iron-uptake regulatory peptide. Journal of Endocrinology. 2008;**197**(2):241-249. DOI: 10.1677/JOE-07-0528

[17] Bekri S, Gual P, Anty R, Luciani N, Dahman M, Ramesh B, et al. Increased adipose tissue expression of hepcidin in severe obesity is independent from diabetes and NASH. Gastroenterology. 2006;**131**(3):788-796. DOI: 10.1053/j.gastro.2006.07.007

[18] Pigeon C, Ilyin G, Courselaud B, Leroyer P, Turlin B, Brissot P, et al. A new mouse liver-specific gene, encoding a protein homologous to human antimicrobial peptide hepcidin, is overexpressed during iron overload. Journal of Biological Chemistry. 2001;**276**(11): 7811-7819. DOI: 10.1074/jbc.M008923200

[19] Nicolas G, Bennoun M, Porteu A, Mativet S, Beaumont C, Grandchamp B, et al. Severe iron deficiency anemia in transgenic mice expressing liver hepcidin. Proceedings of the National Academy of Sciences of the United States of America. 2002;**99**(7):4596-4601. DOI: 10.1073/pnas.072632499

[20] Nemeth E, Preza GC, Jung CL, Kaplan J, Waring AJ, Ganz T. The N-terminus of hepcidin is essential for its interaction with ferroportin: Structure-function study. Blood. 2006;**107**(1):328-333. DOI: 10.1182/blood-2005-05-2049

[21] Knutson MD, Oukka M, Koss LM, Aydemir F, Wessling-Resnick M. Iron release from macrophages after erythrophagocytosis is up-regulated by ferroportin 1 overexpression and down-regulated by hepcidin. Proceedings of the National Academy of Sciences of the United States of America. 2005;**102**(5):1324-1328. DOI: 10.1073/pnas.0409409102

[22] Koskenkorva-Frank TS, Weiss G, Koppenol WH, Burckhardt S. The complex interplay of iron metabolism, reactive oxygen species, and reactive nitrogen species: Insights into the potential of various iron therapies to induce oxidative and nitrosative stress. Free Radical Biology & Medicine. 2013;**65**:1174-1194. DOI: 10.1016/j.freeradbiomed.2013.09.001

[23] Evstatiev R, Gasche C. Iron sensing and signalling. Gut. 2012;**61**(6):933-952. DOI: 10.1136/gut.2010.214312

[24] Krishnamurthy P, Xie T, Schuetz JD. The role of transporters in cellular heme and porphyrin homeostasis. Pharmacology & Therapeutics. 2007;**114**(3):345-358. DOI: 10.1016/j.pharmthera.2007.02.001

[25] Muñoz M, García-Erce JA, Remacha AF. Disorders of iron metabolism. Part 1: Molecular basis of iron homoeostasis. Journal of Clinical Pathology. 2011;**64**(4):281-286. DOI: 10.1136/jcp.2010.079046

[26] Chen H, Attieh ZK, Syed BA, Kuo YM, Stevens V, Fuqua BK, et al. Identification of zyklopen, a new member of the vertebratemulticopper ferroxidase family, and characterization in rodents and human cells. Journal of Nutrition. 2010;**140**(10):1728-1735. DOI: 10.3945/jn.109.117531

[27] Wang J, Pantopoulos K. Regulation of cellular iron metabolism. Biochemical Journal. 2011;**434**(3):365-381. DOI: 10.1042/BJ20101825

[28] Vashchenko G, MacGillivray RT. Multi-copper oxidases and human iron metabolism. Nutrients. 2013;**5**(7):2289-2313. DOI: 10.3390/nu5072289

[29] Soe-Lin S, Apte SS, Andriopoulos Jr B, Andrews MC, Schranzhofer M, Kahawita T, et al. Nramp1 promotes efficient macrophage recycling of iron following erythrophagocytosis in vivo. Proceedings of the National Academy of Sciences of the United States of America. 2009;**106**(14):5960-5965. DOI: 10.1073/pnas.0900808106

[30] Hentze MW, Muckenthaler MU, Galy B, Camaschella C. Two to tango: Regulation of Mammalian iron metabolism. Cell. 2010;**142**(1):24-38. DOI: 10.1016/j.cell.2010.06.028

[31] Nemeth E, Ganz T. The role of hepcidin in iron metabolism. Acta Haematologica. 2009; **122**(2-3):78-86. DOI: 10.1159/000243791

[32] Nemeth E, Tuttle MS, Powelson J, Vaughn MB, Donovan A, Ward DM, et al. Hepcidin regulates cellular iron efflux by binding to ferroportin and inducing its internalization. Science. 2004;**306**(5704):2090-2093. DOI: 10.1126/science.1104742

[33] Kaplan J, Ward DM, De Domenico I. The molecular basis of iron overload disorders and iron-linked anemias. International Journal of Hematology. 2011;**93**(1):14-20. DOI: 10.1007/s12185-010-0760-0

[34] Miyazawa K, Shinozaki M, Hara T, Furuya T, Miyazono K. Two major Smad pathways in TGF-beta superfamily signalling. Genes Cells. 2002;**7**(12):1191-1204

[35] Babitt JL, Huang FW, Xia Y, Sidis Y, Andrews NC, Lin HY. Modulation of boné morphogenetic protein signaling in vivo regulates systemic iron balance. Journal of Clinical Investigation. 2007;**117**(7):1933-1939. DOI: 10.1172/JCI31342

[36] Lin L, Valore EV, Nemeth E, Goodnough JB, Gabayan V, Ganz T. Iron transferrin regulates hepcidin synthesis in primary hepatocyte culture through hemojuvelin and BMP2/4. Blood. 2007;**110**(6):2182-2189. DOI: 10.1182/blood-2007-04-087593

[37] Mleczko-Sanecka K, Casanovas G, Ragab A, Breitkopf K, Müller A, Boutros M, et al. SMAD7 controls iron metabolism as a potent inhibitor of hepcidin expression. Blood. 2010;**115**(13):2657-2665. DOI: 10.1182/blood-2009-09-238105

[38] Rawlings JS, Rosler KM, Harrison DA. The JAK/STAT signaling pathway. Journal of Cell Science. 2004;**117**(8):1281-1283. DOI: 10.1242/jcs.00963

[39] Fleming RE. Hepcidin activation during inflammation: Make it STAT. Gastroenterology. 2007;**132**(1):447-449. DOI: 10.1053/j.gastro.2006.11.049

[40] Pietrangelo A, Dierssen U, Valli L, Garuti C, Rump A, Corradini E, et al. STAT3 is required for IL-6-gp130-dependent activation of hepcidin in vivo. Gastroenterology. 2007;**132**(1):294-300. DOI: 10.1053/j.gastro.2006.10.018

[41] Przybyszewska J, Żekanowska E. The role of hepcidin, ferroportin, HCP1, and DMT1 protein in iron absorption in the human digestive tract. Przegląd Gastroenterologiczny. 2014;**9**(4):208-213. DOI: 10.5114/pg.2014.45102

[42] Salgia RJ, Brown K. Diagnosis and management of hereditary hemochromatosis. Clinical Liver Disease. 2015;**19**(1):187-198. DOI: 10.1016/j.cld.2014.09.011

[43] Quigley P. Hereditary hemochromatosis: Dealing with iron overload. Nursing. 2016;**46**(5): 36-43. DOI: 10.1097/01.NURSE.0000482258.55896.d8

[44] Castiella A, Zapata E, Alústiza JM. Non-invasive methods for liver fibrosis prediction in hemochromatosis: One step beyond. World Journal of Hepatology. 2010;**2**(7):251-255. DOI: 10.4254/wjh.v2.i7.251

[45] Porto G, Brissot P, Swinkels DW, Zoller H, Kamarainen O, Patton S, et al. EMQN best practice guidelines for the molecular genetic diagnosis of hereditary hemochromatosis (HH). European Journal of Human Genetics. 2016;**24**(4):479-495. DOI: 10.1038/ejhg.2015.128

[46] European Association for the Study of the Liver. EASL clinical practice guidelines for HFE hemochromatosis. Journal of Hepatology. 2010;**53**(1):3-22. DOI: 10.1016/j.jhep.2010.03.001

[47] McDonald CJ, Wallace DF, Crawford DH, Subramaniam VN. Iron storage disease in Asia-Pacific populations: The importance of non-HFE mutations. Journal of Gastroenterology and Hepatology. 2013;**28**(7):1087-1094. DOI: 10.1111/jgh.12222

[48] Cukjati M, Vaupotic T, Rupreht R, Curin-Serbec V. Prevalence of H63D, S65C and C282Y hereditary hemochromatosis gene mutations in Slovenian population by na improved high-throughput genotyping assay. BMC Medical Genetics. 2007;**8**:69. DOI: 10.1186/1471-2350-8-69

[49] Cézard C, Rabbind Singh A, Le Gac G, Gourlaouen I, Ferec C, Rochette J. Phenotypic expression of a novel C282Y/R226G compound heterozygous state in HFE hemochromatosis: Molecular dynamics and biochemical studies. Blood Cells, Molecules and Diseases. 2013;**52**(**1**):27-34. DOI: 10.1016/j.bcmd.2013.07.011

[50] Nandar W, Connor JR. HFE gene variants affect iron in the brain. Journal of Nutrition. 2011;**141**(4):729S-739S. DOI: 10.3945/jn.110.130351

[51] Wu XG, Wang Y, Wu Q, Cheng WH, Liu W, Zhao Y, et al. HFE interacts with the BMP type I receptor ALK3 to regulate hepcidin expression. Blood. 2014;**124**(8):1335-1343. DOI: 10.1182/blood-2014-01-552281

[52] Eum KD, Seals RM, Taylor KM, Grespin M, Umbach DM, Hu H, et al,. Modification of the association between lead exposure and amyotrophic lateral sclerosis by iron

and oxidative stress related gene polymorphisms. Amyotrophic Lateral Sclerosis & Frontotemporal Degeneration. 2015;**16**(1-2):72-79. DOI: 10.3109/21678421.2014.964259

[53] Fan G, Du G, Li H, Lin F, Sun Z, Yang W, et al. The effect of the hemochromatosis (HFE) genotype on lead load and iron metabolism among lead smelter workers. PLoS One. 2014;**9**(7):e101537. DOI: 10.1371/journal.pone.0101537

[54] Krivosheev AB, Maximov VN, Voevoda MI, Kuimov AD, Kondratova MA, Tuguleva TA, et al. Alleles c282y and h63d hfe gene, insulin resistance and susceptibility to disturbance of porphyrin metabolism in non-alcoholic fatty liver disease. Eksperimental'naia i Klinicheskaia Gastroenterologiia. 2015;(3):39-44

[55] Shen LL, Gu DY, Zhao TT, Tang CJ, Xu Y, Chen JF. Implicating the H63D polymorphism in the HFE gene in increased incidence of solid cancers: A meta-analysis. Genetics and Molecular Research. 2015;**14**(4):13735-13745. DOI: 10.4238/2015.October.28.36

[56] Yokoyama JS, Bonham LW, Sears RL, Klein E, Karydas A, Kramer JH, et al. Decision tree analysis of genetic risk for clinically heterogeneous Alzheimer's disease. BMC Neurology. 2015;**15**:47. DOI: 10.1186/s12883-015-0304-6

[57] Enein AA, El Dessouky NA, Mohamed KS, Botros SK, Abd El Gawad MF, Hamdy M, et al. Frequency of hereditary hemochromatosis (HFE) gene mutations in Egyptian beta thalassemia patients and its relation to iron overload. Open Access Macedonian Journal of Medical Sciences. 2016;**4**(2):226-231. DOI: 10.3889/oamjms.2016.055

[58] Barbara KH, Marcin L, Jedrzej A, Wieslaw Z, Elzbieta AD, Malgorzata M, et al. The impact of H63D HFE gene carriage on hemoglobin and iron status in children. Annals of Hematology. 2016;**95**(12):2043-2048. DOI: 10.1007/s00277-016-2792-x

[59] Ali-Rahmani F, Schengrund CL, Connor JR. HFE gene variants, iron, and lipids: A novel connection in Alzheimer's disease. Frontiers in Pharmacology. 2014;**5**:165. DOI: 10.3389/fphar.2014.00165

[60] Xia J, Xu H, Jiang H, Xie J. The association between the C282Y and H63D polymorphisms of HFE gene and the risk of Parkinson's disease: A meta-analysis. Neuroscience Letters. 2015;**595**:99-103. DOI: 10.1016/j.neulet.2015.04.010

[61] Duan C, Wang M, Zhang Y, Wei X, Huang Y, Zhang H, et al. C282Y and H63D polymorphisms in hemochromatosis gene and risk of Parkinson's disease: A meta-analysis. American Journal of Alzheimer's Disease & Other Dementias. 2016;**31**(3):201-207. DOI: 10.1177/1533317515602220

[62] Nahon P, Sutton A, Rufat P, Ziol M, Thabut G, Schischmanoff PO, et al. Liver iron, HFE gene mutations, and hepatocellular carcinoma occurrence in patients with cirrhosis. Gastroenterology. 2008;**134**(1):102-110. DOI: 10.1053/j.gastro.2007.10.038

[63] Li M, Wang L, Wang W, Qi XL, Tang ZY. Mutations in the HFE gene and sporadic amyotrophic lateral sclerosis risk: A meta-analysis of observational studies. Brazilian Journal of Medical and Biological Research. 2014;**47**(3):215-222. DOI: 10.1590/1414-431X20133296

[64] Saremi L, Lotfipanah S, Mohammadi M, Hosseinzadeh H, Sayad A, Saltanatpour Z. Association of HFE gene mutations with nonalcoholic fatty liver disease in the Iranian population. Cellular and Molecular Biology. 2016;**62**(12):123-128. DOI: 10.14715/cmb/2016.62.12.21

[65] Zamboni P, Tognazzo S, Izzo M, Pancaldi F, Scapoli GL, Liboni A, et al.Hemochromatosis C282Y gene mutation increases the risk of venous leg ulceration. Journal of Vascular Surgery. 2005;**42**(2):309-314. DOI: 10.1016/j.jvs.2005.04.003

[66] Aranda N, Viteri FE, Montserrat C, Arija V. Effects of C282Y, H63D, and S65C HFE gene mutations, diet, and life-style factors on iron status in a general Mediterranean population from Tarragona, Spain. Annals of Hematology. 2010;**89**(8):767-773. DOI: 10.1007 / s00277-010-0901-9

[67] Roetto A, Papanikolaou G, Politou M, Alberti F, Girelli D, Christakis J, et al. Mutant antimicrobial peptide hepcidin is associated with severe juvenile hemochromatosis. Nature Genetics. 2003;**33**(1):21-22. DOI: 10.1038/ng1053

[68] Delatycki MB, Allen KJ, Gow P, MacFarlane J, Radomski C, Thompson J, et al. A homozygous HAMP mutation in a multiply consanguineous family with pseudo-dominant juvenile hemochromatosis. Clinical Genetics. 2004;**65**(5):378-383. DOI: 10.1111/j.0009-9163.2004.00254.x

[69] Roetto A, Daraio F, Porporato P, Caruso R, Cox TM, Cazzola M, et al. Screening hepcidin for mutations in juvenile hemochromatosis: Identification of a new mutation (C70R). Blood. 2004;**103**(6):2407-2409. DOI: 10.1182/blood-2003-10-3390

[70] Robson KJ, Merryweather-Clarke AT, Cadet E, Viprakasit V, Zaahl MG, Pointon JJ, et al. Recent advances in understanding haemochromatosis: A transition state. Journal of Medical Genetics. 2004;**41**(10):721-730. DOI: 10.1136/jmg.2004.020644

[71] Merryweather-Clarke AT, Cadet E, Bomford A, Capron D, Viprakasit V, Miller A, et al. Digenic inheritance of mutations in HAMP and HFE results in different types of haemochromatosis. Human Molecular Genetics. 2003;**12**(17):2241-2247. DOI: 10.1093/hmg/ddg225

[72] Abdel Rahman HA, Abou-Elew HH, El-Shorbagy RM, Fawzy R, Youssry I. Influence of iron regulating genes mutations on iron status in Egyptian patients with sickle cell disease. Annals of Clinical and Laboratory Science. 2014;**44**(3):304-309

[73] Altès A, Bach V, Ruiz A, Esteve A, Felez J, Remacha AF, et al,. Mutations in HAMP and HJV genes and their impact on expression of clinical hemochromatosis in a cohort of 100 Spanish patients homozygous for the C282Y mutation of HFE gene. Annals of Hematology. 2009;**88**(10):951-955. DOI: 10.1007/s00277-009-0705-y

[74] Matthes T, Aguilar-Martinez P, Pizzi-Bosman L, Darbellay R, Rubbia-Brandt L, Giostra E, et al. Severe hemochromatosis in a Portuguese family associated with a new mutation in the 5′-UTR of the HAMP gene. Blood. 2004;**104**(7):2181-2183. DOI: 10.1182/blood-2004-01-0332

[75] Silva B, Pita L, Gomes S, Gonçalves J, Faustino P. The hepcidin gene promoter nc.-1010C > T; −582A > G haplotype modulates serum ferritin in individuals carrying the common H63D mutation in HFE gene. Annals of Hematology. 2014;**93**(12):2063-2066. DOI: 10.1007/s00277-014-2160-7

[76] Parajes S, González-Quintela A, Campos J, Quinteiro C, Domínguez F, Loidi L. Genetic study of the hepcidin gene (HAMP) promoter and functional analysis of the c.-582A > G variant. BMC Genetics. 2010;**11**:110. DOI: 10.1186/1471-2156-11-110

[77] Pechlaner R, Weiss G, Bansal S, Mayr M, Santer P, Pallhuber B, et al. Inadequate hepcidin serum concentrations predict incident type 2 diabetes mellitus. Diabetes/Metabolism Research and Reviews. 2016;**32**(2):187-192. DOI: 10.1002/dmrr.2711

[78] Berdoukas V, Coates TD, Cabantchik ZI. Iron and oxidative stress in cardiomyopathy in thalassemia. Free Radical Biology & Medicine. 2015;**88**(Pt A):3-9. DOI: 10.1016/j.freeradbiomed.2015.07.019

[79] Crichton RR, Dexter DT, Ward RJ. Brain iron metabolism and its perturbation in neurological diseases. Journal of Neural Transmission. 2011;**118**(**3**):301-314. DOI:10.1007/s00702-010-0470-z

[80] Papanikolaou G, Samuels ME, Ludwig EH, MacDonald ML, Franchini PL, Dubé MP, et al. Mutations in HFE2 cause iron overload in chromosome 1q-linked juvenile hemochromatosis. Nature Genetics. 2004;**36**(1):77-82. DOI: 10.1038/ng1274

[81] Casanovas G, Mleczko-Sanecka K, Altamura S, Hentze MW, Muckenthaler MU. Bone morphogenetic protein (BMP)-responsive elements located in the proximal and distal hepcidin promoter are critical for its response to HJV/BMP/SMAD. Journal of Molecular Medicine. 2009;**87**:471-480.DOI: 10.1007/s00109-009-0447-2

[82] Andriopoulos Jr B, Corradini E, Xia Y, Faasse SA, Chen S, Grgurevic L, et al. L. BMP6 is a key endogenous regulator of hepcidin expression and iron metabolism. Nature Genetics. 2009;**41**(4):482-487. DOI: 10.1038/ng.335

[83] Aguilar-Martinez P, Lok CY, Cunat S, Cadet E, Robson K, Rochette J. Juvenile hemochromatosis caused by a novel combination of hemojuvelin G320V/R176C mutations in a 5-year old girl. Haematologica. 2007;**92**(3):421-422. DOI: 10.3324/haematol.10701

[84] Core AB, Canali S, Babitt JL. Hemojuvelin and bone morphogenetic protein (BMP) signaling in iron homeostasis. Frontiers in Pharmacology. 2014;**5**:104. DOI: 10.3389/fphar.2014.00104

[85] Brakensiek K, Fegbeutel C, Mälzer M, Strüber M, Kreipe H, Stuhrmann M. Juvenile hemochromatosis due to homozygosity for the G320V mutation in the HJV gene with fatal outcome. Clinical Genetics. 2009;**76**(5):493-495. DOI: 10.1111/j.1399-0004.2009.01261.x

[86] Militaru MS, Popp RA, Trifa AP. Homozygous G320V mutation in the HJV gene causing juvenile hereditary haemochromatosis type A. A case report. Journal of Gastrointestinal and Liver Diseases. 2010;**19**(2):191-193

[87] Le Gac G, Scotet V, Ka C, Gourlaouen I, Bryckaert L, Jacolot S, et al. The recently identified type 2A juvenile haemochromatosis gene (HJV), a second candidate modifier of the C282Y homozygous phenotype. Human Molecular Genetics. 2004;**13**(17):1913-1918. DOI: 10.1093/hmg/ddh206

[88] Latour C, Besson-Fournier C, Meynard D, Silvestri L, Gourbeyre O, Aguilar-Martinez, et al. Differing impact of the deletion of hemochromatosis-associated molecules HFE and transferrin receptor-2 on the iron phenotype of mice lacking bone morphogenetic protein 6 or hemojuvelin. Hepatology. 2016;**63**(1):126-137. DOI: 10.1002 /hep.28254

[89] Wu Q, Wang H, An P, Tao Y, Deng J, Zhang Z, et al. HJV and HFE play distinct roles in regulating hepcidin. Antioxidants and Redox Signaling. 2015;22(**15**):1325-1336. DOI: 10.1089/ars.2013.5819

[90] Kent P, Wilkinson N, Constante M, Fillebeen C, Gkouvatsos K, Wagner J, et al. Hfe and Hjv exhibit overlapping functions for iron signaling to hepcidin. Journal of Molecular Medicine. 2015;**93(**5):489-498. DOI: 10.1007/s00109-015-1253-7

[91] Lanktree MB, Sadikovic B, Waye JS, Levstik A, Lanktree BB, Yudin J, et al. Clinical evaluation of a hemochromatosis next-generation sequencing gene panel. European Journal of Haematology. 2017;**98**(3):228-234. DOI: 10.1111/ejh.12820

[92] Hamdi-Rozé H, Beaumont-Epinette MP, Ben Ali Z, Le Lan C, Loustaud-Ratti V, Causse X, et al. Rare HFE variants are the most frequent cause of hemochromatosis in non-c282y homozygous patients with hemochromatosis. American Journal of Hematology. 2016;**91**(12):1202-1205. DOI: 10.1002/ajh.24535

[93] Funakoshi N, Chaze I, Alary AS, Tachon G, Cunat S, Giansily-Blaizot M, et al. The role of genetic factors in patients with hepatocellular carcinoma and iron overload—A prospective series of 234 patients. Liver International. 2016;**36**(5):746-754. DOI: 10.1111/liv.12984

[94] Camaschella C, Roetto A, Calì A, De Gobbi M, Garozzo G, Carella M, et al. The gene TFR2 is mutated in a new type of haemochromatosis mapping to 7q22. Nature Genetics. 2000;**25**(1):14-15. DOI: 10.1038/75534

[95] Del-Castillo-Rueda A, Moreno-Carralero MI, Cuadrado-Grande N, Alvarez-Sala-Walther LA, Enríquez-de-Salamanca R, et al. Mutations in the HFE, TFR2, and SLC40A1 genes in patients with hemochromatosis. Gene. 2012;**508**(1):15-20. DOI: 10.1016/j.gene.2012.07.069

[96] Bardou-Jacquet E, Ben Ali Z, Beaumont-Epinette MP, Loreal O, Jouanolle AM, Brissot P. Non-HFE hemochromatosis: Pathophysiological and diagnostic aspects. Clinics and Research in Hepatology and Gastroenterology. 2014;**38**(2):143-154. DOI: 10.1016/j.clinre.2013.11.003

[97] Brissot P, Bardou-Jacquet E, Jouanolle AM, Loréal O. Iron disorders of genetic origin: A changing world. Trends in Molecular Medicine. 2011;**17**(12):707-713. DOI: 10.1016/j.molmed.2011.07.004

[98] Mehta K, Busbridge M, Renshaw D, Evans RW, Farnaud S, Patel VB. Characterization of hepcidin response to holotransferrin in novel recombinant TfR1 HepG2 cells. Blood Cells, Molecules and Diseases. 2016;**61**:37-45. DOI: 10.1016/j.bcmd.2016.06.008

[99] McDonald CJ, Wallace DF, Ostini L, Subramaniam VN. Parenteral vs. oral iron: Influence on hepcidin signaling pathways through analysis of Hfe/Tfr2-null mice. American Journal of Physiology-Gastrointestinal and Liver Physiology. 2014;**306**(2):132-139. DOI: 10.1152/ajpgi.00256.2013

[100] Schmidt PJ, Fleming MD. Transgenic HFE-dependent induction of hepcidin in mice does not require transferrin receptor-2. American Journal of Hematology. 2012;87(**6**):588-595. DOI: 10.1002/ajh.23173

[101] D'Alessio F, Hentze MW, Muckenthaler MU. The hemochromatosis proteins HFE, TfR2, and HJV form a membrane-associated protein complex for hepcidin regulation. Journal of Hepatology. 2012;**57**(5):1052-1060. DOI: 10.1016/j.jhep.2012.06.015

[102] Girelli D, Trombini P, Busti F, Campostrini N, Sandri M, Pelucchi S, et al. A time course of hepcidin response to iron challenge in patients with HFE and TFR2 hemochromatosis. Haematologica. 2011;**96**(4):500-506. DOI: 10.3324 /haematol.2010.033449

[103] Cazzola M. Genetic disorders of iron overload and the novel "ferroportin disease". Haematologica. 2003;**88**(**7**):721-724

[104] Pietrangelo A. The ferroportin disease. Blood Cells. 2004;**32**:131-138

[105] Callebaut I, Joubrel R, Pissard S, Kannengiesser C, Gérolami V, Ged C, et al. Comprehensive functional annotation of 18 missense mutations found in suspected hemochromatosis type 4 patients. Human Molecular Genetics. 2014;**23**(17):4479-4490. DOI: 10.1093 / hmg/ddu160

[106] Brissot P, Troadec MB, Bardou-Jacquet E, Le Lan C, Jouanolle AM, Deugnier Y, et al. Current approach to hemochromatosis. Blood Reviews. 2008;**22**(4):195-210. DOI: 10.1016 /j.blre.2008.03.001

[107] Mayr R, Janecke AR, Schranz M, Griffiths WJ, Vogel W, Pietrangelo A, et al. Ferroportin disease: A systematic meta-analysis of clinical and molecular findings. Journal of Hepatology. 2010;**53**(5):941-949. DOI: 10.1016/j.jhep.2010.05.016

[108] McNamara L, Gordeuk VR, MacPhail AP. Ferroportin (Q248H) mutations in African families with dietary iron overload. Journal of Gastroenterology and Hepatology. 2005;**20**(12):1855-1858. DOI: 10.1111/j.1440-1746.2005.03930.x

[109] Sham RL, Phatak PD, Nemeth E, Ganz T. Hereditary hemochromatosis due to resistance to hepcidin: High hepcidin concentrations in a family with C326S ferroportin mutation. Blood. 2009;**114**(2):493-494. DOI: 10.1182/blood-2009-04-216226

[110] An P, Jiang L, Guan Y, Wang H, Wang J, Tian Y, et al. Identification of hereditary hemochromatosis pedigrees and a novel SLC40A1 mutation in Chinese population. Blood Cells, Molecules and Diseases. 2017;**63**:34-36. DOI: 10.1016 /j.bcmd.2017.01.002

[111] Sham RL, Phatak PD, West C, Lee P, Andrews C, Beutler E. Autosomal dominant hereditary hemochromatosis associated with a novel ferroportin mutation and unique clinical features. Blood Cells, Molecules and Diseases. 2005;**34**(2):157-161. DOI: 10.1016/j.bcmd.2004.12.002

[112] Détivaud L, Island ML, Jouanolle AM, Ropert M, Bardou-Jacquet E, Le Lan C, et al. Ferroportin diseases: Functional studies, a link between genetic and clinical phenotype. Human Mutation. 2013;**34**(11):1529-1536. DOI: 10.1002/humu.22396

[113] Kono S. Aceruloplasminemia. Current Drug Targets. 2012;**13**(9):1190-1199

[114] Ariza J, Rogers H, Hartvigsen A, Snell M, Dill M, Judd D, et al. Iron accumulation and dysregulation in the putamen in fragile X-associated tremor/ataxia syndrome. Movement Disorders. 2017. DOI: 10.1002 /mds.26902

[115] Johannesson T, Kristinsson J, Torsdottir G, Snaedal J. Ceruloplasmin (Cp) and iron in connection with Parkinson's disease (PD) and Alzheimer's disease (AD). Laeknabladid. 2012;**98**(10):531-537

[116] Vroegindeweij LH, van der Beek EH, Boon AJ, Hoogendoorn M, Kievit JA, Wilson JH, et al. Aceruloplasminemia presents as Type 1 diabetes in non-obese adults: A detailed case series. Diabetic Medicine. 2015;**32**(8):993-1000. DOI: 10.1111/dme.12712

[117] Miyajima H. Aceruloplasminemia. Neuropathology. 2015;**35**(1):83-90. DOI: 10.1111 / neup.12149

[118] Zandman-Goddard G, Shoenfeld Y. Hyperferritinemia in autoimmunity. The Israel Medical Association Journal. 2008;**10**(1):83-84

[119] Adams PC, Barton JC. A diagnostic approach to hyperferritinemia with a non-elevated transferrin saturation. Journal of Hepatology. 2011;**55**(2):453-458. DOI: 10.1016 /j.jhep.2011.02.010

[120] Camaschella C, Zecchina G, Lockitch G, Roetto A, Campanella A, Arosio P, et al. A new mutation (G51C) in the iron-responsive element (IRE) of L-ferritin associated with hyperferritinaemia-cataract syndrome decreases the binding affinity of the mutated IRE for iron-regulatory proteins. British Journal of Haematology. 2000;**108**(3):480-482. DOI: 10.1046/j.1365-2141.2000.01920.x

[121] Giansily-Blaizot M, Cunat S, Moulis G, Schved JF, Aguilar-Martinez P. Homozygous mutation of the 5'UTR region of the L-Ferritin gene in the hereditary hyperferritinemia cataract syndrome and its impact on the phenotype. Haematologica. 2013;**98**(4):e42-e43. DOI: 10.3324/haematol.2012.077198

[122] Levi S, Rovida E. Neuroferritinopathy: From ferritin structure modification to pathogenetic mechanism. Neurobiology of Disease. 2015;**81**:134-143. DOI: 10.1016 /j.nbd.2015.02.007

[123] Curtis AR, Fey C, Morris CM, Bindoff LA, Ince PG, Chinnery PF, et al. Mutation in the gene encoding ferritin light polypeptide causes dominant adult-onset basal ganglia disease. Nature Genetics. 2001;**28**(4):350-354. DOI: 10.1038/ng571

[124] Ayton S, Lei P, Adlard PA, Volitakis I, Cherny RA, Bush AI, Finkelstein DI. Iron accumulation confers neurotoxicity to a vulnerable population of nigral neurons: Implications for Parkinson's disease. Molecular Neurodegeneration. 2014;**9**:27. DOI: 10.1186 /1750-1326-9-27

[125] Heeney MM, Finberg KE. Iron-refractory iron deficiency anemia (IRIDA). Hematology/ Oncology Clinics of North America. 2014;**28**(4):637-652. DOI: 10.1016/j.hoc.2014.04.009

[126] Lehmberg K, Grosse R, Muckenthaler MU, Altamura S, Nielsen P, Schmid H, et al. Administration of recombinant erythropoietin alone does not improve the phenotype in ironrefractory iron deficiency anemia patients. Annals of Hematology. 2013;**92**(3):387-394. DOI: 10.1007/s00277-012-1618-8

[127] Folgueras AR, de Lara FM, Pendás AM, Garabaya C, Rodríguez F, Astudillo A, et al. Membrane-bound serine protease matriptase-2 (Tmprss6) is an essential regulator of iron homeostasis. Blood. 2008;**112**(6):2539-2545. DOI: 10.1182/blood-2008-04-149773

[128] Sørensen E, Rigas AS, Thørner LW, Burgdorf KS, Pedersen OB, Petersen MS, et al. Genetic factors influencing ferritin levels in 14,126 blood donors: Results from the Danish Blood Donor Study. Transfusion. 2016;**56**(3):622-627. DOI: 10.1111/trf.13397

[129] Cau M, Danjou F, Chessa R, Serrenti M, Addis M, Barella S, et al. The V736A TMPRSS6 polymorphism influences liver iron concentration in nontransfusion-dependent thalassemias. American Journal of Hematology. 2015;**90**(12):225-226. DOI: 10.1002/ajh.24193

[130] De Falco L, Silvestri L, Kannengiesser C, Morán E, Oudin C, Rausa M, et al. Functional and clinical impact of novel TMPRSS6 variants in iron-refractory iron-deficiency anemia patients and genotype-phenotype studies. Human Mutation. 2014;**35**(11):1321-1329. DOI: 10.1002 /humu.22632

[131] Xiong Y, Wu Z, Yang W, Zhao X, Peng G, Tang K, et al. A novel splicing mutation of TMPRSS6 in a Chinese child with iron-refractory iron deficiency anaemia. British Journal of Haematology. 2015;**171**(4):647-649. DOI: 10.1111/bjh.13416

[132] Altamura S, D'Alessio F, Selle B, Muckenthaler MU. A novel TMPRSS6 mutation that prevents protease auto-activation causes IRIDA. Biochemical Journal. 2010;**431**(3):363-371. DOI: 10.1042/BJ20100668

[133] Yilmaz-Keskin E, Sal E, de Falco L, Bruno M, Iolascon A, Koçak U, Yenicesu I. Is the acronym IRIDA acceptable for slow responders to iron in the presence of TMPRSS6 mutations? The Turkish Journal of Pediatrics. 2013;**55**(5):479-484

[134] Poggiali E, Andreozzi F, Nava I, Consonni D, Graziadei G, Cappellini MD. The role of TMPRSS6 polymorphisms in iron deficiency anemia partially responsive to oral iron treatment. American Journal of Hematology. 2015;**90**(4):306-309. DOI: 10.1002/ajh.23929

[135] Rombout-Sestrienkova E, van Kraaij MG, Koek GH. How we manage patients with hereditary haemochromatosis. British Journal of Haematology. 2016;**175**(5):759-770. DOI: 10.1111 /bjh.14376

[136] Blanchette NL, Manz DH, Torti FM, Torti SV. Modulation of hepcidin to treat iron deregulation: Potential clinical applications. Expert Review of Hematology. 2016;**9**(2):169-186. DOI: 10.1586/17474086.2016.1124757

[137] Ramos E, Ruchala P, Goodnough JB, Kautz L, Preza GC, Nemeth E, et al. Minihepcidins prevent iron overload in a hepcidin-deficient mouse model of severe hemochromatosis. Blood. 2012;**120**(18):3829-3836. DOI: 10.1182//blood-2012-07-440743

[138] Casu C, Oikonomidou PR, Chen H, Nandi V, Ginzburg Y, Prasad P, et al. Minihepcidin peptides as disease modifiers in mice affected by β-thalassemia and polycythemia vera. Blood. 2016;**128**(2):265-276. DOI: 10.1182/blood-2015-10-676742

[139] Chua K, Fung E, Micewicz ED, Ganz T, Nemeth E, Ruchala P. Small cyclic agonists of iron regulatory hormone hepcidin. Bioorganic & Medicinal Chemistry Letters. 2015;**25**(21):4961-4969. DOI: 10.1016/j.bmcl.2015.03.012

[140] Fung E, Chua K, Ganz T, Nemeth E, Ruchala P. Thiol-derivatized minihepcidins retain biological activity. Bioorganic & Medicinal Chemistry Letters. 2015;**25**(4):763-766. DOI: 10.1016 /j.bmcl.2014.12.094

[141] Silvestri L. Inhibiting the hepcidin inhibitor for treatment of iron overload. Blood. 2013;**121**(7):1068-1069. DOI: 10.1182/blood-2012-12-472597

[142] Schmidt PJ, Toudjarska I, Sendamarai AK, Racie T, Milstein S, Bettencourt BR, et al. An RNAi therapeutic targeting Tmprss6 decreases iron overload in Hfe(−/−) mice and ameliorates anemia and iron overload in murine β-thalassemia intermedia. Blood. 2013;**121(**7):1200-1208. DOI: 10.1182/blood-2012-09-453977

[143] Schmidt PJ, Racie T, Westerman M, Fitzgerald K, Butler JS, Fleming MD. Combination therapy with a Tmprss6 RNAi-therapeutic and the oral iron chelator deferiprone additively diminishes secondary iron overload in a mouse model of β-thalassemia intermedia. American Journal of Hematology. 2015;**90**(4):310-313. DOI: 10.1002/ajh.23934

[144] Corradini E, Schmidt PJ, Meynard D, Garuti C, Montosi G, Chen S, et al. BMP6 treatment compensates for the molecular defect and ameliorates hemochromatosis in Hfe knockout mice. Gastroenterology. 2010;**139**(5):1721-1729. DOI: 10.1053 /j.gastro.2010.07.044

[145] Hashizume M, Uchiyama Y, Horai N, Tomosugi N, Mihara M. Tocilizumab, a humanized anti-interleukin-6 receptor antibody, improved anemia in monkey arthritis by suppressing IL-6-induced hepcidin production. Rheumatology International. 2010;**30**(7):917-923. DOI: 10.1007/s00296-009-1075-4

[146] Isaacs JD, Harari O, Kobold U, Lee JS, Bernasconi C. Effect of tocilizumab on haematological markers implicates interleukin-6 signalling in the anaemia of rheumatoid arthritis. Arthritis Research & Therapy. 2013;**15**(6):204

[147] Song SN, Iwahashi M, Tomosugi N, Uno K, Yamana J, Yamana S, et al. Comparative evaluation of the effects of treatment with tocilizumab and TNF-α inhibitors on serum hepcidin, anemia response and disease activity in rheumatoid arthritis patients. Arthritis Research & Therapy. 2013;**15**(5):R141. DOI: 10.1186/ar4323

[148] Casper C, Chaturvedi S, Munshi N, Wong R, Qi M, Schaffer M, et al. Analysis of inflammatory and Anemia-Related biomarkers in a randomized, Double-Blind, Placebo-Controlled study of siltuximab (Anti-IL6 Monoclonal Antibody) in patients with multicentric castleman disease. Clinical Cancer Research. 2015;**21**(19):4294-4304. DOI: 10.1158/1078-0432.CCR-15-0134

[149] Fatih N, Camberlein E, Island ML, Corlu A, Abgueguen E, Détivaud L, et al. Natural and synthetic STAT3 inhibitors reduce hepcidina expression in differentiated mouse hepatocytes expressing the active phosphorylated STAT3 form. Journal of Molecular Medicine. 2010;**88**(5):477-486. DOI: 10.1007/s00109-009-0588-3

[150] Zhang SP, Wang Z, Wang LX, Liu SJ. AG490: An inhibitor of hepcidin expression in vivo. World Journal of Gastroenterology. 2011;**17**(45):5032-5034. DOI: 10.3748/wjg.v17.i45.5032

[151] Schwoebel F, van Eijk LT, Zboralski D, Sell S, Buchner K, Maasch C, et al. The effects of the anti-hepcidin Spiegelmer NOX-H94 on inflammation-induced anemia in cynomolgus monkeys. Blood. 2013;**121**(12):2311-2315. DOI: 10.1182 /blood-2012-09-456756

[152] Van Eijk LT, John AS, Schwoebel F, Summo L, Vauléon S, Zöllner S, et al. Effect of the antihepcidin Spiegelmer lexaptepid on inflammation-induced decrease in serum iron in humans. Blood. 2014;**124**(17):2643-2646. DOI: 10.1182/blood-2014-03-559484

[153] Vater A, Klussmann S. Turning mirror-image oligonucleotides into drugs: Theevolution of Spiegelmer(®) therapeutics. Drug Discovery Today. 2015;**20**(1):147-155. DOI: 10.1016/j.drudis.2014.09.004

[154] Boyce M, Warrington S, Cortezi B, Zöllner S, Vauléon S, Swinkels DW, et al. Safety, pharmacokinetics and pharmacodynamics of the anti-hepcidin Spiegelmer lexaptepid pegol in healthy subjects. British Journal of Pharmacology. 2016;**173**(10):1580-1588. DOI: 10.1111/bph.13433

[155] Mayeur C, Kolodziej SA, Wang A, Xu X, Lee A, Yu PB, et al. Oral administration of a bone morphogenetic protein type I receptor inhibitor prevents the development of anemia of inflammation. Haematologica. 2015;**100**(2):e68-e71. DOI: 10.3324 /haematol.2014.111484

[156] Sun CC, Vaja V, Chen S, Theurl I, Stepanek A, Brown DE, et al. A hepcidin lowering agent mobilizes iron for incorporation into red blood cells in an adenine-induced kidney disease model of anemia in rats. Nephrology Dialysis Transplantation. 2013;**28**(7):1733-1743. DOI: 10.1093/ndt/gfs584

[157] Theurl M, Nairz M, Schroll A, Sonnweber T, Asshoff M, Haschka D, et al. Hepcidin as a predictive factor and therapeutic target in erythropoiesis-stimulating agent treatment for anemia of chronic disease in rats. Haematologica. 2014;**99**(9):1516-1524. DOI: 10.3324 /haematol.2013.099481

[158] Steinbicker AU, Bartnikas TB, Lohmeyer LK, Leyton P, Mayeur C, Kao SM, et al. Perturbation of hepcidin expression by BMP type I receptor deletion induces iron overload in mice. Blood. 2011;**118**(15):4224-4230. DOI: 10.1182/blood-2011-03-339952

[159] Böser P, Seemann D, Liguori MJ, Fan L, Huang L, Hafner M, et al. Anti-repulsive guidance molecule C (RGMc) antibodies increases serum iron in rats and cynomolgus monkeys by hepcidin downregulation. American Association of Pharmaceutical Scientists Journal. 2015;**17**(4):930-938. DOI: 10.1208/s12248-015-9770-4

[160] Tesfay L, Clausen KA, Kim JW, Hegde P, Wang X, Miller LD, et al,. Hepcidin regulation in prostate and its disruption in prostate cancer. Cancer Research. 2015;**75**(11):2254-2263. DOI: 10.1158/0008-5472.CAN-14-2465

[161] Theurl I, Schroll A, Sonnweber T, Nairz M, Theurl M, Willenbacher W, et al. Pharmacologic inhibition of hepcidin expression reverses anemia of chronic inflammation in rats. Blood. 2011;**118**(18):4977-49784. DOI: 10.1182/ blood-2011-03-34506

[162] Fung E, Nemeth E. Manipulation of the hepcidin pathway for therapeutic purposes. Haematologica. 2013;**98**(11):1667-1676. DOI: 10.3324/haematol.2013.084624

[163] Sasu BJ, Cooke KS, Arvedson TL, Plewa C, Ellison AR, Sheng J, et al. Antihepcidin antibody treatment modulates iron metabolism and is effective in a mouse model of inflammation-induced anemia. Blood. 2010;115(**17**):3616-3624. DOI: 10.1182/blood-2009-09-245977

[164] Xiao JJ, Krzyzanski W, Wang YM, Li H, Rose MJ, Ma M, et al. Pharmacokinetics of anti-hepcidin monoclonal antibody Ab 12B9m and hepcidin in cynomolgus monkeys. American Association of Pharmaceutical Scientists Journal. 2010;**12**(4):646-657. DOI:10.1208/s12248-010-9222-0

[165] Cooke KS, Hinkle B, Salimi-Moosavi H, Foltz I, King C, Rathanaswami P, et al. A fully human anti-hepcidin antibody modulates iron metabolism in both mice and nonhuman primates. Blood. 2013;**122**(17):3054-3061. DOI: 10.1182/blood-2013-06-505792

[166] Poli M, Girelli D, Campostrini N, Maccarinelli F, Finazzi D, Luscieti S, et al. Heparin: A potent inhibitor of hepcidin expression in vitro and in vivo. Blood. 2011;**117**(3):997-1004. DOI: 10.1182/blood-2010-06-289082

[167] Poli M, Asperti M, Ruzzenenti P, Mandelli L, Campostrini N, Martini G, et al. Oversulfated heparins with low anticoagulant activity are strong and fast inhibitors of hepcidin expression in vitro and in vivo. Biochemical Pharmacology. 2014;**92**(3):467-475. DOI: 10.1016/j.bcp.2014.09.007

[168] Asperti M, Naggi A, Esposito E, Ruzzenenti P, Di Somma M, Gryzik M, et al. High sulfation and a high molecular weight are important for Anti-hepcidin activity of heparin. Frontiers in Pharmacology. 2016;**6**:316. DOI: 10.3389/fphar.2015.00316

[169] Poli M, Asperti M, Ruzzenenti P, Regoni M, Arosio P. Hepcidin antagonists for potential treatments of disorders with hepcidin excess. Frontiers in Pharmacology. 2014;**5**:86. DOI: 10.3389/fphar.2014.00086

[170] Jiang F, Yu WJ, Wang XH, Tang YT, Guo L, Jiao XY. Regulation of hepcidina through GDF-15 in cancer-related anemia. Clinica Chimica Acta. 2014;**428**:14-19. DOI: 10.1016/j.cca.2013.10.015

[171] Fujiwara T, Ikeda T, Nagasaka Y, Okitsu Y, Katsuoka Y, Fukuhara N, et al. A low-molecular-weight compound K7174 represses hepcidin: Possible therapeutic strategy against anemia of chronic disease. PLoS One. 2013;**8**(9):e75568. DOI: 10.1371 /journal.pone.0075568

[172] Kautz L, Jung G, Valore EV, Rivella S, Nemeth E, Ganz T. Identification of erythroferrone as an erythroid regulator of iron metabolism. Nature Genetics. 2014;**46**(**7**):678-684. DOI: 10.1038/ng.2996

[173] Kautz L, Jung G, Du X, Gabayan V, Chapman J, Nasoff M, et al. Erythroferrone contributes to hepcidin suppression and iron overload in a mouse model of β-thalassemia. Blood. 2015;**126**(**17**):2031-2037. DOI: 10.1182/blood-2015-07-658419

[174] Wittrup A, Lieberman J. Knocking down disease: A progress report on siRNA therapeutics. Nature Reviews Genetics. 2015;**16**(9):543-552. DOI: 10.1038/nrg3978

Section 2

Genetic Polymorphisms in Animal Metabolism

Chapter 12

Genes Involved Litter Size in Olkuska Sheep

Urszula Kaczor

Additional information is available at the end of the chapter

http://dx.doi.org/10.5772/intechopen.69205

Abstract

Major genes increasing litter size were identified in certain sheep breeds. These genes include *BMPR-1B*, *BMP15*, *GDF9* and *B4GALNT2*, *FecX2*. Polish Olkuska sheep is a high-fecundity sheep breed; while some animals might give birth to just one or two lambs, there are Olkuska ewes which have six or even seven lambs/lambing. Fertility of this breed is caused by mutation in the major gene $FecX^{O}$ (*BMP15* gene), but analysis of polymorphism at the locus *GDF9* revealed presence of four polymorphisms: G447A (L159L), A978G (G326G), G994A (V332I) and G1111A (V371M). Substitutions V371 and V332I are missense mutations found in the sequence encoding active GDF9 protein. V371 polymorphism has also an effect on litter size in Olkuska breed ewes. Study of genes associated with litter size in Olkuska sheep is of high importance, as they could be used in breeding programmes as selection markers for increasing production efficiency.

Keywords: fecundity, genes, litter size, Olkuska sheep

1. Introduction

Currently, more than 1200 sheep breeds differing in many production features, including fertility, are known globally. Ewes usually give birth to one or two lambs/litter. However, there are certain highly prolific breeds—such as *inter alia* Cambridge, Thoka, Javanese, Belclare, Lacaune, Woodland, Booroola, Aragonesa, Romney (Inverdale and Hanna), Garole (Bengal), Belle-ile, small-tailed Han, Hu and Kendrapada—whose litter size ranges from three to six lambs. Genetically conditioned differences in number of maturing and ovulating follicles in different breeds of sheep have been researched already since 1980 [1], when an attempt was made to explain the genetic basis for multiple births within a litter in various breeds around the world. It has been shown that sheep fertility depending on breed may be determined either polygenic or by a major segregating gene named the *Fec* gene.

Most mutations increasing ovulation levels and the number of lambs born to an ewe were identified in genes encoding proteins belonging to the family of transforming growth factors TGF-β: BMPR1B (bone morphogenetic protein receptor-1B), BMP15 (bone morphogenetic protein 15) and GDF9 (growth differentiation factor 9). In addition, mutations $FecL^{L}$ in Lacaune breed on chromosome 11 and FecX2W (fecundity gene *X2*) in Woodland sheep were identified. $FecX^{L}$ locus contains two genes *IGF2BP1* (insulin-like growth factor 2 mRNA binding protein1) and *B4GALNT2* (beta-1, 4-N-acetyl-galactosaminyl transferase 2). It has been shown that *B4GALNT2* is responsible for high prolificacy of Lacaune sheep [2]. The mechanism of action of the gene FecX2 on X chromosome in Woodland sheep is not yet exactly understood [3].

1.1. FecB mutation in the bone morphogenetic protein receptor 1B (*BMPR1-B*) gene

Booroola was the first major gene (FecB) significantly influencing level of ovulation and litter size in sheep to be identified [4]. The effect of FecB mutation (Q249R) identified in Booroola Merino breed in the gene of bone morphogenetic protein receptor *BMPR1-B* on chromosome 6 is an increase in ovulation level and litter size in carriers of one or two copies of the gene FecB. This mutation was also identified in Asian breeds: Garole, Javanese, thin-tail Hu and Han. With regard to level of ovulation, the observed increase is additive in nature, while as concerns litter size—it is partly dominant. In ewes with heterozygous $FecB^{B+}$ ovulation level increased by 1.3 CL (corpus luteum), while in ewes with $FecB^{BB}$, the observed increase was up to 3.6 CL. The effect on litter size between homozygous++ and BB was +0.8 [6].

Many authors have shown high fertility of carriers of $FecB^{B+}$ genotype, among others in Garole-223% lamb production [6], Hu-210%, Han-240% [7] and Javanese breeds-259% [8]. Research results in Indian sheep of Muzaffarnagari breed engendered some discussion, as presence of ewes with FecB gene that still had single births was proven, and share of sheep with genotypes $FecB^{BB}$and $FecB^{B+}$ was identified as 3.47 and 41.73%, respectively [9].

In antral follicles of $FecB^{B+}$ ewes, a decrease in granulosa cell proliferation and premature expression of LH receptors were observed [10]. Appearance of FecB mutation in sheep compared with ewes devoid of mutation is associated with higher number of growing small cavitary (antral) follicles on the ovaries. Both total number of granulosa cells and total secretion of estradiol and inhibins in the ovaries of $FecB^{BB}$ ewes still remain the same as in ewes with $FecB^{++}$ genotype. Significant impact of gene FecB on development of ovaries during foetal life is also observed, including, *inter alia*, a reduced number of oocytes from the 35th to the 50th day of gestation, a smaller number of class 1 follicles from 75th to 90th day of gestation and class 2 follicles (on 135th day). A small number of class 2 follicles were also observed in early neonatal life of $FecB^{BB}$ sheep [10, 11]. Significant effect of FecB gene on function of the hypothalamic-pituitary system has been proven as well. It has been found that it may lead to increased secretion of follicle-stimulating hormone (FSH) in $FecB^{BB}$ homozygotes, although it has not been confirmed in all of the animals investigated. No FecB influence on release of luteinizing hormone (LH) has been found [12].

1.2. Mutations in the gene of bone morphogenetic protein 15 (*BMP15*)

1.2.1. Protein BMP15

BMP15 protein together with growth factor 9 (GDF9) plays an important role in folliculogenesis [13, 14]. Its paracrine action affects granulosa cells, theca cells and the oocyte itself [15]. *In vitro* cultures indicate that recombinant protein BMP15 is a potent stimulator of granulosa cell proliferation, suggesting that both cell growth and their subsequent division and differentiation require BMP15 action [16]. The protein inhibits expression of FSH and LH receptors, as decrease in activity of BMP15 increases cell sensitivity to action of gonadotropins [17]. The conducted experiments showed that BMP15 inhibits expression of StAR protein, responsible for transport of cholesterol—specifically low density lipoprotein (LDL)—into cells. LDL is the substrate for production of steroid hormones. In rats, BMP may modulate the process of steroidogenesis in granulosa cells, modifies biological effects of FSH by inhibition of progesterone-induced FSH secretion, without affecting production of estradiol [16]. BMP15 mRNA transcripts are observed from the primary follicle stage, in secondary, tertiary and dominant follicles stages, ending with atretic antral follicles [18]. In sheep, BMP15 affects proliferation rate and inhibits baseline and FSH-mediated secretion of progesterone by granulosa cells of small antral follicles [11]. Presence of BMP15 mRNA was determined in the oocytes (class 1, 2, 3, 4 and 5 follicles), but it has not been demonstrated in granulosa cells and follicle theca [19].

1.2.2. Polymorphism in the BMP15 gene

In mammals, formation of BMP15 protein is determined by action of a single gene on chromosome X [20]. An encoded sequence with a length of 1179 bp is contained in two exons separated by an intron of 5400 bp in length. mRNA translation produces a peptide built of 393 amino acids, and the resulting mature protein has a length of 125 amino acids [21]. Mutations identified in the *BMP15* locus ($FecX^I$, $FecX^H$, $FecX^L$, $FecX^G$, $FecX^B$ and $FecX^R$) result in appearance of the same phenotype in different sheep breeds, and have different molecular basis. Heterozygous ewes give birth to more lambs, while homozygotes with two copies of a gene are infertile. Action of mutations marked $FecX^O$ and $FecX^{Gr}$ identified in Olkuska and Grivette breeds differs from the above-mentioned, as in the case of ewes with both one and two copies of the gene, an increase in prolificacy is observed (**Table 1**).

Substitution of $FecX^H$ detected in Hanna sheep causes introduction of a stop codon in place of glutamine in position 23 of amino acid residue of mature protein. Transition C>T observed in the case of $FecX^G$ in Galoway and Cambridge breeds, also introduces a premature stop codon in place of glutamine at position 31 of the polypeptide chain. As concerns carriers of these mutations, heterozygotes show increased levels of ovulation, while homozygotes with two copies of the gene are infertile [17].

A similar phenotype is observed for $FecX^I$ mutation, where hydrophobic valine is substituted for asparagine at position 31 of mature protein. This leads to changes in electrostatic potential of the region involved in formation of dimers—this, in turn, interferes with dimerization and

Variant	Base change	Coding base bp	Coding residue*	Amino acids change	Mutation/reference
V299D	T>A	897	299	Val>Asp	*FecX*^{I}/[12]
Q291-	C>T	873	291	Gln>STOP	*FecX*^{H}/[12]
C321Y	G>A	963	321	Cys>Tyr	*FecX*^{L}/[24]
Q239STOP	C>T	718	239	Gln>STOP	*FecX*^{G}/[21]
S367I	G>T	1100	367	Ser>Izo	*FecX*^{B}/[21]
Del	Deletion	525–541	175–180		*FecX*^{R}/[26]
175–180	17 bp				
T317I	C>T	950	317	Thr>Ile	FecX^{Gr}/[27]

*Position of the coding residue in the *Ovis aries* bone morphogenic protein 15; BMP15 protein GenBank accession number AAF81688.1.

Table 1. Mutations identified in sheep at the *BMP-15* gene locus.

consequently leads to the elimination of biological effects of BMP15. Homozygous ewes are infertile due to folliculogenesis being arrested at initial stage of the process [10].

FecX^{B} mutation found in *BMP15* gene locus in Belclare sheep is a result of polar serine being substituted for non-polar isoleucine at position 99. This substitution has a significant impact on the ability of a protein to bind to type II membrane receptor; it determines the structure of the ligand-receptor complex with BMP2, BMP7, activin A proteins. This polymorphism abolishes biological activity of BMP15, most likely by prejudicing the binding of protein and receptor [21]. Homozygous ewes are infertile due to hypoplasia of ovaries. Admittedly, presence of antral follicles was observed, but with oocytes of anomalous size, surrounded by a single layer of abnormal granulosa cells. Morphology of ovaries of such sheep is similar to image of ovaries of FecX^{I} Inverdale ewes.

One copy of the allele FecX^{I} (Inverdale) or FecX^{H} (Hanna) results in ovulation level increase of +0.8–1.0 CL, significantly affecting size of the litter by +0.6 lamb. Homozygous FecX^{II} and FecX^{HH} Hanna ewes are sterile; in their small and poorly developed ovaries, follicles are provided with a single layer of granulosa cells [22]. In FecX^{I+} sheep, follicles were determined to be of a smaller diameter than those produced in ovaries of homozygotes devoid of mutation. However, FecX^{I+} ewes present a greater number of mature preovulatory dominant follicles of smaller diameter, and therefore do not differ in the level of estradiol and inhibin from non-mutated ones [23]. Preovulatory follicles are also characterized by early maturation, which determines greater secretion of FSH and early formation of LH receptors [12].

Studies by Bodin et al. [24] on prolific sheep of Lacaune breed showed presence of FecX^{L} mutation, leading to substitution of cysteine for tyrosine at position 53 of the BMP15 chain. Just as observed in the case of polymorphisms (FecX^{I}, FecX^{H}, FecX^{G} and FecX^{B}), also this change in gene structure causes increased level of ovulation in heterozygous ewes and infertility in homozygotes. *In vitro* studies revealed that the mutation FecX^{L} is responsible for defective secretion of both precursors and active forms of BMP15. It is believed that this may be caused by damage to structure of one of the disulphide bonds whose formation involves cysteine, and that play an important role in stabilizing the structure of BMP15 [24]. In the case of presence of one copy of $FecX^L$ in ewes, ovulation level increase of +1.9–2.17 CL is observed [2, 25].

Lacaune sheep are, next to Hanna, Inverdale, Cambridge, Belclare and small-tail Han breeds, an example where increase in litter size is determined by the presence of two major genes: $FecX^L$ and FecL on autosomal chromosome 11 [2].

In Aragonesa $FecX^R$ ewes, a 17 bp deletion results in a frameshift and appearance of a stop codon, even before the coding region of mature protein. The consequence of this mutation is an 85% modification in the propeptide sequence, specifically limitation of its size to 45 amino acids out of 245 present in the original propeptide. Heterozygous ewes are very highly fecund, while the presence of two copies of the mutated gene leads to a blockage of follicular development at initial growth state and female infertility. $FecX^{R+}$ ewes have an average of 2.66 lamb/litter compared to flock average of 1.36. Presence of one copy of the gene resulted in litter size increase of +1.3 lamb [26].

A mutation in the gene *BMP15* changing the amino acid sequence in the amino acid chain p.T317I was identified in French Grivette sheep. Ewes of $FecX^{GrGr}$ genotype have 2.5 lamb/litter, while $FecX^{++}$ and $FecX^{Gr+}$give birth to 1.83 and 1.93 lamb in a litter, respectively. Sterilization of homozygotes with the $FecX^{GrGr}$ mutation has not been identified in the studied population [27].

Recent research in phenomenon of high fertility of ewes of the African breed Barbarine (167% annual lamb crop) showed presence of another substitution in the gene encoding *BMP15*, resulting in A119T mutation in the coding sequence of mature protein. Frequency of the mutated allele in the population of these sheep, or its impact of prolificacy are unknown [28].

1.2.3. Mutations in the growth differentiation factor 9 (GDF9) gene

1.2.3.1. Protein GDF9

Growth differentiation factor 9 (GDF9) is another protein belonging to TGF-β family. This peptide regulates development of ovarian follicles in rodents and ruminants (sheep), as well as humans [12, 29]. It has been shown that its synthesis, similarly as in the case of BMP15, occurs in the oocyte [30]. Mice lacking functional protein GDF9 (GDF9KO) were infertile, their follicle growth was arrested at primary follicle stage, with granulosa cells layer not properly formed, and changes in the zona pellucida. Oocytes were excessively enlarged and surrounded by a single layer of deformed granulosa cells, or oocyte was not observed in the follicle whatsoever [30, 31]. Growth differentiation factor 9 as a multi-functional protein is responsible for follicular growth from its early stage—it initiates and regulates folliculogenesis and oocyte development. It has autocrine effects on oocytes, plays a role in their development and maturation, and paracrine effects on somatic cells, inhibits expression of luteinizing hormone receptor gene and stimulating synthesis of hyaluronic acid [32, 33]. *GDF9* gene expression in sheep occurs in oocytes, with the presence of the transcript and protein demonstrated in the oocyte during formation of the follicle, in class 1 primary follicles as well as in follicles in the phase of intensive growth. *In vitro* experiments demonstrated that GDF9 is also found in degraded oocytes and in malformed follicular structures [34, 35]. In humans, GDF9 plays an important role in pathogenesis of polycystic ovary syndrome and premature ovarian failure [36].

1.2.3.2. Polymorphism in the GDF9 gene

The gene encoding protein GDF9 was found to be located in sheep on chromosome 5 [37]. The gene consists of two exons, with length of 397 and 968 bp, respectively. Its total length is 5644 bp, with coding sequence comprised of 1359 nucleotides [35].

A number of mutations (**Table 2**) were identified in gene *GDF9*; it was determined that the mutation FecG^H (G8, Ser1184Phe) causes sterility in homozygous ewes. Impact of the mutations G1 (G260A, R87H), G2 (C471T), G3 (G477A), G4 (G721A, E241K), G5 (A978G), G6 (G994A, V332I) and G7 (G1111A, V371M) on fertility of sheep had not been initially analysed, but fertile homozygous animals with G1, G4 and G7 mutations were found [21, 30]. Effects of FecG^H mutation are due to lack of active form of the protein, leading to arrest of follicular growth in the early stages of development [38, 39] (**Table 2**).

Mutation FecG^H (G8) occurs within the sequence responsible for coupling a protein to the receptor and is a missense mutation. As a result, synthesized protein exhibits less affinity for the cell surface receptor. Ewes with one copy of the gene with FecG^H mutation have higher ovulation level. Early maturation of small secondary follicles, inhibition of their growth and earlier ovulation of a larger number of oocytes were noted [21]. Most likely, early maturation of the developing follicles is associated with inhibition of FSH receptor expression at mRNA level due to the absence of biologically active GDF9 [19]. The fact that the FecG^H mutation

Variant	Base change	Coding base bp	Coding residue*	Amino acids change	Mutation/reference
A87H	G>A	260	87	Ala>His	G1/[21]
V157V	C>T	471	157	Val>Val	G2/[21]
L159L	G>A	477	159	Leu>Leu	G3/[21]
Q241L	G>A	721	241	Gln>Leu	G4/[21]
Q326Q	A>G	978	326	Gln>Gln	G5/[21]
V332I	G>A	994	332	Val>Ile	G6/[21]
V371M	G>A	1111	371	Val>Met	G7/[21]
S395F	C>T	1184	395	Ser>Phe	G8 (*FecG^H*)/[21]
F345C	T>G	1034	345	*Phe>Cys*	*FecG^E*/[41]
S109R	A>C	1279	109	*Ser>Arg*	*FecG^T*/[40]

*Position of the coding residue in the *Ovis aries* growth differentiation factor 9; GDF9 protein GenBank accession number AAC28089.2.

Table 2. Mutations identified in sheep at the *GDF9* gene locus.

determines the decrease in quantity of active form of GDF9 was confirmed by immunization of ewes, which caused increase in ovulation level [30]. Presence of $FecG^{H}$ resulted in increased litter size in Belclare sheep, from 1.98 in animals lacking the mutation to 2.67 lamb/litter in heterozygotes; for Cambridge sheep, the litter size surged from 2.27 to 4.28 lamb/litter.

Phenotypic effect similar to $FecG^{H}$ was observed for $FecG^{T}$ mutation in Icelandic Thoka sheep breed [40].

The results of research conducted on Brazilian Santa Ines breed indicate that presence of a mutation called $FecG^{E}$ (Embrapa) in *GDF9* gene has a completely different phenotypic effect than the mutations in the locus of this gene listed above, because ewes with identified two copies of the gene are prolific [41].

2. Genes determining litter size in Olkuska sheep

2.1. Mutations in the *BMP15* gene

Analysing reasons behind high fertility of the prolific Olkuska sheep breed, neither $FecX^{I}$ mutation in *BMP15* gene nor $FecB^{B}$ mutation in gene *BMPR-1B* was identified [42]. However, a number of new mutations were detected in the *BMP15* gene locus: A77A, L110L, P101, V135G [27] and N237K and N337H, defined as $FecX^{O}$ (synonyms: N69H or A1009C or p.Asn69His) (**Table 3**) [27, 43].

Substitution of N237K was identified outside the coding region of mature peptide in most studied ewes, and no connection with their fertility was demonstrated. $FecX^{O}$ was located in exon 2, in the coding sequence of mature protein (position 69 aa), right next to the sites of the mutations $FecX^{I}$, $FecX^{H}$, $FecX^{L}$ and $FecX^{B}$ found, respectively, at positions 39, 23, 53 and 99 aa of mature protein.

Two alleles (A and C) and three genotypes (AA, AC and CC) were found for the A1009C mutation identified in the sequence encoding BMP15 mature protein. The C allele (with

Variant	Base change	Coding base (bp)	Coding residue (bp)	Amino acid change	Reference
A77A	T>G	231	77	Ala>Ala	[27]
P101A	G>C	301	101	Pro>Ala	[27]
L110L	C>T	330	110	Leu>leu	[27]
V135G	T>G	404	135	Val>Gly	[27]
$FecX^{O}$	**A>C**	**1009**	**337**	**Asn>His**	[27]
N337H					[43]
N237K	A>T	711	237	Asn>Lys	[43]

Table 3. Mutations identified in **Olkuska sheep** in the *BMP15* gene.

N337H mutation) had a frequency of 0.55 and ewes with one (AC) and two (CC) copies of the gene constituted 56 (AC) and 27% (CC) of the animals, respectively [43].

2.1.1. *Effects of N337H mutation on litter size of Olkuska sheep*

Analysis of effects of mutation N337H on litter size of ewes showed a significant impact of polymorphism on prolificacy, which in sheep of genotype $FecX^{++}$ was 1.74 ± 0.55 lamb/litter, with 2.47 ± 0.77 and 2.98 ± 1.50 lamb/litter for $FecX^{+O}$ and $FecX^{OO}$ genotypes, respectively [43]. Very similar results showed Demars et al. [27] for genotypes $FecX^{++}$, $FecX^{+O}$ and $FecX^{OO}$ namely, 1.84, 2.46 and 3.05, respectively.

Changes in litter size in subsequent lambings of Olkuska ewes show an increase in fecundity correlated with increasing age of a mother. The maximum size of litter in $FecX^{OO}$ ewes was noted in their third lambing, with ewes giving birth to an average of 3 lambs/litter. However, for mothers with genotype $FecX^{++}$, litter size continued to increase up to their fourth lambing, when the litter size reached 2.25 lambs [43]. Increase in the number of lambs in the first three consecutive lambings, and then subsequent decrease in litter size has been demonstrated in studies on other highly prolific sheep breeds. Liu et al. [44] showed that average litter size for $FecB^{BB}$ homozygotes in small-tail Han sheep was 2.47 in the first lambing of an ewe, and 3.17 for older mothers. Increase in litter size as ewes were aging was also observed in Chinese Hu breed. Carriers of *FecB* gene bore an average of 1.92 lamb/litter in their first lambing, compared to 2.56 lamb in the third lambing [45]. The number of lambs in a litter was also positively affected by the number of prior lambings, an ewe has undergone in hybrids Garole × Marpura; heterozygous mothers gave birth into 1.51 ± 0.06, 1.55 ± 0.07, 1.70 ± 0.09 lamb/litter in their first, second and third lambing, respectively [46].

2.1.2. *Litter size in Olkuska sheep population*

In all herds of sheep breeds with a segregating major gene, distribution of litter size similar to the one determined in Olkuska sheep, that is, with high proportion of twin births and large share of triplets and larger litters, was determined. Distribution analysis of litters of Olkuska ewes showed that 29% of $FecX^{OO}$ mothers gave birth to four or more lambs in a litter, including sextuplets and septuplets. In the most numerous group of $FecX^{+O}$ ewes, only 14% of animals showed similar litter size, and among sheep of genotype $FecX^{++}$ no litters of such size were observed (**Table 4**).

In the case of $FecX^{++}$, the proportion of triplets was also only 11.2% [43]. A much smaller share of quadruplet and lager litters was found in Javanese $FecB^{BB}$ ewes (16%) [8]. The most common litter sizes in Garole $FecB^{B+}$ sheep were twins, single births and triplets; accounting for, respectively, 65, 21 and 5% of the total [47]. In turn, share of quadruplet and triplet litters in $FecB^{BB}$ ewes of Javanese breed was, 34 and 20%, respectively, with an average litter size of 2.5 lamb/litter [48]. Interestingly, in the flock of Olkuska sheep, for mothers with genotypes $FecX^{OO}$ and $FecX^{+O}$ singleton births were twice less frequent than for $FecX^{++}$ ewes (16 vs. 33%). Share of twin births decreased along with appearance of additional alleles with the mutation; among $FecX^{++}$ewes they accounted for 55% of litters, and for genotype $FecX^{OO}$

Gene/genotype	Litter size of ewes (lambs)				
	1	2	3	4	5, 6, 7
BMP15 **gene-N337H (%)**					
FecX^{++} (AA)	37	51.8	11.2		
FecX^{+O} (AC)	15.6	40.8	29.8	8.3	5.2
FecX^{OO} (CC)	18.6	23.9	28.3	9.7	19.4
GDF9 **gene-V371M (%)**					
GG	20.8	40.6	26.8	6.6	5.2
GA	8.3	20	28.3	15	33.2
GDF9 **gene-V332I (%)**					
GG	17.4	39	28.9	7	7.3
GA	25.7	37	21.9	9	6.7

Table 4. Percentage of litter types of ewes with N337H (*BMP15* gene) and V371M, V332I (*GDF9* gene) mutations.

only for 27%. In the population of Olkuska sheep with average annual lamb production of 218%, the distribution of litters of various sizes was: 21.7% of singletons, 41% of twins, 24.6% of triplets and 12.7% of quadruplets and larger. Thus, the share of litters larger than triplet is as high as 37.1%. In Garole sheep, characterized by slightly lower prolificacy (168–187%), the proportion of mothers with twins, triplets and quadruplets was 65, 21 and 5%, respectively [6]. Similar differences in distribution of litter size were observed in a herd of Chevoit-Thoka sheep [49]. With an average litter size of 2.23 lamb/litter, the authors found similar share of twin litters (56.5%) in this population, but noted a much smaller share of births with quadruplet and larger litters (3.1%). High frequency of twin births, reaching 47% of the studied population, was demonstrated in Thoka-Chevoit sheep; this breed was also characterized by a high share of singleton births (35%) [50]. A much smaller share of multiple births in comparison with data collected for Olkuska sheep was demonstrated in Aragonese breed with 120–150% fecundity: 66.4% of singleton litters, 28.4% of twin ones, but only 1.9% of triplets. It should be noted that among more than 2000 ewes studied, only three gave birth to quadruplets and only one to quintuplets. For sheep lacking the FecX^R mutation, only singleton births were noted [26].

2.1.3. *Effect of mutation N337H on litter size*

In studies on effects of mutation N337H (FecX^O) on litter size, it was shown that the effect on ovulation levels in O+ and OO ewes was an increase of +2 and +3.3 CL [27]. Effect of the O+ copy of the gene was measured at +0.73 lamb, with the effect of two copies of the gene estimated at +1.07 lamb/litter. Analysing litter size over three first lambings of an ewe, the effect on O+ ewes was +0.62 lamb/litter, and +1.07 lamb for the OO genotype (**Table 5**) [43].

Litter size of ewes	Genotype *BMP15* (N337H)			Mutation effect [43]
	AA	CA	CC	
Reproductive life span	1.74	2.47	2.98	O+: +0.73
				OO: +0.34
Lambings: I–III	1.74	2.36	2.81	O+: 0.62
				OO: +0.45
I	1.76	2.36	2.51	O+: +0.60
				OO: +0.15

Table 5. Estimated mutation effect for number of lambs born to ewes.

Comparative analysis carried out on the basis of studies by many authors between litter size for carriers of one copy of the gene versus wild sheep genotypes for populations with a major segregating gene revealed that the data vary depending on breed, age and environment. In the presence of one copy of the gene ($FecB^{B+}$), effect varies from +0.48 in Booroola × Dorset hybrids in Australia [5] to +1.16 lamb/litter for offspring of Booroola × Romney and Booroola × Perendale hybrids in New Zealand [51]. Ewes with two copies of the gene had litters larger by +0.64 lamb for the Israeli Affec × Awassi hybrids, +1.61 for Chinese Merino meat strain [52, 53]. Garole × Malpura ewes of genotypes $FecB^{B+}$ and $FecB^{BB}$ gave birth to, on average, 1.73 and 2.17 lamb, respectively, while litter size of $FecB^{++}$ sheep was 1.03 lamb. Litter size for $FecB^{B+}$ and $FecB^{BB}$ ewes compared to sheep of $FecB^{++}$ genotype was higher by +0.70 and +1.14, respectively. The effect of one copy of the gene was increasing in consecutive lambings, from +0.52 in the first lambing to +1.03 in the ewes' third lambing [46, 54].

2.2. Mutations in the gene *GDF9*

Identification of variations in the gene sequence of *GDF9* revealed presence of point mutations G3, G5, G6 and G7—detected in 2004 in Belclare and Cambridge sheep by a team led by Hanrahan et al. [21]—also in Olkuska sheep (**Table 6**).

Presence of $FecG^{H}$ (G8) mutation was excluded [43]. Thus, the Polish Olkuska breed can be classified as one of the few breeds in the world, where presence of polymorphisms has been confirmed both in the gene *BMP15* and the autosomal gene. Next to the N337H mutation in *BMP15* gene, missense mutations V371M (G7) and V332I (G6) have been identified in the region encoding mature protein GDF9. It should be noted that in Olkuska sheep, the allele with mutation V371M occurs with very low frequency of 0.06, but GA heterozygotes demonstrate high annual lamb production of 346%, with the same for GG ewes at 236% (**Table 7**) [43].

Analysis of litter size distribution in sheep with GG and GA genotypes in the locus V371M (G7) revealed that the most frequently occurring litter size in GG ewes was twins (40.6%), followed by singletons (20.8%). Litters of quadruplets and larger accounted for 11.8% of all births. Among mothers with identified one allele with the GA mutation, the share of twin

Mutation	Base change	Coding base (bp)	Coding residue (bp)	Amino acid change (aa)	Reference
G3	G→A	477	159	Leu>Leu	[43]
G5	A→G	978	326	Gly>Gly	[43]
G6	G→A	994	332	Val>Ile	[43]
G7	G→A	1111	371	Val>Met	[43]

Table 6. Mutations identified in Olkuska sheep in the *GDF9* gene.

Variant	Allele		Genotype	
	G	A	GG	AG
V371M	0.94	0.06	0.89	0.11
V332I	0.83	0.17	0.69	0.29

Table 7. Allele and genotype frequencies in the population of Olkuska sheep, (mutations V371M, V332I) in *GDF-9 gene.*

litters was twice smaller (20%), while litters with four and more lambs accounted for almost 50%. The share of single births was only 8.3% [43].

Also mutation V332I (G6) was found to be present in Olkuska sheep; with two alleles (G and A) and three genotypes (GG, AG and AA) found (**Table 7**).

The G allele appeared with a very high frequency of 0.84, and ewes of genotype GG accounted for 70% of all animals. Mothers with the GG genotype did not differ in average litter size from GA sheep, both over total duration of their productive life (2.24 ± 0.87 vs. 2.13 ± 0.91 lamb), and in the first three lambings (2.39 ± 0.90 vs. 2.30 ± 0.87) [43].

2.2.1. *Effect of mutation V371M (G7) on litter size*

Ewes with one allele with V371M substitution showed an increase in litter size of +0.55 lamb, while those with the V332I mutation showed a decrease of 0.18 lamb/litter [43]. Thus, only in the presence of the A allele, the mutation V371M resulted in an increase in litter size. Mutations described earlier by Hanrahan et al. [21], namely: G3, G4, G5 and G6 were also detected in the case of Olkuska breed. However, impact of these mutations on prolificacy of ewes has not been studied.

In ewes of the Brazilian breed Santa Ines, a mutation that does not cause infertility has been identified in gene *GDF9*. Melo et al. [55] and Silva et al. [41] identified substitution F345C ($FecG^{E}$) to a significant degree determining fecundity of sheep. Alleles $FecG^{+}$ and $FecG^{E}$of frequencies 0.48 and 0.52, and genotypes $FecG^{++}$, $FecG^{+E}$ and $FecG^{EE}$ with frequencies 0.17, 0.61 and 0.22, respectively, have been identified. Association between the genotype and level of ovulation and litter size has been confirmed. $FecG^{EE}$ ewes bore an average of 1.78 lambs/litter, $FecG^{+E}$ sheep 1.44 and $FecG^{++}$ mothers 1.13 lambs/litter. Level of ovulation in $FecG^{EE}$ ewes (2.22 ± 0.12) was 82% higher than that observed for the $FecG^{++}$ genotype. No statistically significant difference was identified between $FecG^{+E}$ heterozygotes and $FecG^{++}$ ewes (1.34 ± 0.08 vs. 1.22 ± 0.11). As concerns litter size distribution, share of twin litters for ewes with the identified three genotypes was 44 and 12% for $FecG^{EE}$ and $FecG^{+E}$ ewes, respectively, while no twin litters were noted for $FecG^{++}$ sheep [41].

Presence of the mutation G1 was also confirmed in Iranian Moghani and Ghezel breeds. Presence of three possible genotypes was identified, and all the ewes were fertile. Infertility was found in only one sheep, carrying also an additional copy of the gene $FecX^{G}$ in gene *BMP15*. Ewes with heterozygous genotype were more prolific compared to those with wild sheep genotype. Share of twin litters was small (6.3%) also among animals with the wild sheep genotype, while among heterozygotes twin births amounted to as much as 53.8%. Four homozygotic mothers with two copies of the gene G1 were fertile, but gave birth to singletons [56]. Mutation G1 was als identified in Indian Garole sheep, and frequency of the wild allele and of that carrying G1 mutation was, G-0.82 and A-0.18, respectively, with respective genotype frequency of 0.64 for GG and 0.36 for AG ewes [57]. Also in this case, presence of genotype with two copies of the AA gene was not detected. Mutation in the gene *GDF9* was accompanied by the presence of *FecB* gene. In Chinese breeds, similar to the case of Olkuska sheep, several mutations in several different genes have been identified. In addition to gene FecB, also presence of mutations G2 (C471T) [58], and G3 (G477A) was revealed. Entirely new mutations G729T (Q243H) and T692C [59] were identified. The authors, however, found no impact of G3 on the number of lambs bore by ewes. While identifying mutation G729T outside the region coding mature protein, the researchers have found the allele T (0.091) as well as genotypes GG and GT (respective frequency of 0.817 and 0.183). In GT ewes, estimated litter size was 2.88 ± 0.19, while for GG sheep, it was only 2.11 ± 0.11. Effect on litter size was also recorded for the T692C mutation, where litters of CC mothers were larger by 0.63 lamb than litters of CG ewes [59]. In Hu sheep, A154G mutation at position 51 of the amino acid located outside the region coding mature protein GDF9 (Asn51Asp) was identified [60].

3. Effect of N337H and V371M (G7) mutations on litter size

Determining effect of simultaneous presence of N337H (A1009C) and V371M (G7) mutations on fertility of Olkuska breed ewes showed that the largest number of lambs was born to $FecX^{OO}$ mothers that were carriers of V371M mutation (3.32 ± 0.26 lamb/litter) (**Table 8**).

Effect of presence of both the allele N337H and V371M in ewes was similar to how presence of two copies of gene N337H affected the sheep, and amounted to +0.92 lambs/litter [43].

Studies conducted so far on interaction and potential interdependencies between different mutations within the loci of genes encoding transforming growth factors TGF-β have shown that presence of one copy of the gene with a mutation in the locus of *BMP15* led to an increase in litter size; the result was sterilization in the case of homozygous genotype with two copies of the gene. This issue has thus far been researched only within a very narrow range. Presence of several alleles of various genes in the same animal was demonstrated by Hanrahan et al.

Trait	Combined genotype in *BMP15* and *GDF9* loci				
	AA^{BMP-15}/GG^{GDF-9}	CA^{BMP-15}/GG^{GDF-9}	CA^{BMP-15}/GA^{GDF-9}	CC^{BMP-15}/GG^{GDF-9}	CC^{BMP-15}/GA^{GDF-9}
Litter size of ewes (LSM ± SE) (reproductive life span)	1.64 ± 0.11	2.26± 0.08	2.56 ± 0.19	2.64 ± 0.08	3.32 ± 0.26

Table 8. Estimated effect of N337H mutation in the *BMP15* gene and V371M mutation in the *GDF9* gene on number of lambs born to Olkuska ewes (combined genotype) [43].

[21] and Davis et al. [42], sheep carrying a copy of both $FecX^B$ and $FecX^G$or $FecX^H$ and $FecX^I$ were infertile. Sheep carrying one copy of any of the above mutations on chromosome X and the mutation FecB (*BMPR-1B*) had fully functional ovaries and ovulation levels higher than observed when these factors were occurring independently. The effect of simultaneous presence of one copy of FecX in *BMP15* and one copy of $FecG^H$ (*GDF9*) was varied. Most observations showed that the effect of these two genes was additive, but in some cases the demonstrated impact of *GDF9* was weakened when the FecX mutation was present alongside it. Estimated effect on level of ovulation due to the presence of $FecX^G$ in Belclare and Cambridge sheep amounted to 0.77 and 1.18 CL, respectively, while presence of $FecX^B$ in Belclare sheep resulted in 2.38 CL. The effect of carrying one copy of $FecG^H$ in Belclare and Cambridge ewes was much higher, and amounted to 1.79 and 2.35 CL, respectively. Generally, it can be assumed that the average stimulating effect on level of ovulation in case of mutations $FecX^G$, $FecX^B$ and $FecG^H$was 0.70, 0.97 and 1.39 CL, respectively. Simultaneous appearance of different copies of a gene with a mutation in one animal resulted in a much greater increase in the observed number of corpora lutea in the ovaries. In sheep with genotypes $FecG^H/FecX^G$ and $FecG^H/FecX^B$, the number of ovulatory follicles was 5.8 and 6.09, respectively, while for carriers of only one copy of the gene $FecX^G$ it was estimated at 2.69 CL, with 3.26 CL for $FecX^B$ ewes, and 2.67 CL for $FecG^H$ genotype [21]. Presence of $FecX^I$ and FecB genes in ewes resulted in high level of ovulation (4.4 CL), suggesting multiplicative effect of these mutations resulting from interactions between the genes *BMP15* and *BMPR-1B* [20].

4. Effect of N337H, G6 and G7 mutations on body weight

Mutations N337H, G6 and G7 detected in Olkuska sheep have no effect on body weight at 2, 28 and 56 days after birth [43]. These results are consistent with observations conducted for sheep breeds with the major gene FecB, such as hybrids Rambouillet × Booroola [61]. No effect of FecB on body weight at birth and weaning was identified for this population. Also, Kleemann et al. [62] and Abella et al. [63] found no impact of FecB on body weight and daily gains in the initial period of a lamb's life. Visscher et al. [64] identified the weak effect of the gene FecB on initial and final body weight of lambs from 7 to 12 weeks of age in Booroola × Texel hybrids. In contrast to these observations, in nine breeds of Chinese sheep with FecB gene, its significant impact on litter size, body weight and body size has been identified. On day 90 after birth, the body weight of lambs with genotypes $FecB^{BB}$ and $FecB^{B+}$ was higher than those of lambs with the genotype $FecB^{++}$. However, these differences were age dependent and have not been detected with respect to weight measured at 2 and 120 days of age [45]. Gootwine et al. [65] have demonstrated lower body weight in lambs that were carriers of $FecB^{B+}$ gene compared to $FecB^{++}$ lambs that did not carry the mutation. Body weight at birth for lambs with various genotypes, but from the same birth type differed significantly; $FecB^{BB}$ lambs compared to $FecB^{++}$ and $FecB^{B+}$ ones had lower body weight. Comparing weight of Assaf breed sheep with different genotypes, lower body weight was identified in the case of lambs with two copies of the gene FecB [66]. Studies on Garole-Malpura sheep aimed at assessing the impact of FecB genotype on body weight have shown that this gene significantly affects body weight at birth and at 12 months of age, as well as weight gains up to 3 months of life of a lamb. There was no effect on body weight at 3 and 9 months of age [46].

5. G617A polymorphism in inhibin-α gene (*INHA*)

Proteins encoded by the genes *GDF9* and *BMP15*, necessary for an oocyte to gain cytoplasmic maturity, are a group of more than 35 proteins in the transforming growth factor β family. Inhibin A and B is one of these proteins. A missense-type substitution 617G > A—not causing amino acid substitution of proline—was identified in Olkuska sheep in exon 2 of the inhibin-α gene (*INHA*) [43]. The highest frequency was found for allele G (0.86) and genotype GG (0.71), and no ewes with genotype AA were identified. No effects of the mutation on litter size were determined; while the difference between mothers of GG and AG genotypes did indeed amount to +0.3 lamb/litter, it was not statistically significant. The impact of the mutation was dependent on the age of the animals, and for an ewe's first litter was only +0.1 lamb. This result confirms conclusions from other studies, which demonstrated the association among INHA, INHBA and INHBB and litter size of sheep [67]. Influence of variation in the inhibin gene on litter size of Merino and Friesian sheep at the level of, respectively, +0.04 and +0.09 lamb had been demonstrated previously [68]. The effect of *Taq*I/*INHA* polymorphism on the number of offspring has also been confirmed for Merino, East-Friesian and Romanowska breeds [69]. After comparing frequency of allele A in sheep with varying prolificacy, the above authors found that with increasing fertility, an increase in the frequency of allele A could be observed as well. *Ovis ammon* and *Ovis vignei* presented only allele B, while high frequency of allele A (0.65) has been determined in romanowska sheep. Studies in fecund small-tail Han and Hu breeds, as well as in low fecundity breeds Dorset, Texel and German Mountain Merino showed presence of polymorphism in the locus of inhibin βB A276G, in the untranslated region 3'-UTR, only in Hu sheep. Presence of genotypes AA, AB and BB with respective frequencies of 0.636, 0.046 and 0.318, as well as alleles A (0.659) and B (0.341), has been identified. Evaluation of genotype influence on litter size of Hu ewes showed that sheep with genotype BB gave birth to +0.58 lambs more than sheep with AA genotype [59].

6. Conclusions

To summarize, Olkuska sheep are among the few breeds with significant polymorphisms in genes coding proteins of the TDF-beta family. Fecundity of this breed is determined not only by the presence of major gene FecXO (N337H,1009 > C) in *BMP15* locus, but also by the presence of a missense mutation V371M (1111G>A) in the gene locus of *GDF9*. Considerable polymorphism in *GDF9* locus —where three other, low-frequency mutations G3, G5 and G6 can be found—is particularly noteworthy. Ewes of Olkuska breed are highly prolific, both in the case of carriers as well as $FecX^{OO}$ animals, in contrast to sterilization observed in the majority of known homozygotes with mutations in the *BMP15* gene. Research in genes determining prolificacy is an important factor for increasing fecundity of ewes and thus profitability of sheep production as well.

Acknowledgements

This work was supported by projects DS/KBZ/3242/2017.

Author details

Urszula Kaczor

Address all correspondence to: rzkaczor@cyf-kr.edu.pl

Department of Animal Biotechnology, Agriculture University in Krakow, Poland

References

[1] Davis GH. Fecundity genes in sheep. Animal Reproduction Science. 2004;**82-83**:247-253

[2] Drouilhet L, Lecerf F, Bodin L, Fabre S, Mulsant P. Fine mapping of the FecL locus influencing prolificacy in Lacaune sheep. Animal Genetics. 2009;**40**(6):1-9

[3] Feary ES, Juengel JL, Smith P, French MC, O'Connel AR, Lawrence SB, Galloway SM, Davis GH, McNatty KP. Patterns of expression of messenger RNAs encoding GDF9, BMP15, TGFBR1, BMPR1B and BMPR2 during follicular development and characterization of ovarian follicular populations in ewes carrying the Woodlands FecX2W mutation. Biology of Reproduction. 2007;**77**:990-998

[4] Davis GH, Montgomery GW, Allison AJ, Kelly RW, Bray AR. Segregation of major gene influencing fecundity in progeny of Booroola sheep. New Zealand Journal of Agricultural Research. 1982;**25**:525-529

[5] Fogarty NM. Enviromental modulation of FecB expession. Use of the FecB (Booroola) gene in sheep breeding programs. In: Proceedings of International Workshop ACIAR; 11-12 November 2008; Maharashtra. India, Pune: ACIAR; 2009;133. pp. 66-69.

[6] Fhamy MH, Mason IL. Less known and rare breeds. In: Fahmy MH, editor. Prolific Sheep. Willingford, UK: CAB International; 1996. pp. 178-186

[7] Feng W, Ma Y, Zhang Z, Zhou D. Prolific breeds of China. In: Fahmy MH, editor. Prolific Sheep. Willingford, UK: CAB International; 1996. pp. 146-151

[8] Inounu I, Iniguez L, Bradford GE, Subandriy O, Tiesnamurti B. Production performance of prolific Javanese ewes. Small Ruminant Research. 1993;**12**:243-257

[9] Singh RV, Sivakumar A, Sivashankar S, Das G. Evaluation of the Booroola FecB gene in Muzaffarnagari sheep. In: Proceedings of International Workshop ACIAR; 11-12 November 2008; Maharashtra. India-Pune: ACIAR; 2009;133. pp. 223-224

[10] Monget P, Fabre S, Mulsant P, Lecerf F, Elsen JM, Mazerbourg S, Pisselet C, Monniaux D. Regulation of ovarian folliculogenesis by IGF and BMP system in domestic animals. Domestic Animal Endocrinology. 2002;**23**(1-2):139-154

[11] Fabre S, Pierre A, Mulsant P, Bodin L, Di Pasquale E, Persani L, Monget P, Monniaux D. Regulation of ovulation rate in mammals: Contribution of sheep genetic models. Reproductive Biology and Endocrinology. 2006;**4**:20

[12] Montgomery GW, Galloway SM, Davis GH, McNatty KP. Genes controlling ovulations rate in sheep. Reproduction. 2001;**121**:843-852

[13] Moore RK, Shimasaki S. Molecular biology and physiological role of the oocyte factor BMP15. Molecular and Cellular Endocrinology. 2005;**234**:67-73

[14] Yan C, Wang P, DeMayo J, DeMayo FJ, Elvin JA, Carino C, Prasad CV, Skinner SS, Dunbar BS, Dube JL, Celeste AJ, Matzuk MM. Synergistic roles of bone morphogenetic protein 15 and growth differentiation factor 9 in ovarian function. Molecular Endocrinology. 2001;**15**(6):854-866

[15] Rybak-Krzyszkowska M, Grzyb A, Milewicz T, Krzaczkowska-Sendrakowska M, Krzysiek J. Primary ovarian insufficiency in infertility clinic. Polish Journal of Endocrinology. 2004;**6**:766-768

[16] Otsuka F, Yamamoto S, Erickson GF, Shimasaki S. Bone morphogenetic protein-15 inhibits follicle-stimulating hormone (FSH) action by suppressing FSH receptor expression. The Journal of Biological Chemistry. 2001;**276**:11387-11392

[17] Moore RK, Erickson GF, Shimasaki S. Are BMP15 and GDF9 primary determinants of ovulation quota in mammals? Trends in Endocrinology and Metabolism. 2004;**15**:356-361

[18] Shimasaki S, Moore RK, Otsuka F, Erickson GF. The bone morphogenetic protein system in mammalian reproduction. Endocrinology Reviews. 2004;**25**:72-101

[19] McNatty KP, Smith P, Moore LG, Reader K, Lun S, Hanrahan JP, Groome NP, Laitinen M, Ritvos O, Juengel JL. Oocyte-expressed genes affecting voulation rate. Molecular and Cellular Endocrinology. 2005;**234**:57-66

[20] Carabatsos MJ, Sellitto C, Goodenough DA, Albertini DF. Oocyte-granulosa cell heterologous gap junctions are required for the coordination of nuclear and cytoplasmic meiotic competence. Developmental Biology. 2000;**226**:167-179

[21] Hanrahan JP, Gregan SM, Mulsant P, Mullen M, Davis G, Powell R, Galloway SM. Mutations in the genes for oocyte-derived growth factors GDF9 and BMP15 are associated with both increased ovulation rate and sterility in Cambridge and Belclare sheep (*Ovis aries*). Biology of Reproduction. 2004;**70**:900-909

[22] Davis GH, Bruce GD, Dodds KG. Ovulation rate and litter size of prolific Inverdale (Fec^I) and Hanna ($FecX^H$) sheep. Proceedings of Association for the Advancement of Animal Breeding and Genetics. 2001;**14**:175-178

[23] Shackell GH, Hudson NL, Heath NL, Lun S, Shaw L, Condell L, Blay LR, McNatty KP. Plasma gonadotropin concentrations and ovarian characteristics in Inverdale ewes that are heterozygous for major gene $FecX^I$ on the X chromosome that influences ovulation rate. Biology of Reproduction. 1993;**48**:1150-1156

[24] Bodin L, Di Pasquale E, Fabre S, Bontoux M, Monget P, Persani L, Mulsant P. A novel mutation in the bone morphogenetic protein 15 gene causing defective protein secretion is associated with both increased ovulation rate and sterility in Lacaune sheep. Endocrinology. 2007;**148**(1):393-400

[25] Bodin L, Lecerf F, Bessicre M, Mulsant P. Features of major genes for ovulation in the Lacaune population. In: Proceedings of the 8th World Congress on Genetics Applied to Livestock Production WCGALP, Belo Horizonte; 13-18 August 2006, Belo Horizonte, MG, Brazil; 2006; 04-04. pp. 1-4.

[26] Monteagudo LV, Ponz R, Tejedor MT, Laviña A, Sierra I. A 17 bp deletion in the Bone Morphogenetic Protein 15(BMP15) gene is associated to increased prolificacy in the Rasa Aragonesa sheep breed. Animal Reproduction Science. 2009;**110**:139-146

[27] Demars J, Fabre S, Sarry J, Rossetti R, Gilbert H, Persani L, Tosser-Klopp, Mulsant P, Nowak Z, Drobik W, Martyniuk E, Bodin L. Genome-wide association studies identify two novel BMP15 mutations responsible for an atypical hyperprolificacy phenotype in sheep. PLos Genetics. 2013;**9**(4):e1003482. DOI: 1010.1371/journal.pgen.1003482

[28] Vacca GM, Dhaouadi A, Rekik M, Carcangi, Pazzola M, Dettori ML. Prolificacy genotypes at BMPR 1R, BMP15 and GDF9 genes in North African sheep breeds. Small Ruminant Research. 2010;**88**:67-71

[29] McNatty KP, Galloway SM, Wilson T, Smith P, Hudson NL, O'Connell A, Bibby AH, Heath DA, Davis GH, Hanrahan JP, Juengel JL. Physiological effects of major genes affecting ovulation rate in sheep. Genetique Selection Evolution. 2005;**37**:25-38

[30] Juengel JL, Hudson NL, Heath DA, Smith P, Reader KL, Lawrence SB, O'Connell AR, Laitinen MPE, Cranfield M, Groome NP, Ritvos O, McNatty KP. Growth Differentiation Factor 9 and one Morphogenetic Protein 15 are essential for ovarian follicular development in sheep. Biology of Reproduction. 2002;**67**:1777-1789

[31] Elvin JA, Yan Ch, Wang P, Wolfman NM, Matzuk MM. Paracrine actions of growth differentiation factor-9 in the mammalian ovary. Molecular Endocrinology. 1999;**13**:1035-1048

[32] Hayashi M, McGee EA, Min G, Klein C, Rose UM, Duin M, Hsueh AJW. Recombinant growth differentiation factor-9 (GDF9) enhances growth and differentiation of cultured early ovarian follicles. Endocrinology. 1999;**3**:1236-1244

[33] Gilchrist RB, Ritter LJ, Cranfield M, Jeffery LA, Amato F, Scott SJ, Myllymaa S, Kaivo-Oja N, Lnakinen H, Mottershead DG, Groome NP, Ritvos. Immunoneutralization of growth differentiation factor 9 reveals it partially account for mouse oocyte miogenic activity. Biology of Reproduction. 2004;**71**:732-739

[34] Bodensteiner KJ, McMNatty KP, Clay CM, Moeller CL, Sawyer H. Expression of growth differentiation factor-9 in the ovaries of fetal sheep homozygous or heterozygous for the Inverdale Prolificacy Gene ($FecX^I$). Biology of Reproduction. 2000;**62**:1479-1485

[35] McNatty KP, Moore LG, Hudson NL, Quirke LD, Lawrnce SB, Reader K, Hanrahan JP, Smith P, Groome NP, Laitinen M, Ritvos O, Juengel JL. The oocyte and its role in regulating ovulation rate: a new paradigm in reproductive biology. Reproduction. 2004;**128**:379-386

[36] Teixeira Filho FL, Baracat EC, Lee TH. Aberrant expression of growth differentiation factor-9 in oocytes of women with polycystic ovary syndrome. The Journal of Clinical Endocrinology and Metabolism. 2002;**87**:1337-1344

[37] Sadighi M, Bodensteiner KJ, Beattie AE, Galloway SM. Genetic mapping of ovine growth differentiation factor 9 (GDF9) to sheep chromosome 5. Animal Genetics. 2002;**33**:224-248

[38] Liao WX, Moore RK, Otsuka F, Shimasaki S. Effect on intracellular interactions on the processing and secretion of bone morphogenetic protein-15 (BMP15) and growth and differentiation factor-9—implication of the aberrant ovarian phenotype of BMP15 mutant sheep. The Journal of Biological Chemistry. 2003;**278**:3713-3719

[39] Liao WX, Moore RK, Shimasaki S. Functional and molecular characterization of naturally occurring mutation in oocyte-secreted factors BMP15 and GDF9. The Journal of Biological Chemistry. 2004;**279**(17):17391-17396

[40] Nicol L, Bishop S, Pong-Wong R, Bendixen Ch, Holm LE, Rhind SM, McNeilly MS. Homozygosity for a single base-pair mutation in the oocyte-specific GDF9 gene results in sterility in Thoka sheep. Reproduction. 2009;**138**:921-933

[41] Silva BDM, Castro EA, Souza CJH, Paiva SR, Sartori R, Franco MM, Azevedo HC, Silva TASN, Vieira AMC, Neves JP, Melo EO. A new polymorphism in the Growth Differentiation Factor 9 **(**GDF9**)** gene is associated with increased ovulation rate and prolificacy in homozygous sheep. Animal Genetics. 2011;**42**(1):89-92

[42] Davis GH, Galloway SM, Ross IK, Gregan SM, Ward J, Nimbkar BV, Ghalsasi PM, Nimbkar C, Gray GD, Subandriyo Inounu I, Tiesnamurti B, Martyniuk E, Eythorsdottir E, Mulsant P, Lecerf F, Hanrahan JP, Bradford GE, Wilson T. DNA tests in prolific sheep from eight countries provide new evidence on origin of the Booroola (FecB) mutation. Biology of Reproduction. 2002;**66**: 1869-1874

[43] Kaczor U. 2011. Identyfikacja markerów plenności owiec olkuskich na podstawie polimorfizmu genów kodujących białka z rodziny TGF-β [tesis]. Uniwersytet Rolniczy w Krakowie. Zeszyty Naukowe 479; 2011

[44] Liu SF, Jiang YL, Du LX. Study of BMPR-IR and BMP15 as candidate gene for fecundity in little tailed Han sheep. Acta Genetica Sinica. 2003;**30**(8):755-760

[45] Guan F, Liu SR, Shi GQ, Ai JT, Mao DG, Yang LG. Polymorphism of Fec B gene in nine sheep breeds or strains and its effects on litter size, lamb growth and development. Acta Genetica Sinica. 2006;**33**(2):117-124

[46] Kumar S, Mishra AK, Kolte AP, Arora AL, Singh D, Singh VK. Effects of the Booroola (FecB) genotypes on growth performance, ewe's productivity efficiency and litter size in Garole x Malpura sheep. Animal Reproduction Science. 2008;**105**(3-4):19-31

[47] Kumar S, Mishra AK, Kolte AP, Dash SK, Karim SA. Screening for Booroola FecB and Galway FecXG mutation In Indian sheep. Small Ruminant Research. 2008;**80**:57-61

[48] Roberts VJ, Barth S, El-Roeiy A, Yen SSC. Expression of inhibin/activin subunits and follistatin messenger ribonucleic acids and proteins in ovarian follicles and the corpus luteum during the human menstrual cycle. The Journal of Clinical Endocrinology and Metabolism. 1993;**77**:1402-1410

[49] Adalsteinsson S, Jonmundson JV, Eythorsdottir E. The high fecundity Thoka gene in Icelandic sheep. Proceedings of the 40th Meeting of the European Association for Animal Production; 27-31 August 1989. Dublin, Ireland: EAAP; 1989;1.pp. 61-62

[50] Walling GA, Bishop SC, Pong-Wong R, Russel AJF, Rhind SM. Detection of a major gene for litter size in Thoka Cheviot sheep using Bayesian segregation analyses. Animal Science. 2002;**75**:339-347

[51] Meyer HH, Baker RL, Harvey TG, Hickey SM. Effects of Booroola merino breeding and the Fec(B) gene on performance of crosses with long wool breeds. 2. Effects on reproductive performance and weight of lamb weaned by young ewes. Lives Production Science. 1994;**39**:191-200

[52] Gootwine E, Reicher S, Rozov A. Prolificacy and lamb survival at birth in Awassi and Assaf sheep carrying the FecB (booroola) mutation. Animal Reproduction Science. 2008;**108**:402-411

[53] Guan F, Liu SR, Shi GQ, Yang LG. Polymorphism of FecB gene in nine sheep breeds or strains and its effects on litter size, lamb growth and development. Animal Reproduction Science. 2007;**99**:44-52

[54] Kumar S, Kolte A, Mishra AK, Arora AL, Singh V. Identification of Fecb mutation in Garolex Malpura sheep and its effect on litter size. Small Ruminant Research. 2006;**64**:305-310

[55] Melo EO, Silva BDM, Castro EA, Silva TASN, Paiva SR, Sartori R, Franco MM, Souza CJH, Neves JP. A novel mutation in the growth and differentiation factor 9 (GDF9) gene is associated, in homozygosis, with increased ovulation rate in Santa Ines sheep. Biology of Reproduction. 2008;**78**:371

[56] Barzegari A, Atashpaz S, Ghabili K, Nemati Z, Rustaei M, Azarbaijani R. Polymorphism in GDF9 and BMP15 associated with fertility and ovulation rate in Moghani and Ghezel sheep in Iran. Reproduction in Domestic Animals. 2010;**45**:666-669

[57] Polley S, De S, Brahma B, Mukherjee A, Vinesh PV, Batabyal S, Arora JS, Pan S, Samanta AK, Datta TK, Goswami SL. Polymorphism of BMPR1B, BMP15 and GDF9 fecundity genes in prolific Garole. Tropical Animal Health and Production. 2010;**42**:985-993

[58] Chang JT, Luo YZ, Hu J. Polymorphism of GDF9 as a candidate gene for fecundity in sheep. Journal of Gansu Agricultural University. 2009;**44**(2):30-33

[59] Chu M, Zhuang H, Zhang Y, Jin M, Di X, Cao G, Feng T, Fang L. Polymorphism of inhibin βB gene and its relation sheep with liter size in sheep. Animal Science. 2011;**82**:57-61

[60] Li BX, Chu MX, Wang JY. PCR-SSCP analysis on growth differentiation factor 9 gene in sheep. Yi Chuan Xue Bao. 2003;**30**:307-310

[61] Willingham TD, Wardon DW, Thompson PV. Effect of FecB allele on birth weight and post-weaning production traits of Rambouillet-Booroola cross wethers. Texas Agriculture Experimental Station Research Report. Sheep and Goat, Wool and Mohair CpR; 2002. pp. 1-6.

[62] Kleemann DO, Ponzoni RW, Stafford JE, Cutten IN, Grimson RJ. Growth and carcass characters of South Australian Merino and its crosses with the Booroola and Trangie Fertility Merino. Australian Journal of Experimental Agriculture. 1985;**25**:750-757

[63] Abella DF, Cognie Y, Thimonier J, Seck M, Blank MR. Effects of the FecB gene on birth weight, postnatal growth rate and puberty in Booroola x Merinos d'Arles ewe lambs. Animal Research. 2005;**54**:283-288

[64] Visscher AH, Dijkstra M, Lord EA, Suss R, Rosler HJ, Heylen K, Veerkamp RF. Maternal and lamb carrier effects of the Booroola gene on food intake growth and carcass quality of male lambs. Animal Science. 2000;**71**:209-217

[65] Gootwine E, Braw-Tal R, Shalhevet A, Bor A, Zenou A. Reproductive performance of Assaf and Booroola-assaf crossbred ewes and its association with plasma FSH levels and induced ovulation rate measured at prepuberty. Animal Reproduction Science. 1993;**31**:69-81

[66] Gootwine E, Rozov A, Bor A, Richer S. Carring the FecB (Booroola) mutation is associated with lower birth weight and slower post-weaning growth rate for lambs, as well as a lighter mature body weight for ewes. Reproduction Fertility and Development. 2006;**18**(4):433-437

[67] Hiendleder S, Lewalski H, Jaeger H, Pracht P, Erhardt G. Nucleotide sequence of ovine α-inhibin (INHA) gene and evaluation of RFLP marker effects on reproductive performance. Animal Genetics. 1996;**27**(2):91-92

[68] Hiendleder S, Lewalski H, Jaeger H, Pracht P, Erhardt G. Genomic cloning and comparative sequence analyses of different alleles of the ovine β_A inhibin/activin INHA gene as a potential QTL for litter size. Animal Genetics. 1996;**27**(2):119

[69] Leyhe B, Hiendleder S, Jaeger C, Wassmuth R. Pronounced differences in the frequency TaqIβ_A inhibin allele between sheep breeds with different reproductive performance. Animal Genetics. 1994;**25**(1):41-43